Interviewing and Helping Skills for Health Professionals

L. Sherilyn Cormier
William H. Cormier
Roland J. Weisser, Jr.
West Virginia University

with contributed chapters by Jean Elder, Cabrillo College

Jones and Bartlett Publishers, Inc.
Boston   Portola Valley

Jones and Bartlett Publishers, Inc.

Sales and customer services: 20 Park Plaza, Boston, MA 02116

Editorial offices: 30 Granada Court, Portola Valley, CA 94025

Printed in the United States of America

10   9   8   7   6   5   4   3

Library of Congress Cataloging in Publication Data

Cormier, L. Sherilyn (Louise Sherilyn),
    Interviewing and helping skills for health professionals.

    Includes bibliographies and index.
       1. Medical personnel and patient.   2. Health counseling.
3. Interpersonal communication.   I. Cormier, William H.
(William Henry), [date].   II. Weisser, Roland J., Jr.
[date].   III. Title. [DNLM: 1. Interviews – Methods.
2. Counseling – Methods.   3. Professional – Patient relations.   W 21.5 C822i]
R727.3.C68 1983   610.69′6   83-14596

ISBN 0-86720-363-3

Sponsoring Editor: *Aline Faben*
Production Services Coordinator: *Marlene Thom*
Production: *Stacey C. Sawyer, San Francisco*
Interior and Cover Design: *John Edeen*
Illustrations: *Cyndie Clark-Huegel*
Typesetting: *Graphic Typesetting Service, Los Angeles*
Printing and Binding: *The Maple Press Co.*

Following are the credits for the chapter-opening photographs: Chapter 1 – Frank Siteman, Jeroboam, Inc.; Chapter 2 – Laimute Druskis, Jeroboam, Inc.; Chapter 3 – Mitchell Payne, Jeroboam, Inc.; Chapter 4 – Michael Rothstein, Jeroboam, Inc.; Chapter 5 – Bruce Kliewe, Jeroboam, Inc.; Chapter 6 – Kit Hedman, Jeroboam, Inc.; Chapter 7 – Robert Foothorap, Jeroboam, Inc.; Chapter 8 – Karen Preuss, Jeroboam, Inc.; Chapter 9 – Kit Hedman, Jeroboam, Inc.; Chapter 10 – Suzanne Arms, Jeroboam, Inc.; Chapter 11 – Michael Rothstein, Jeroboam, Inc.; Chapter 12 – Bruce Kliewe, Jeroboam, Inc.; Chapter 13 – Hank Lebo, Jeroboam, Inc.; Chapter 14 – William Thompson, Jeroboam, Inc.

To Christiane and Lisanne
W. H. C. and L. S. C.

and

To Roland, Dorothy, and Elsie
Amy, Jimmy, and Jon
and especially Lydia
R. J. W., Jr.

In Memoriam
Clark Kendall Sleeth, M.D.
April 10, 1913–November 30, 1982

Preface

The fundamental purpose of this book is to teach health professionals basic interviewing and communication skills that can help improve the quality of patient care as well as relationships with patients, their families, and other health care team members. We have attempted to present a pragmatic approach for applying communication techniques to the process of health care interviewing. The time required to conduct an interview that both satisfies the needs of the patient and provides the professional with the necessary information required for care varies directly with the skill of the interviewer. In addition to time savings, beginning interviewers who have training in communication skills are more confident and less apprehensive during initial contacts with patients than are students who have not had the opportunity to learn and practice established interview techniques.

Scope of the Book

This book reflects a communication skills model rather than a particular theoretical orientation. This model derives from the works of Truax and Carkhuff (1967), Carkhuff (1969 a, b), Ivey (1971), Hackney and Nye (1973), Egan (1975, 1982), Ivey and Authier (1978), Carkhuff and Anthony (1979), Hackney and Cormier (1979), and Cormier and Cormier (1979). The model emphasizes fundamental relationship tools and interviewing skills that are basic to effective communication and are generally accepted by persons of all theoretical orientations. The book also reflects the premise that health professionals are part of a larger health care system that we view as a helping process (discussed further in Chapter 2). Chapter 1 discusses communication skills. Chapters 3 through 10 describe a variety of interviewing and information-gathering skills to be used in communicating with and eliciting data from patients. Chapters 11 and 12 discuss reactions of patients in illness and patients in crisis and were written by a nurse educator, Jean Elder. Intervention strategies to promote health maintenance are presented in Chapter 13. And, finally, Chapter 14 discusses patient rights and other ethical and legal issues.

Intended Audience

We present a wide range of skills that are essential for all persons involved in the health care field, regardless of their particular roles. Thus the book is intended to be used by different types of health care worker, including nurses, physicians, dentists, dental hygienists, physical therapists, X-ray technicians, medical technologists, pharmacists, and any other health care providers who have frequent contact with patients. We believe that the communication problems and patient situations experienced by one group of health professionals do not differ significantly from those encountered by other groups of health professionals. The book's relevance for a variety of health professionals highlights the collaborative effort or team approach that is so important to effective patient care.

We present a variety of clinical examples throughout the book. Some of these examples may be pertinent to nurses, others to dental hygienists, still others to physicians, and so on. A unique advantage of this approach is that it acquaints each particular group of health professionals with some of the patient situations other members of the health care team will encounter during patient interviewing.

Format of the Book

We have designed a learning format to help the reader acquire, demonstrate, and assess interviewing and communication skills in a systematic fashion. The format of the book is flexible; it may be used as a self-instructional device, as a reference in an organized course, or with an in-service or continuing education program.

The format of each chapter is the same. The chapter begins with chapter objectives and a brief introduction, followed by content material interspersed with clinical examples, learning activities with feedback or self-assessments, a chapter summary, and suggested readings. People involved in field testing this book discovered that these features helped them to get involved and interact with the content material. We will explain each component briefly.

Objectives

In each chapter, certain major concepts and skills are defined. These concepts and skills are outlined as "Objectives" at the beginning of each chapter. The objectives highlight the most important concepts to be learned from the chapter and serve as benchmarks or standards by which progress can be assessed.

Learning Activities and Feedback

Learning activities related directly to the chapter objectives are interspersed throughout each chapter. These activities, which are intended to provide both practice and feedback, consist of transcripts of model interviews, exercises, and feedback. There

are several ways in which the learning activities can be used. Many of the exercises suggest written responses. Written responses may help students and instructors alike to check accuracy and specificity. If, however, writing is not a workable learning strategy, you may prefer to work through an activity and just think about the responses. Whichever technique you employ, it is important to work through each learning activity successfully before proceeding to the next topic.

Another kind of learning activity involves direct rehearsal of certain skills. These "overt rehearsal" exercises are designed to help you apply and assess skills in simulated interactions with a role-play patient. Role-play activities involve three people or roles: an interviewer, a patient, and an observer. Roles should be traded successively so that each person can experience the role play from each of the three different perspectives. Performance checklists are included in most role-play activities to assist the observer in making an accurate and objective assessment of the interviewer's skills. The person who role plays the patient may also wish to participate in the assessment.

Most of the chapter learning activities are followed by some form of feedback. For example, if a learning activity involves identifying positive and negative examples of the use of silence in a patient interview, feedback will indicate which examples are positive and which are negative. The feedback immediately follows the learning activity. Our intention is to have you complete the learning activity first and then use the feedback as a guide to check responses. Some readers, however, may learn more easily if they study the feedback while doing the activity.

We attempt in most of our feedback to give some rationale for the responses. In many feedback sections, we include several possible responses. These responses are intended as guidelines for you to judge your own responses, and you should view them as providing information and alternatives. We do not anticipate that you will generate identical responses. Other responses may be as good as or superior to the examples given in the feedback. Space does not permit listing all the potentially useful responses in the feedback for each learning activity.

One of our concerns involves the way you approach the examples and practice opportunities in this book. Obviously, reading an example or participating in a role-play interview is not as authentic as seeing an actual patient or engaging in a real patient interaction. However, some practice is necessary in any new learning program. Even if the exercises seem contrived and artificial, they will encourage the development of effective interviewing and communication skills for patient care. The structured practice opportunities in the book may require a great deal of discipline in performance. But the degree to which you generalize your skills from practice to an actual patient interview may depend on how much you invest and participate in the practice opportunities. This participation is particularly important with respect to the learning activities that involve role play or simulation. It has been our experience that both beginning and experienced health professionals sometimes approach role playing with a degree of apprehension, defensiveness, or discomfort. Acknowledging such emotions is healthy, but omitting the role play because of them would be counterproductive. It is just not possible to learn to swim without first jumping in the water!

Chapter Summary

At the end of each chapter, a short summary succinctly reviews the major principles, concepts, and skills presented in the chapter. The purpose of the summary is to highlight the key points of the chapter and to help you review and recall the primary concepts. Some people find it useful to read the summary before reading the chapter as an overview or cueing device to help them discriminate key points as they work through the chapter. Others may choose to read the summary after completing the chapter and use it primarily for synthesis and review.

Suggested Readings

Following the chapter summary is a list of suggested readings. Each reading is annotated and suggests one or more chapters or article for you to consult. The suggested readings have been selected for their relevance to the particular content of each chapter. They are intended to acquaint you with other timely references and to provide additional sources for readers who may wish to develop a greater understanding of a specific topic or skill.

Acknowledgments

We want to acknowledge the contributions of some persons to the preparation and development of this book. They include Edward Murphy, who helped us develop the original plans for the manuscript; Aline Faben, editor, Wadsworth Health Sciences Division, who served as project editor for the book; Adrian Perenon, senior editor, Wadsworth Health Sciences Division, who consulted with us about the manuscript; Jean Elder, Director, Vocational Nursing Program, Cabrillo College, who authored two important chapters in the book; and Anne Drake and Lydia Weisser, who typed the manuscript and provided invaluable editorial consultation. We are also grateful for the helpful suggestions made by our reviewers: Jean R. Miller, University of Utah; Myrna Jean Moffett, San Diego State University; Virgil Parsons, San Jose State University; and Mark G. Perlroth, M.D., Stanford University Medical Center.

The manuscript preparation was also facilitated by those persons who participated in its field testing and by the support of the West Virginia University Family Practice Department.

L. Sherilyn Cormier
William H. Cormier
Roland J. Weisser, Jr.

Contents

3

The Health Care Interview: Stages and Special Problems   46

7

Action-Oriented Responses: Questions and Confrontation   124

8

Obtaining a Health History   148

9

Instructions, Information Giving, and Patient Compliance   *184*

10

Dealing with Defensive Reactions   *203*

13

Intervention Strategies   254

14

Ethical and Legal Issues in Health Care Interviewing   296

List of Learning Activities

Communication in Health Care Interviewing

Objectives

After completing this chapter you will be able to do the following:

1. Identify in conversations with friends and colleagues the context and the verbal and nonverbal levels of the sender's messages.

2. Identify in conversations with friends and colleagues occasions when the verbal and nonverbal messages of the sender are consistent or congruent and occasions when they are inconsistent or incongruent.

3. Identify in writing situations that are difficult to handle in dealing with patients, families, and other colleagues.

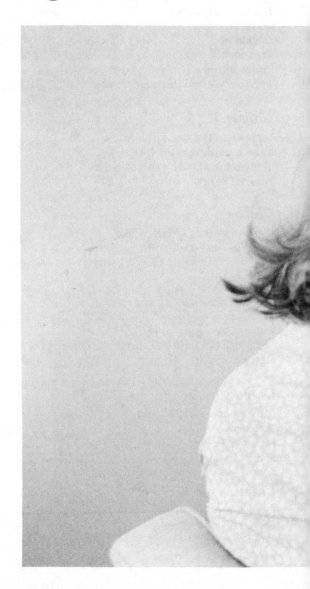

1

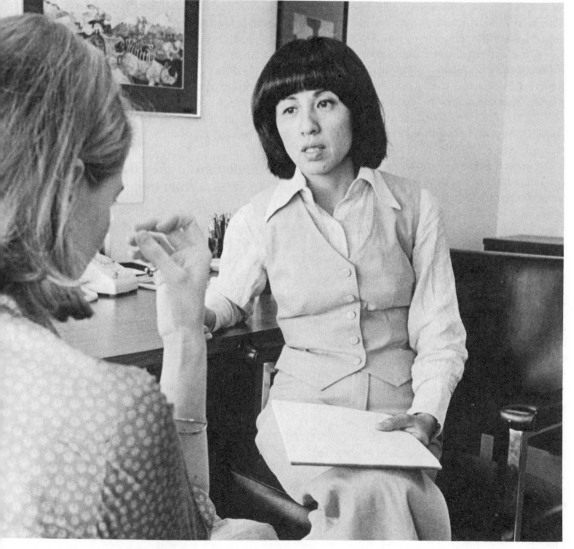

"Clinical medicine should be regarded neither as an art nor as a science in itself, but as a special kind of relationship between two people..." (Ashley Montague).

In the last decade, there has been increasing recognition of the psychosocial and environmental aspects of illness and wider acceptance of the premise that health care is more effective when given in the context of a positive relationship between patients and health care providers. Communication is the medium through which this relationship develops, and the quality of the communication influences the quality of the health care relationship. Effective communication skills are at the core of any effective interpersonal relationship.

A recent study assessed the degree of stress associated with hospitalization by having a large number of medical and surgical patients rate aspects of their hospitalization in terms of perceived stressfulness (Volicer, Isenberg, & Burns, 1977). Many of the events or circumstances rated as most stressful were related not to physical comfort or environmental aspects of hospitalization but rather to communication or the absence of good communication between patients and hospital staff. The following were perceived as highly stressful for many patients: not being told their diagnosis, having their questions ignored, not knowing the reasons for or the results of treatment, and perceiving the staff as using medical jargon and being in a constant rush. Bakal (1979), in reviewing these events, concluded that "[such] problems are easy to solve by improving communication between the health professional and the patient" (p. 99).

Communication is the basis for information exchange and processing and cannot be turned on and off like a water faucet. In fact, it is impossible not to communicate: Even a unilateral decision to terminate communication with someone automatically communicates. As Hein (1980) observes, any health care procedure is preceded

---

Before you read this chapter it is important that you read the preface, which explains the purpose and format of the book.

by a form of communication, and during an interaction between health professionals and patients, communication is ongoing. All communication has some degree of impact on the patient (p. 12).

In health care settings, communication occurs in the context of verbal exchanges or interviews. Kahn and Cannell (1957) define an interview as *a specialized pattern of verbal and nonverbal interaction initiated for a specific purpose and focused on a specific content area*. An interview may be formal or informal, short or long, and it may occur face-to-face or over the telephone. Regardless of the characteristics, the interview is the primary setting in which patients and health professionals become acquainted, exchange information, and interact in various ways. The health professional has at his or her disposal a number of methods of obtaining information, some based on observation and others on instrumentation and laboratory procedures, but the most important one is the interview (Enelow & Swisher, 1979, p. 5).

Functions of the Health Care Interview

The importance of the interview contact in patient care cannot be overemphasized. Engel and Morgan (1973) regard a well-conducted patient interview as "the most powerful, the most sensitive, and the most versatile instrument available" (p. vii). These authors have described six functions of a good health care interview:

1. *To establish a relationship.* The interview serves as the primary vehicle through which a health care relationship is initiated, developed, and sustained. Often this relationship must be developed between two persons who begin as total strangers (p. viii).

2. *To define roles and responsibilities.* The interview provides an opportunity for the respective roles and responsibilities of the health professional and the patient to be clarified and defined. Such information is conveyed by "direct or [by] subtle messages" during the interaction (p. 3). Roles and responsibilities may vary according to the set-

ting and the nature of the contact, and such clarification is vital for a successful interviewer/patient interaction. Frequently patients are uncertain about their own role and are puzzled by that of the health professional. Confusion may exist about the formality or informality of the relationship and the expectations regarding the patient's involvement in his or her own health care. Defining roles involves informing the patient about the responsibilities associated with your job and about any tasks for which the patient is responsible. Defining roles does not mean emphasizing your role and status so much that the patient perceives you as distant or arrogant.

3. *To collect data.* The interview serves as the primary vehicle for data collection. Data collection may include identifying the nature of the patient's health problems, delineating disease processes, describing the patient's emotions, behaviors, and interpersonal style, defining the patient's past and current life circumstances, and establishing the patient's biological, psychological, and environmental resources (assets) and deficits (pp. viii–ix). The health professional's interpersonal competence and skill in interviewing can affect the accuracy and completeness of the data obtained.

4. *To process data.* The interview also provides the forum for data processing, so that the interviewer can interpret and evaluate what a patient reports. Accurate information processing involves "the ability to organize the information, to recognize its meaning, to test its significance, and yet remain open and receptive to that which resists interpretation" (p. ix). The ability to process information depends not only on the interviewer's knowledge but also on her or his skill in getting the patient to provide unbiased information (p. ix).

5. *To establish a contract.* Through the interview process a contract emerges between the health professional and the patient; this contract defines the mutually acceptable conditions for continuing care (p. x). In this context the term *contract* refers to the ground rules or agreements about their relationship—explicit or implicit—that exist between two individuals. According to Froelich

and Bishop (1977), there should be agreement to three kinds of contracts in a patient interview: (1) to interact; (2) to exchange information; and (3) to give and receive treatment (p. 11).

Contracts should be clarified and defined at the outset of the health care relationship. The patient and the health professional should discuss their expectations of each other and of the interaction. If expectations are not clarified, misunderstanding and resentment may develop, and as a consequence, inaccurate or incomplete information may be relayed by the patient and an erroneous assessment made by the health professional. The health professional must determine whether the patient's expectations are realistic and whether he or she will be able to fulfill those expectations.

6. *To achieve compatible communication.* The interview process enables both the health professional and the patient to identify what is required in order to communicate effectively. Some of the benefits of compatible communication include the receipt of more complete and accurate information from a patient, more complete patient cooperation, the reduced likelihood of patient hostility and suspiciousness, and the reduction of patient stress because of inappropriate demeanor and behaviors (Kagan, 1979).

Effective Communication Skills

In the past, the view that good communicators or interviewers were "born and not made" was a common one. However, a substantial body of evidence now supports the view that good communication skills can be learned (Medio, 1980; Stillman, Sabers, & Redfield, 1976; Vaughn & Marks, 1976). People who appear to be "born interviewers" have, in fact, observed, learned, and practiced successful communications skills in other aspects of their lives and have adapted, integrated, and used those skills in patient care. The ability to communicate effectively is a learned skill, involving recognition of elements, levels, and patterns of communication.

Five Elements of Communication

There are five commonly recognized elements of a communication exchange (see Figure 1-1): *sender, receiver, message, feedback,* and *context*. Any time one person in the interaction delivers or gives information, that person is referred to as a *sender*. The person to whom the message or information is delivered is the *receiver*.

A communication can be interpreted on two levels: the spoken word or the *verbal message,* and the nonverbal behaviors or the *nonverbal message*. After receiving a message, the receiver makes a response to the message. This response is referred to as *feedback*. Like a message, feedback also occurs at two levels: verbal and nonverbal. Thus, due to the continual exchange of nonverbal information, all persons involved in the information exchange are both senders and receivers simultaneously. As Froelich and Bishop (1977) note, "without the constant nonverbal feedback the interaction may enter into mutual monologues" with persons expressing themselves as though the others were absent (p. 57).*

The sender and the receiver send and react to messages within a *context*. The context is the physical setting or the time and place in which the communication takes place and is a very important element in interpreting the meaning of the communication exchange. For example, if a person states "My leg hurts," the meaning of this statement can vary greatly depending on the context in which it is expressed. A receiver would interpret this statement differently if the sender were a runner who had just finished a marathon than if he or she were a patient in a hospital emergency room.

Although this explanation may make a communication exchange seem relatively cut-and-dried, communication rarely occurs so easily. Not only

_____

*From *Clinical interviewing skills,* 3rd ed., by R. E. Froelich and F. M. Bishop. Copyright ©1977 by The C. V. Mosby Co. This and all other quotations from the same source are reprinted by permission.

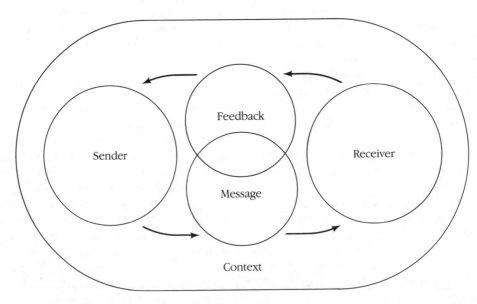

Figure 1-1

Five Elements of Communication

does the meaning of a message depend on the context of the interaction; it is also subject to the way in which the message is delivered and interpreted. As Froelich and Bishop (1977) note, there is often a vast discrepancy between the message a person intends to send, the manner in which he or she sends it, and the receiver's interpretation of the message. For example, if a health professional tells a patient to "take one of these pills when the pain becomes severe," a patient could interpret this in many ways, including some of the following:

The pills are powerful so don't take very many of them.

Never take two pills at one time.

The pills only work on severe pains.

Don't take the pills unless you have to.

Take only these pills, no others, for pain (Froelich & Bishop, 1977, p. 57).

Another important element of a communication exchange has to do with discrepancies between the sender and receiver concerning which part of the message is most important. Generally the most significant aspect of a message is that part of the message that is assimilated by the receiver. Unfortunately, in many cases this may not be the part of the message that is critical to the sender. For instance, a patient may describe a number of signs and symptoms to an interviewer and reveal that, as a result of the symptoms, she has become anxious about her health. The interviewer may concentrate on the description of the symptomatology and neglect the patient's expression of anxiety, which for the patient may have been the more critical part of the message.

Two Levels of Communication

Senders and receivers (or patients and health professionals) communicate simultaneously on two levels during speech and during silence—the verbal and the nonverbal levels. The health professional must be aware of what and how the patient is communicating on both these levels. The verbal

level of communication refers to the words or objective report of the patient (sometimes referred to as the *content* of the communication or what the patient talks about). Verbal communication is denotative in function; that is, a patient uses words to denote, designate, or make known a particular idea or piece of information.

The nonverbal level of communication refers to the body language or subjective expression of the patient. It may be defined to include all the unspoken communication that occurs between two persons and includes such elements as voice inflection, tone, volume, gestures, posture, touch, demeanor, mood, appearance, physical distance, and facial expressions (Froelich & Bishop, 1977). Sometimes the nonverbal level of communication is referred to as the *process* of the communication or how the patient talks and acts. Nonverbal communication is *connotative* in function; that is, a patient uses body language to connote, imply, or suggest the presence of an idea or piece of information.

Unfortunately, the verbal report of patients is the level that many health professionals notice the most, perhaps because it is easier to be attentive to objective reports than to subjective elements. However, oral self-report can be "limited by embarrassment, hostility, fear, lack of knowledge and so forth" (Enelow & Swisher, 1979, p. 16). In disregarding a patient's nonverbal communication, therefore, the health professional may be missing a very important and accurate source of information.

Patients' nonverbal communication can provide important behavioral signs that may betray various difficulties or problems; thus the importance of "reading" patient nonverbal messages cannot be overemphasized. Nonverbal messages are usually more spontaneous than verbal messages and may provide a patient's instantaneous reaction to the interviewer's last message (Froelich & Bishop, 1977). Reading the patient's nonverbal messages requires the interviewer to observe the patient carefully during all phases of the interaction. Yet, as Enelow and Adler (1979) observe: "Taking notes and looking at one's chart or clipboard while writing is a common barrier to 'reading' body language. Even more frequent, however, is the simple failure to observe the patient carefully, and to heed the communication that is not being provided in words" (p. 56).

Both verbal and nonverbal communication are important for understanding patient messages. These two levels of communication are interdependent. The probability of interpreting a message reliably is increased if both channels of communication are used. As Froelich and Bishop (1977) note, "when touch, sounds, words, body language, gestures, and facial expressions are all considered together, the true meaning of a communication is rarely missed" (p. 57).

Two Patterns of Communication

Sometimes the nonverbal behavior of patients may contradict the verbal message. Satir (1972) describes two patterns of communication: _congruent_ and _incongruent_. In a congruent communication pattern everything the person says and does is consistent; the verbal and nonverbal messages sent to the receiver "match" each other. For example, a patient displays congruent communication when stating "I _hate_ the idea of having to be in the hospital" with special emphasis on the word "hate" and with a facial expression that is appropriate to the type and intensity of the emotion. A congruent communication pattern indi-

cates that the speaker has insight and awareness into his or her feelings, attitudes, and concerns.

It is not uncommon, however, for patients to exhibit incongruent communication, in which the verbal message and the body language contradict each other. For example, a patient may state "I've just accepted the fact that we won't have any children" with a tremble in the voice and a quiver of the lips. In this situation, the nonverbal message is different from the spoken words. It is important for health professionals to be alert to incongruent communication patterns. As Enelow and Adler (1979) observe, "any nonverbal message from the patient that suggests something other than the content of the verbal message or seems to be in conflict with it should be given special attention. . . . Lack of congruence between verbal and nonverbal messages may indicate that something is being omitted, whether deliberately or unconsciously" (p. 60). (Incongruent messages and ways of responding to them are discussed in greater detail in Chapter 7.)

Given all the elements that are inherent in a communication exchange and the possible inconsistencies among these elements, it is not difficult to understand why effective communication requires a complex set of skills and why failures in good communication are so common. The following exercises present opportunities for you to observe and practice the elements of effective communication.

=== _LEARNING ACTIVITIES_ ===

Communication   This learning activity presents two exercises to give you practice in identifying context, levels (verbal and nonverbal), and patterns (incongruent and congruent) of communication. Each exercise takes place during actual conversations with others. Although we do not provide any feedback following these exercises, you may want to solicit reactions from the people involved in the conversations or jot down your reactions and discuss them with an instructor or colleague.

Exercise 1: Context and levels of communication

In conversations with friends, family members, and colleagues:

1. Identify the context and the verbal and nonverbal levels of the other person's messages (Chapter Objective 1).
2. Identify what information each level of communication gives you.
3. Observe which level of communication (verbal or nonverbal) is consistently easier for you to notice and speculate why.
4. Note how the context of the communication affects your interpretation of the messages received.

Exercise 2: Patterns of communication

According to Chapter Objective 2, in conversations with friends, family members, and colleagues:

1. Identify occasions in which the verbal and nonverbal messages of the sender are consistent or congruent.
2. Identify situations in which the verbal and nonverbal messages are inconsistent or incongruent. In this case, identify what information the incongruent communication pattern gives you about the person with whom you are interacting.

Common Concerns of Health Professionals

Health professionals in a variety of settings have similar concerns and common difficulties in communicating and dealing with patients. Most of these concerns center directly on patient care. Other concerns relate to dealing with families of patients or with other health care team members.

McGuire (1979) conducted an analysis of patient interviewing techniques among senior-level students. He found that most of the students demonstrated six problem tendencies in their interviews:

1. To avoid discussion of personal or affective matters. Interview time was spent primarily in the discussion of objective parameters such as "How long have you had this illness?" or "How many flights of stairs can you climb?" or "Do you have fluoride in your drinking water?" to the exclusion of subjective matters such as "How do you feel about this illness?" or "What effect has your illness had on your earning capacity?";

2. To fail to explain the purpose of the interview to the patient;

3. To fail to seek clarification of vague or ambiguous patient messages;

4. To be imprecise in certain areas of assessment (for example, in reporting dates, onset of illness, and previous treatments);

5. To be unable to keep the patient focused on the subject;

6. To assume the patient had only one problem and neglect to explore additional possible problem areas.

Other analyses and discussions with health care professionals have revealed the following problem areas: defining the nature of the patient/health professional relationship and one's professional role; maintaining control of the interview; being systematic; developing an effective and efficient question style; dealing with silence comfortably; and attending to patients' feelings.

In a survey the authors conducted with nursing, dental, medical, and physical therapy students, the following areas were reported by most of the students as areas of major concern in patient care: values conflict with a patient; cultural or language barriers; depressed patients; angry and hostile patients; seductive patients; noncompliant patients; overly dependent and demanding patients; and chronic complainers. These students also reported having difficulty with patients who rambled, changed the subject, asked personal questions, or had extreme emotional reactions to illness. Several areas of concern surfaced regarding relationships with other team members, including working with an angry, hostile, or noncooperative team member and dealing with errors or misunderstandings in orders or directions given by a colleague. Concerns were reported about dealing with families and visitors who were dogmatic, broke the rules, were inconsiderate of the rights of others, refused to disclose a diagnosis to their child, or argued with the health professional over care and treatment of a family member or close friend.

These problematic areas can be summarized into eight major areas of concern for many health professionals:

1. Developing a systematic and precise interviewing style;

2. Defining the nature of the health professional/patient relationship and respective roles;

3. Maintaining control of the interview;

4. Responding to patients' feelings or emotions;

5. Discussing personal or sensitive issues with patients;

6. Responding effectively to extreme emotional reactions of patients;

7. Dealing effectively with families, visitors, and other health care team members; and

8. Incorporating interviewing skills with health care skills in patient care.

Some of the issues found in each of these eight areas of concern will be described in the following section.

Developing a Systematic and Precise Interviewing Style

Beginning health professionals often feel at a loss when they start to talk to or interview a patient.

They are unsure exactly how to begin and what topics to pursue. As a result their interviewing style may not be "cost effective," and they may forget to ask for or report important data. They can solve these problems by better understanding the typical sequence of an interview, by recalling messages accurately, by responding to patient communication selectively, and by developing a systematic approach for using appropriate questions to obtain a patient's history. These skills are discussed in Chapters 3, 5, and 8.

Defining the Health Professional/Patient Relationship and Roles

Some health professionals report difficulty in communicating to patients the nature of the health professional/patient relationship and the respective roles of each party. Consequently patients may misinterpret or misconstrue the purpose of the interaction and some of the health professionals' behaviors and actions. It is easier to communicate with patients when interviewers understand the context of the interaction and the nature of their role in the interaction. It is also important for health professionals to feel comfortable with their defined role and to use it to the best advantage. These skills are discussed in greater detail in Chapters 2 and 3.

Maintaining Control of the Interview

A common complaint among health professionals is "I didn't get anything accomplished in that session" or "It's so tiring to talk to Mrs. X. She always tells stories and rambles and I can't get the information I need." Health professionals must learn to listen to patients and at the same time not relinquish control of the interview. Retaining control of the interview is also called "focusing" the interview (see Chapter 4). Sometimes a summarization or confrontation response is useful with patients who continually ramble or change the subject. These responses are described in Chapters 6 and 7.

Responding to Patient Feelings

Health professionals with varying degrees of experience express concern about responding to patients' feelings or emotions. Patients often have difficulty expressing their feelings, and many health professionals feel it is far easier to respond to objective information than to subjective or affective information. Patients' feelings, however, can have a significant role in contributing to, exacerbating, or improving the course of an illness. It is essential for health professionals to be able to recognize and help patients discuss their feelings about illness.

Health professionals should also realize that some patients may seek health care ostensibly for physical symptoms but actually to relieve emotional distress. In other words, psychological discomfort may be concealed by the more obvious presentation of somatic complaints (Anstett & Collins, 1982). In a study of health care users conducted by Follette and Cummings (1967), patients who experienced emotional distress were higher-than-average users of both in-patient and out-patient health care facilities. This finding supports the contention of Bernstein and Bernstein (1980) and others that often when patients seek health care "they do not complain of difficult or intolerable life circumstances but of physical symptoms which they, as well as professionals, view as acceptable bases for seeking care"* (p. 118). Unfortunately many of these patients may be terminated from treatment because diagnostic measures do not reveal any organic basis for their symptoms. Skilled and sensitive interviewers usually are able to discover whether patients need relief from emotional distress if the symptoms continue for no apparent reason and, upon such discovery, can provide appropriate support and treatment. Chapters 4, 6, and 11 discuss in further detail the impor-

tance of dealing with subjective or affective information.

Discussing Personal or Sensitive Issues with Patients

Health professionals are aware of discomfort not only in responding to patient feelings but also about discussing personal or sensitive issues with patients. Some interviewers feel very uncomfortable when patients bring up topics such as marital and sexual adjustment, value-laden issues, or effects of illness. Other interviewers believe it is important to discuss such issues but do not know how to initiate such a discussion with patients. These topics, however, often cannot be avoided. Exploring marital and sexual issues, for example, is an important part of patient assessment and history taking. Often, too, the perceived effects of illness may have the greatest impact on the patient's marital and sexual adjustment.

On the reverse side of this issue, some health professionals do feel comfortable discussing personal issues concerning the patient but are at a loss when the patient asks them personal questions about themselves or their lives. Generally, the interviewer must discriminate the purpose of such questions and respond accordingly.

Another aspect of health care that may be a sensitive or uncomfortable experience for patients is the physical examination. For some patients the act of disrobing or being disrobed produces feelings ranging from mild disconfort to embarrassment or humiliation. The examination also may reveal anxieties a patient has about certain areas of his or her body. A few patients may view the physical exam as an opportunity to be affectionate, flirtatious, or openly seductive. Enelow and Swisher (1979) assert that patient feelings of anxiety and embarrassment will be lessened if rapport has been established before the examination and if the interview and exam are not two separate processes. They believe "the interview is still in process during the physical exam" (Enelow & Swisher, p. 185). Chapters 8, 10, and 11 discuss these issues in greater depth.

---

*From *Interviewing: A guide for health professionals,* by L. Bernstein and R. Bernstein. Copyright © 1980 by Appleton-Century-Crofts. This and all other quotations from the same source are reprinted by permission.

Responding to Extreme Emotional Reactions to Illness

Patients who are faced with chronic disabling illness or with critical illness and patients in some crisis situations may have extreme emotional reactions to their situations. For example, instead of discouragement, such patients may experience severe depression. Instead of irritation or resentment, some may express anger or hostility. Strong feelings may be evident in patient behaviors, as in the case of a patient who becomes seductive, noncompliant, demanding, or overly dependent. Depression and anxiety are common reactions in patients recovering from a myocardial infarction (Hackett, Cassem, & Wishnie, 1968; Wishnie, Hackett, & Cassem, 1971), and secondary emotional reactions are quite common among burn victims (Andreasen, Norris, & Hartford, 1971; Andreasen & Norris, 1972). According to Rosen and Wiens (1979), "modern medical and surgical treatments may prolong life but may have iatrogenic psychological complications" (p. 421). These authors cite depression during hemodialysis and following open-heart surgery as examples of this problem.

Blum (1960) has described ten major reactions, one or more of which is likely to describe a person's response to illness. These include depression and self-rejection; fear; counterphobia; anxiety; frustration and anger; withdrawal or apathy; exaggeration of symptoms; repression; dependency; and self-centeredness. It should be noted that the way a person reacts to illness is characteristic of that person's typical response to any stressful or anxiety-provoking situation (Enelow & Swisher, 1979).

Health professionals report having difficulty responding to highly emotional patients in an objective manner. Often it is easier to respond in like fashion and become abrupt, defensive, or angry. Yet, as Bernstein and Bernstein (1980) assert, "responsible care of patients must recognize, understand, and deal appropriately with emotional reactions if optimal benefits are to be obtained" (p. 125). Chapters 10, 11, and 12 discuss some emotional reactions to illness and describe possible ways that health professionals can be of help to such patients.

Health professionals, like patients, may have particular biases, prejudices, or personal problems and concerns of their own. All health professionals may, at times, have difficulty responding to patient needs because of overwhelming or unsatisfied needs of their own. Although there is no easy solution to this problem, it needs to be emphasized that the personal well-being of the health professional is often a significant factor in relating to patients effectively. Health professionals need to take care of themselves first in order to provide effective care for others. Sometimes this may mean taking a day off, getting a good night's sleep, or letting off steam by talking, crying, exercising, and so on.

Dealing Effectively with Families, Visitors, and Other Health Care Team Members

Sometimes it is not the patient but the "significant others" who pose the greatest challenge to the health professional. For example, whereas a critically ill patient may make very few demands on the health professional, families, relatives, and close friends may make a great many demands. Families, often responding to the stress of illness in their loved one, may be dogmatic, argumentative, or inconsiderate of the rights of the patient or of others. Family members also may disagree on what the health professional should tell the patient about the illness or about impending procedures. Although there is not one "right" way to handle such dilemmas, generally it is better to confront such issues directly with the family. On the other hand, the family is often ignored in health care practice. Understanding the reasons for the family's reactions will help the health professional to avoid becoming personally defensive, angry, or upset and to involve the family in important decisions about the patient's illness and self-care.

Problems may also flare during interactions with other health care team members, making professional relationships less than satisfying. Short staffing, long hours, and great numbers of patients to care for can create short tempers and reluctance to cooperate and can lead to misunderstandings of orders and directives. Unfortunately, when such problems arise among members of the health care team, the patient is directly affected. Patient care may be in jeopardy because of lingering or unresolved problems in the relationships among health care team members. It is important for all health professionals to use the principles of effective communication and interpersonal relationships in their interactions with colleagues as well as with patients. Whether assisting subordinates to maintain or improve job performance or interacting with supervisors or colleagues, effective communication can improve staff relationships and enhance patient care. Although it is not the major emphasis in this book, communication with families and other health care team members is discussed briefly in Chapters 5, 7, 9, and 10.

Incorporating Interviewing Skills with Health Care Skills

A constant and difficult challenge facing a concerned health professional is how to incorporate interviewing skills with health care skills. For most health professionals, training in health care skills has been or will be a predominant part of their curriculum. Above all, most health care curricula attempt to ensure that graduates have mastered the necessary technical or medically related skills. Unfortunately, training in interpersonal skills is sometimes neglected entirely or appended as an afterthought to some other course. Consequently, many health professionals never learn good interpersonal skills and thus relate ineffectively to their patients. The patient, as a consumer of health care services, demands both technical and interpersonal competence on the part of the attending professionals. As Froelich and Bishop (1972) note, in the minds of most patients the two attributes (technical competence and interest in the patient as a person) are inseparable (p. 1). They assert that disinterest in the patient implies that the professionals also are not motivated to exercise their scientific competence (p. 2). Chapters 2 and 13 describe some ways in which health care and interviewing skills can be integrated in the overall treatment and care of patients.

The following learning activity provides an opportunity for you to identify situations involving patient care, family contacts, and interactions with colleagues that may be especially difficult for you.

══════════════ LEARNING ACTIVITIES ══════════════

Common Concerns of Health Professionals

In this learning activity you are to identify particularly troublesome situations in dealing with patients, families, and health care team members, using a communication experience survey (Chapter Objective 3). The instructions for completing this survey follow.

Instructions

Listed on the following pages are a number of different patient types and patient-interaction situations that have been shown to provoke frustration or anxiety in health professionals and health profession students. There is also a list of circumstances involving interactions with professional colleagues and families of patients that have been shown to be equally disconcerting.

For each of the 39 items, indicate the degree of difficulty you experience in talking with each type of patient or in each circumstance. Rate the items using the 5-point rating scale, where 1 means you experience no difficulty and 5 means you experience extreme difficulty.

If you have not yet encountered all the situations described, base your answer on the degree of difficulty you would expect to have, given your current vantage point—that is, second-year medical student, third-year nursing student, and so on. If you feel that the item will not or does not apply to you, you may leave it blank.

	Not difficult	A little difficult	Moderately difficult	Very difficult	Extremely difficult
Communicating with Patients					
1. Communicating with depressed patients is ...	1	2	3	4	5
2. Communicating with angry or hostile patients is ...	1	2	3	4	5
3. Communicating with dependent patients is ...	1⁻	2	3	4	5
4. Communicating with patients who deny their illness is ...	1	2	3	4	5
5. Communicating with seductive patients is ...	1	2	3	4	5
6. Communicating with patients who are terminally ill or dying is ...	1	2	3	4	5
7. Communicating with patients who are chronically ill is ...	1	2	3	4	5
8. Communicating with noncompliant patients (for example, who refuse medication) is ...	1	2	3	4	5
9. Communicating with handicapped patients is ...	1	2	3	4	5
10. Communicating with patients who ask personal questions is ...	1	2	3	4	5
11. Communicating with patients who make excessive demands is ...	1	2	3	4	5
12. Communicating with patients who continually complain about all aspects of their care is ...	1	2	3	4	5
13. Communicating with patients who are homosexual is ...	1	2	3	4	5
14. Communicating with patients of the opposite sex is ...	1	2	3	4	5
15. Communicating with pre-operative patients is...	1	2	3	4	5
16. Communicating with post-operative patients is ...	1	2	3	4	5

	Not difficult	A little difficult	Moderately difficult	Very difficult	Extremely difficult
17. Communicating with patients who constantly change the subject is . . .	1	2	3	4	5
18. Communicating with patients who constantly ask questions or request information about their health problem is . . .	1	2	3	4	5
19. Communicating with patients who ramble a lot is . . .	1	2	3	4	5
20. Communicating with patients who exhibit cultural or language barriers is . . .	1	2	3	4	5
21. Communicating with patients to explain your role is . . .	1	2	3	4	5
22. Communicating with patients who are reluctant to speak and who create long silences is . . .	1	2	3	4	5
23. Communicating with patients who discuss personal values (such as religion, education, sexual preference, socioeconomic level, and the like) is . . .	1	2	3	4	5
24. Communicating with patients who exhibit extreme emotional reactions is . . .	1	2	3	4	5

Communicating with Families

	Not difficult	A little difficult	Moderately difficult	Very difficult	Extremely difficult
25. Communicating with a family member who is dogmatic or arrogant toward you is . . .	1	2	3	4	5
26. Communicating with a family member who is inconsiderate of the rights of others is . . .	1	2	3	4	5
27. Communicating with a family member who tells the patient a certain painful procedure won't hurt is . . .	1	2	3	4	5
28. Communicating with a family member who breaks the rules such as bringing in food for a patient on a special diet is . . .	1	2	3	4	5
29. Communicating with a family member who argues with you about aspects of the patient's care is . . .	1	2	3	4	5
30. Communicating with a family member who is angry or extremely upset is . . .	1	2	3	4	5

	Not difficult	A little difficult	Moderately difficult	Very difficult	Extremely difficult
Communicating with Colleagues					
31. Communicating with a colleague who is dogmatic and arrogant is . . .	1	2	3	4	5
32. Communicating with a colleague who is not as committed to patient care as you are is . . .	1	2	3	4	5
33. Communicating with a colleague who is noncooperative is . . .	1	2	3	4	5
34. Communicating with a colleague who is hostile is . . .	1	2	3	4	5
35. Communicating with a colleague who feels that you have a lighter workload is . . .	1	2	3	4	5
36. Communicating with a colleague who constantly complains is . . .	1	2	3	4	5
37. Communicating with a colleague who is called about a sudden change in a patient and responds "I don't know why you called—I can't do anything about it" is . . .	1	2	3	4	5
38. Communicating with a colleague about misunderstandings in directions given by another colleague is . . .	1	2	3	4	5
39. Communicating with a colleague for an "error" such as an infiltrated I.V. is . . .	1	2	3	4	5

Feedback

There are no "correct" or "incorrect" answers to this survey. Your responses may differ greatly from those of a friend or a colleague. We suggest you examine your responses for each of the three areas listed in the survey—patients, families, and colleagues—particularly noting which situations you rated as 1 or 2 and which you rated as 3, 4, or 5. From these ratings you can determine the situations you handle with ease and comfort and those that present the greatest difficulty and anxiety for you. What types of persons or situations seem to be more difficult for you than others? How might these situations interfere with your being an effective health professional? Consider how you might have felt five years ago and compare your present reactions. You may wish to discuss your reactions with an instructor, supervisor, or a colleague.

Chapter Summary

We have attempted to define the skills presented in this book as precisely as possible to help you develop a systematic framework and methodology for patient interviewing. However, we caution against using the book as a prescriptive device, prescribed automatically and without prior thought or assessment.

The clinical examples given in this book and the guidelines described for dealing with certain situations are simply guidelines. It is not possible or desirable to describe every kind of patient or difficult situation that arises in actual practice. This book will describe a variety of tools that you may apply not only to patient situations that are similar to the examples given but also to patients whose concerns and problems may be quite diverse.

As experience in working with patients accumulates, it becomes apparent that all patients are not alike. Even those with similar health histories or illnesses present a variety of challenges to the health professional. The interviewing and communication skills presented in this book cannot always be used in the same way, at the same pace, or even with similar results for all patients. The effective health professional is the one who is best able to adapt the ingredients of effective interviewing and good communication to each new situation.

Suggested Readings

Enelow, A. J., & Swisher, S. N. *Interviewing and patient care*. New York/Oxford: Oxford University Press, 1979. Chapter 1, "The Interview in Clinical Medicine," describes some of the features and advantages of interviewing in health care.

Engel, G. L., & Morgan, W. L. *Interviewing the patient*. London: W. B. Saunders, 1973. The introduction of this book, pp. vii–xv, describes succinctly the role and functions of a well-conducted patient interview.

Froelich, R. E., & Bishop, F. M. *Clinical interviewing skills*. St. Louis: Mosby, 1977. Chapter 8, "Nonverbal Communication," provides an excellent discussion of the parameters of patient nonverbal behavior. Sample illustrations of various nonverbal messages also are given.

Hein, E. C. *Communication in nursing practice*. Boston: Little, Brown, 1980. This book represents an excellent source for more detailed information about the role and content of communication in interactions with patients. Chapter 4, "The Nursing Interview," and Chapter 13, "The Criteria for Sending Effective Messages," are particularly relevant for understanding the purpose of health care interviews and effective communication with patients.

Kagan, N. Counseling psychology, interpersonal skills, and health care. In G. C. Stone, F. Cohen, & N. E. Adler (Eds.), *Health psychology—A handbook*. San Francisco, Calif.: Jossey-Bass, 1979, pp. 465–486. This chapter emphasizes some of the reasons why health care providers are interested in the interpersonal aspects of patient care.

McGuire, P. Teaching essential interviewing skills to medical students. In P. J. Oborne, M. M. Gruneberg, & J. R. Eiser (Eds.), *Research in psychology and medicine*. London: Academic Press, 1979. This chapter provides an excellent overview of the author's study of interviewing deficiencies among medical students and the need to overcome such limitations.

Medio, F. *Teaching interpersonal communication skills to medical students: A comparison of four methods*. Unpublished doctoral dissertation, West Virginia University, 1980. Medio's research demonstrated that formal training in the use of communication skills provided substantial improvement in interviewing performance and cognitive learning.

Stillman, P., Sabers, D., & Redfield, D. The use of paraprofessionals to teach interviewing skills. *Pediatrics*, 1976, *57*, 769–774. This article describes how paraprofessionals were used to improve the interviewing skills of medical students. The article includes a very specific interview checklist that can be used to assess a variety of interviewing skills including content, questions, and rapport.

Volicer, B. J., Isenberg, M. A., & Burns, M. W. Medical-surgical differences in hospital stress factors. *Journal of Human Stress*, 1977, *3*, 3–13. This article emphasizes the importance of staff/patient communication in reducing the stress level of hospitalized patients.

The Helping Process in Patient Interactions

Objectives

After completing this chapter you will be able to do the following:

1. Identify in writing an empathic or nonempathic response from a series of eight written statements between patients and health professionals.

2. After reading a description of four patient situations, write an example of an "appreciation of differences" statement to be used as a response to the patient.

3. After reading four statements by a health professional and a description of the health professional's actions, identify in writing whether verbal and nonverbal messages are congruent or incongruent.

4. Identify in writing an expert or an inexpert interviewer from a written description of eight interviewer behaviors.

5. Identify in writing a characteristic suggesting trustworthiness or nontrustworthiness from written descriptions of eight health professional actions.

6. After reading a series of six written patient situations, write at least two examples of trait structuring and two examples of role structuring that could be used appropriately to prepare patients to meet and work therapeutically with new health professionals.

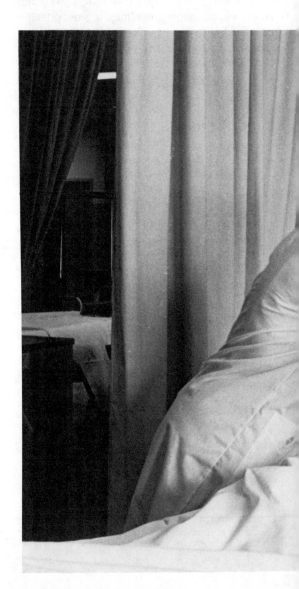

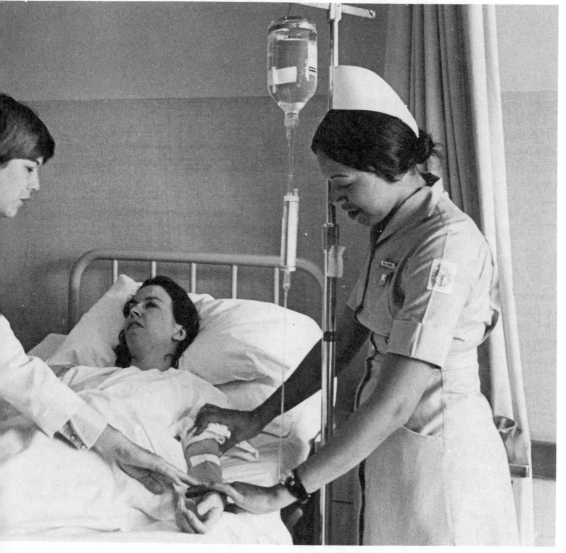

2

A basic premise of this book is that all health professionals, in interacting with patients, are part of a helping process. Whether or not the health professional is aware of it, patients tend to cast the health care provider into the role of a helper and thus have certain beliefs and expectations about the nature of the relationship and the attitudes and behaviors of the attending professional. Patients expect health professionals not only to remove their discomfort but also to induce a state of comfort and well-being for them (Enelow & Swisher, 1979, p. 3).

According to Leigh and Reiser (1980), patients engage in help-seeking behavior whenever they decide to do something about symptoms or distress (p. 4). Such symptoms and distress may include both medical and nonmedical problems. Depending on the nature of the symptoms, patients may expect health professionals to provide medically oriented treatment for relief of medical symptoms or to establish a supportive interpersonal relationship for resolution of interpersonal problems. Effective health care not only promotes recovery from illness but also helps patients maintain health and achieve wellness.

Okun (1982) describes a helper as "anyone who assists persons to overcome or to deal with problems" (p. 4). Helping has been described by various other writers (Blackham, 1977, p. 7; Patterson, 1980; Pepinsky & Pepinsky, 1954) as a confidential and interactional relationship between a person with a problem and a skilled helper who provides conditions that facilitate problem management and resolution in a way that is consistent with the person's values. By virtue of their training, assigned role, and setting, some health professionals may interact directly with patients who view the primary relationship between themselves and the health care provider as helping or therapeutic in nature. For many other health professionals, the helping relationship is an indirect one, secondary to some other role such as providing oral hygiene or obtaining laboratory specimens. In both instances, helping, in a therapeutic sense, is part of the overall health professional/patient interaction. As Long and Prophit (1981) suggest,

the way that health care providers "listen to and interact with patients is a factor in both patient recovery and patient comfort" (p. xi).

The purposes of this chapter are to describe some differences between helping, crisis intervention, and psychotherapy; to delineate a helping model that health professionals can use in patient interactions; to discuss the role of the health care provider within that helping model; and to describe some characteristics of an effective helping relationship.

Differences Between Helping, Crisis Intervention, and Psychotherapy

Helping, crisis intervention, and psychotherapy represent different ways of working with patients to promote effective problem management or resolution. A helping interaction has four components: (1) someone seeking help and (2) someone willing to give help who is also (3) capable of or trained to help (4) in a setting that permits help to be given and received (Hackney & Cormier, 1979, p. 25).

Crisis intervention, on the other hand, has been compared by Belkin (1980) to the use of first aid in medicine. Crisis intervention is viewed as the temporary but immediate relief of an emergency situation presented by an incapacitated person. Like first aid procedures, crisis intervention procedures are "specific and clear cut" (Belkin, 1980, p. 239).

Psychotherapy has been defined as an intensive self-understanding and reconstruction of the dynamics that account for particular life crises and long-standing personality traits (Ivey & Simek-Downing, 1980, pp. 13–14). The primary focus of psychotherapy is the alleviation of pathological problems and conditions (Brammer & Shostrom, 1982; Ivey & Simek-Downing, 1980).

In summary, helping, crisis intervention, and psychotherapy are related ways of assisting people in need. The similarities among them are depicted by the overlapping bell curves in Figure 2-1. However, the three approaches also differ substantially with regard to the nature of the problems presented by the patients, the goals of the interaction, the duration of the interaction, and the methods utilized. These differences are listed in Figure 2-1 below the curves. These differences and similarities are examined in detail in the following section.

Differences in the Nature of Patients' Problems

Patients seen in the context of a helping framework may present problems related to coping with emotional responses to illness; managing occupational, financial, social, and psychological effects of their illness; deciding on treatment alternatives; and making lifestyle changes that are preventive in nature. Patients for whom crisis intervention is most appropriate usually are confronted by a problem in which familiar methods of coping are either not applicable or not effective in resolving the situation (Brockopp, 1973, p. 74). Such patients may experience a great deal of stress, feel panicky or defeated, report a diminished ability to concentrate, and require immediate relief (Puryear, 1979, p. 6). If crisis intervention is not readily available, psychological deterioration may result and psychotherapy may be required.

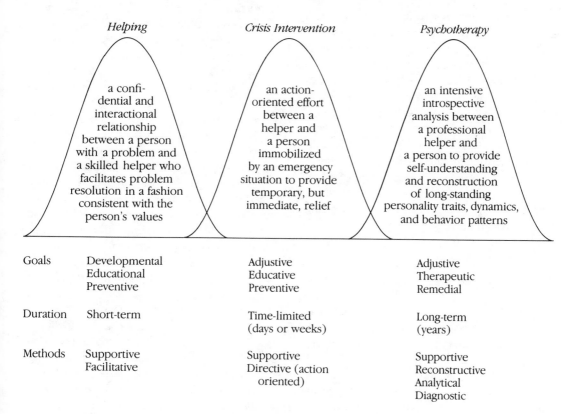

	Helping	Crisis Intervention	Psychotherapy
	a confidential and interactional relationship between a person with a problem and a skilled helper who facilitates problem resolution in a fashion consistent with the person's values	an action-oriented effort between a helper and a person immobilized by an emergency situation to provide temporary, but immediate, relief	an intensive introspective analysis between a professional helper and a person to provide self-understanding and reconstruction of long-standing personality traits, dynamics, and behavior patterns
Goals	Developmental Educational Preventive	Adjustive Educative Preventive	Adjustive Therapeutic Remedial
Duration	Short-term	Time-limited (days or weeks)	Long-term (years)
Methods	Supportive Facilitative	Supportive Directive (action oriented)	Supportive Reconstructive Analytical Diagnostic

Figure 2-1

Definitions, Characteristics, and Comparisons of Helping, Crisis Intervention, and Psychotherapy (Adapted from *Therapeutic psychology: Fundamentals of counseling and psychotherapy,* 4th ed., p. 7, by L. M. Brammer and E. L. Shostrom. Copyright © 1982 by Prentice-Hall, Inc. Reprinted by permission.)

Patients who require psychotherapy usually have problems that are more severe, disabling, or pathological than those described above. These patients may have extreme emotional reactions to illness, such as prolonged and severe depression or psychotic incapacitation, or they may present health-related problems that are psychological rather than organic in etiology.

Differences in Goals

The goals of helping have been described generally by Blocher (1966) as developmental, educative, and preventive in nature. Other goals of a helping interaction include promoting effective decision making, resolving problems, and enhancing the person's ability to cope more successfully. Crisis intervention has a very specific goal: to help the patient resolve the crisis and return to his or her level of functioning before the onset of the crisis (Belkin, 1980; Puryear, 1979). According to Blocher (1966), psychotherapy goals are adjustive, therapeutic, and remedial in nature. Personality and behavior change are appropriate outcomes of psychotherapy. Stated another way, psychotherapy attempts to modify long-standing personality traits such as coping styles and defense mechanisms, as well as learned, self-defeating behavior patterns.

Differences in Duration

The professional may be called in for a consultation or may interact with a patient on only one occasion; this is a very short-term interaction. The duration of contact is more extended between a health professional and a patient with a chronic illness or for a health care provider who has repeated but intermittent contacts with a patient over a longer period, such as a family physician, dentist, home health nurse, or nurse's aide.

Crisis intervention is time limited. A crisis is, by definition, a situation lasting no more than six weeks (Puryear, 1979). Crisis intervention is designed to provide immediate relief from and resolution of the crisis. It is not uncommon for a health professional to have only one contact, or,

at the most, several contacts, with a patient in a crisis situation. Because of its duration, intervention must be rapid and direct.

Psychotherapy is frequently intensive and long term. The specific duration depends on the nature and severity of the patient's problems, the setting (out-patient or in-patient), and the role and theoretical orientation of the attending professional. Normally patients in psychotherapy are seen on a regular weekly or intermittent basis over a period ranging from several months to several years.

Differences in Methods

The methods used in a helping framework are supportive and educational in nature. There is an emphasis on problem solving. Talking and interviewing are the primary interactional methods used by the helper, but on occasion ancillary methods such as simulation and role playing may be used. The helper relies primarily on listening, understanding, and other facilitative verbal and nonverbal communication skills.

The methods used in crisis intervention are supportive and directive in nature. There is an emphasis on focused problem solving, with most of the discussion related directly to the immediate crisis. The crisis intervention worker uses action-oriented methods to provide immediate relief and resolution. These methods include listening and understanding, information giving, instructions, and, when appropriate, advice giving.

The methods used by psychotherapists are supportive, reconstructive, and analytical in nature. There is emphasis on in-depth analysis and unconscious as well as conscious dynamics and awareness. In addition to treatment and intervention methods, psychotherapy makes use of traditional psychiatric diagnostic categories, such as those described in DSM III (the *Diagnostic and Statistical Manual of Mental Disorders,* 1980, published by the American Psychiatric Association). Talking and interviewing may be supplemented with other therapeutic procedures such as psychological testing, dream analysis, biofeedback, and hypnosis. In addition, some psychotherapists such as psychiatrists may use medically oriented treatments and prescribe medication for their patients' psychological problems.

Health professionals frequently become involved as helpers as they assist patients to cope with and resolve problems about short-term, chronic, or severe illness. Health professionals also function in various types of crisis situations, including (but not limited to) those precipitated by chronic or critical illness, death, sexual assault, and child and spouse abuse. Health professionals may assist individual patients and/or their families in dealing with the specific crisis situation effectively. Generally, health professionals do not become involved in promoting the extensive personality and behavior changes expected by psychotherapy unless they have had specialized, supervised training in counseling, psychology, or psychiatry. Typically, patients who want help primarily for psychological problems or who present severe or long-standing pathological conditions are referred to other helping professionals such as social workers, counselors, psychologists, and psychiatrists.

We agree with Bernstein and Bernstein (1980) that health professionals should not try to be psychotherapists in their interactions with patients. However, the use of helping skills is always appropriate in providing medical care "when problems in personal, familial, or social life either cause physical symptoms or interfere with the treatment of these symptoms" (Bernstein & Bernstein, 1980, p. 108). In the following section we describe a helping model we believe is useful for health professionals who are not psychotherapists but are interested in learning to respond effectively both to the emotional and the physical needs of their patients.

A Helping Model for the Health Professions

A variety of helping models exist, and there are two that we believe are particularly useful for health professionals. The first is the *human relations skills training model.* This model has its origins in the writings of Carl Rogers (1951; 1957),

although it has been refined by others, including Truax and Carkhuff (1967), Egan (1975; 1982), Ivey (1971), and Ivey and Authier (1978).

The basic assumptions of the human relations training model are:

1. A helping relationship is critical to an effective helping interaction. A helping relationship is characterized by three conditions, often referred to as *core* or *facilitative conditions*; empathy (accurate understanding), respect (positive regard), and genuineness (congruence).

2. The attitudes and the behaviors of the helping person (health care personnel) must reflect these three core conditions. That is, helping persons must communicate the presence of these three conditions to those seeking help by functioning therapeutically in the relationship and by utilizing effective communication skills.

3. Behavioral ways of communicating the core conditions of empathy, respect, and genuineness include verbal and nonverbal skills such as paying attention, paraphrasing, reflecting feelings, clarifying, confronting, instructing, and so on.

The second helping model we consider very useful is the *social influence model.* This model is founded on principles of social psychology, but its application to the helping professions has been developed by Strong (1968) and Strong and Schmidt (1970).

The two basic assumptions of the social influence model are the following:

1. The helper must establish power or a base of influence with the patient through a relationship comprising three characteristics or relationship enhancers: competence (expertness), trustworthiness (credibility), and attractiveness (liking).

2. The helper must actively use this base of influence to effect opinion and behavior change in the patient.

This chapter—and the book as a whole—are based on a helping model that combines the skills and ideas inherent in the human relations skills training model and the social influence model. We believe that health professionals involved in patient interactions should use such a helping framework for several reasons. First, some health professionals find it hard to conceptualize how they are part of a helping process. A helping framework may facilitate this understanding and conceptualization process. Second, a helping model provides a system or a methodology that health professionals can use in their work with patients. In other words, a framework provides a rationale for what one does with patients. Finally, the two helping models described above are the basis for the relationship and communication skills described in this book. You may find it easier to acquire and apply these skills if you first understand their theoretical origins.

As we saw in the description of the human relations skills training model, there are three core or facilitative conditions—empathy, respect, and genuineness—and three relationship enhancers—competence, trustworthiness, and attractiveness—in an effective helping relationship. These six factors not only represent subjective qualities or attitudes of health professionals but also are apparent in the skillful use of verbal and nonverbal communication skills. We describe these six characteristics in more detail in the following sections.

Empathy

One definition of empathy is "the capacity to respond to another's feelings and experiences as if they were your own." It means, as the phrase goes, "putting yourself in the other person's shoes." According to Brammer and Shostrom (1982), responding empathically to a person is an "attempt to think *with,* rather than *for* or *about*" the person (p. 160).

Empathy is a critical variable in influencing the quality and effectiveness of a helping relationship. Empathy helps establish rapport with and elicit information from a patient. Egan (1982) views empathy as "both a relationship-establishing skill and a data-gathering or problem-clarification skill" (p. 88). He observes that being empathic also shows understanding and support and is a "tool of civility" (p. 99).

Empathy is both an attitude and a skill. The desire to understand and to be with a patient reflects an empathic attitude on the part of the interviewer. This attitude, however, must be translated into actions or skills and be *communicated* to the patient. Ideally, a patient will sense not only that the health professional *wants* to understand but also that he or she *does* understand. Truax and Carkhuff (1967) describe empathy as a variable that exists on a continuum. At one end of the continuum, lack of empathy implies that the interviewer either totally misses or has no awareness or understanding of even the most obvious patient messages. At the other end, empathy involves being "tuned in to the patient's wavelength," implying a oneness with and comprehension of the patient's innermost thoughts and feelings even though they may remain unspoken.

Carkhuff (1969a) and Egan (1982) have suggested several guidelines for learning to communicate empathically. These guidelines are summarized in Table 2-1. First, concentrate with intensity on the patient's messages, both verbal and nonverbal. This concentration will help you become "tuned in" to the patient. Second, allow time to think. Use silence judiciously to give yourself time to assimilate material before responding too hastily. Third, formulate a verbal response that is interchangeable with the patient's message. According to Carkhuff, Pierce, and Cannon (1977), an interchangeable response is one that reflects the same level of intensity as the patient's message and neither adds to nor subtracts from the patient's communication. The truly empathic response is also accurate—it represents exactly what the patient has said, no more and no less. Verbal responses that reflect empathy include verbal attentiveness (minimal verbal encouragers and verbal tracking), paraphrasing, reflecting feelings, clarifying, and summarizing (see also Chapters 5 and 6).

Fourth, make the verbal response short and concise. The impact of empathy is lost or hidden in longwindedness. Fifth, use language that is similar to that used by the patient. Sixth, respond in a nonverbal manner that is appropriate to the feelings expressed by the patient. It would be inappropriate, for example, to respond with smiling if

Table 2-1
Core or Facilitative Conditions (Empathy, Respect, and Genuineness)

Condition	Definition	Purposes	Guidelines for Use
Empathy	The capacity to respond to the patient's feelings and experiences as if they were your own; the ability to communicate accurate understanding of the patient.	1. To establish rapport; 2. To show understanding and support; 3. To demonstrate civility; 4. To clarify problems; 5. To collect information.	1. Concentrate with intensity on the patient's verbal and nonverbal messages. 2. Use silence to assimilate the material before responding. 3. Formulate and deliver a verbal response that is equivalent to the message expressed by the patient. 4. Make the verbal response concise. 5. Use language that is similar to that used by the patient. 6. Respond in a nonverbal manner that is congruent with the patient's feelings.
Respect	The ability to see a patient as a person with worth and dignity; consists of commitment, understanding, a nonjudgmental attitude, and warmth.	1. To communicate a willingness to work with the patient; 2. To communicate interest in the patient as a person; 3. To communicate acceptance of the patient; 4. To communicate caring to the patient; 5. To provide an outlet for and to diminish the patient's angry feelings.	1. Reserve specified amount of time and energy for patient's use. 2. Interact with patient without "hurrying." 3. Indicate, with questions or comments, interest in and efforts to understand the patient. 4. Convey understanding of patient without overt approval or disapproval. 5. Comment on positive aspects or attitudes of patient. 6. Express differences of opinion with comments that support rather than criticize patient's ideas.

Table 2-1 (cont'd)

Condition	Definition	Purposes	Guidelines for Use
Respect (continued)			7. Support verbal expressions with appropriate nonverbal behaviors of respect and warmth.
Genuineness	The ability to be yourself, without presenting a facade.	1. To reduce the emotional distance between interviewer and patient; 2. To increase the identification process between interviewer and patient, thereby providing rapport and trust.	1. Be congruent; make sure verbal messages, nonverbal behavior, and feelings are consistent. 2. Be aware of any inconsistencies in your messages and behaviors. 3. Avoid overemphasizing your role, position, status, or authority. 4. Be spontaneous—do not constantly ponder what to say, and yet at the same time be tactful. 5. Express genuineness with supporting nonverbal behaviors, such as direct eye contact, smiling, and leaning toward the patient.

the patient has expressed sadness or even seriousness. Finally, as Egan (1982) observes, *indigenous* helpers—those who are similar to patients in occupational, cultural, and educational background and so on—may be perceived as more empathic simply because of these similarities.

Goldstein (1980) has provided some useful examples of the verbal communication of empathy in a dialogue between an elderly patient and a home aide. In the dialogue, note that explicit statements of empathy made by the home aide are different from mere "parroting." An empathic interchangeable response is not just a restatement of what the patient has said.

Dialogue*

Patient: The old age home was really different from this apartment building. All my

*From "Relationship-Enhancement Methods," by A. P. Goldstein. In F. H. Kanfer and A. P. Goldstein (Eds.), *Helping people change,* pp. 36–37. Copyright © 1980 by Pergamon Publishers. Reprinted by permission.

friends are still there. I don't even know anyone here.

Home Aide: Sounds like you're lonely in your new home. Kind of like a stranger in a new place. I can see how it's pretty depressing missing all your friends.

Patient: I sure am lonely. Every friend I have is still at the home and it's so hard living all alone with three whole rooms to myself. I even get sad listening to people's voices in the other apartments.

Home Aide: You'd like to get out of your three lonely rooms and meet some of the other people in the building. You'd be happier if you made some new friends.

Patient: I don't like . . . It makes me feel silly for you to wash and feed me.

Aide: It makes you uncomfortable when someone takes care of you. You feel like you should be doing things on your own and you shouldn't need me.

Patient: Mmhmm. I feel like a baby when someone's helping me. But I know I can't do stuff myself now because I've tried.

Aide: You feel foolish when you have to rely on other people since you should be helping yourself. But you know that you need other people's help now for your own well-being.

Patient: I think about things like falling down the stairs, or dropping my cigarette in bed, or a stranger coming to my house late at night. . . . I don't really know what I'd do. . . .

Aide: You're worried about whether you could handle an emergency all alone.

Patient: Yeah, I worry, *a lot.* . . . I remember how scary it was the time I fainted and nobody was here to help me.

Aide: It would be nice to be able to count on somebody's help when something goes wrong and you're not sure you can take care of things all by yourself.

Egan (1982) observes that the use of explicit statements of empathy such as those used in this dialogue may be unnecessary with a more established relationship. He states:

> I also realize that people who grow close to each other do not often use explicit statements of empathy in their conversations. That, I believe, is not because empathy doesn't exist or is unimportant. It is rather that the relationship itself has grown empathic, and the need for explicit statements of empathy lessens (p. 99).

The explicit communication of empathy appears to be most critical and useful during the early phases of interacting with patients. The helper should bear in mind that what is experienced as empathic for one person may not be construed as empathic by someone else. The guidelines presented in this section for empathy reflect an understanding of empathy in a predominantly western culture. Patients from other cultures may not interpret empathy in the same way. (Now complete the learning activity for empathy on pages 26 and 27.)

Respect

Respect, also referred to as *positive regard,* means the ability to prize or value the patient as a person with worth and dignity (Rogers, 1957). Like empathy, respect is an attitude, an inner quality that reflects a way of considering people or patients, and, like empathy, this attitude must be translated into actions to affect the helping relationship. According to Egan (1982), "respect is not often communicated directly in words in helping situations. Actions speak louder than words. . . . Respect is communicated principally by the ways helpers *orient* themselves *toward* and *work with* [patients]" (p. 121).

LEARNING ACTIVITIES

Empathic Responding

In this learning activity, we present eight patient/health professional statements. Your task is to identify in writing whether each health professional statement is an empathic or a nonempathic response (Chapter Objective 1). Do not try to judge whether the response is the best possible one but simply whether it is empathic or nonempathic. The first one is completed as an example. Check your responses with those found in the feedback following the learning activity.

1. *Patient:* I don't know how much longer I can keep coming in for these periodic checkups. It's getting awfully expensive. I'm not sure how much these checkups really help anyway.

   Health Professional: Of course you should continue these checkups as much as possible. Otherwise we may not be able to detect a small problem and it may get out of hand.

   _____ Empathic   __✓__ Nonempathic (the health professional responds paternalistically)

2. *Patient:* I don't understand why I'm being discharged so early. With no one at home to help me, I'm not sure how I'll manage.

   Health Professional: You sound as if you aren't certain you're ready to leave the hospital yet.

   _____ Empathic   _____ Nonempathic

3. *Patient:* It's just great that this clinic is available for folks like me. Otherwise I couldn't afford to get care for my kids.

   Health Professional: You sound really pleased about having the clinic available for you and your family.

   _____ Empathic   _____ Nonempathic

4. *Patient:* I've been on this medicine for almost a year now, and I'm getting sort of tired of having to take it.

   Health Professional: Well, you'd better keep taking it for as long as you live, for your own good.

   _____ Empathic   _____ Nonempathic

5. *Patient:* I don't know if I want braces or not. My mom wants me to get them, but my friends who have them say braces are a real pain.

   Health Professional: You appear to be in a dilemma about whether or not getting braces is the best thing for you to do.

   _____ Empathic   _____ Nonempathic

6. *Patient:* This operation is frightening to me. I've never had any kind of surgery before.

   Health Professional: Well, don't worry about it. It really won't be that bad.

   _____ Empathic   _____ Nonempathic

7. *Patient:* Have you ever had to undergo all these tests? It is a lot more painful than I thought it would be.

   Health Professional: I'm sorry you've noticed so much pain. I guess I should have made it a point to mention the discomfort so you would have been better prepared.

   _____ Empathic   _____ Nonempathic

8. *Patient:* I just don't see why you're making such a fuss because my blood sugar is high. It's a lot lower than it has been in the past.

   Health Professional: Well, maybe it is lower, but it's still not where I want it to be.

   _____ Empathic   _____ Nonempathic

Feedback

2. Empathic. The health professional responds directly to the patient's feelings of doubt about being discharged.
3. Empathic. The health professional reflects the patient's feelings of satisfaction about the clinic.
4. Nonempathic. The health professional completely misses the patient's feelings of doubt and simply urges the patient to continue the medication.
5. Empathic. The health professional is aware of and responds to the patient's dilemma.
6. Nonempathic. The health professional avoids the patient's feelings of fear and offers false reassurance instead.
7. Empathic. The health professional responds to the impact of the tests on the patient.
8. Nonempathic. The health professional responds defensively.

Raush and Bordin (1957) and Egan (1982) have identified four components of respect: having a sense of commitment to the patient; making an effort to understand the patient; suspending critical judgment; and expressing a reasonable amount of warmth (see also Table 2-1).

Commitment

Commitment to the patient implies some degree of willingness and interest in working with the patient. Like empathy and respect, the attitude of commitment must be felt by the patient. Scheduling a specified amount of time to see the patient, reserving time for the patient's exclusive use, ensuring relative privacy and confidentiality during sessions, and applying professional skills to help the patient—all these aid in communicating commitment.

Bernstein and Bernstein (1980) have observed the serious and negative consequences that result when such commitment on the part of the health professional is missing. They state:

> From the point of view of the patient, then, the most serious barriers to a good relationship (and consequently better diagnosis and treatment) are the professional's lack of time, his seeming lack of concern, and his failure to tell the patient what he needs to know and can understand about his illness. Repeatedly in studies and surveys when patients are asked their opinion about medical care they respond critically and often bitterly about the doctor's or nurse's hurry when taking care of them. This "hurry" is apt to be interpreted—and resented—not as a lack of time, but as a lack of humane interest in the sick individual (p. 6).

Health professionals who don't make such a commitment are doing a great disservice to their patients and, ultimately, to themselves.

Understanding

Patients will feel respected to the degree that they *feel* the health care provider is attempting to understand them and to treat their complaints with seriousness and concern. Health professionals can demonstrate their efforts to understand by being empathic, by asking questions designed to elicit information important to the patient, and by indicating with comments or actions their interest in understanding the patient (Raush & Bordin, 1957, p. 352). Respect and empathy are mutually reinforcing and work "hand in hand." The two characteristics are synergistic—the overall effect of both is greater than the effect of either one alone.

Nonjudgmental Attitude

A nonjudgmental attitude refers to the interviewer's capacity to suspend judgment of the patient's actions or motives and to avoid condemning or condoning the patient's personality or behavior. It implies the ability to be accepting rather than critical of patients. It does not necessarily mean that the health professional supports or agrees with all the patient does or says. Rather, the interviewer

is able to create an atmosphere in which the patient feels safe and nondefensive and can ultimately be more responsive to the interviewer's opinions and suggestions when they are introduced. An interviewer conveys a nonjudgmental attitude by warmly accepting the patient's expressions and experiences as part of that person without imposing conditions (Goldstein, 1980, p. 39). In contrast, whenever an interviewer expresses dislike or disapproval regarding the motives, actions, personality, or behavior of a patient, he or she is conveying a judgmental attitude.

Consider the differences in the way Interviewers A and B respond to the following patient:

Patient: I suppose I should stay at home to care for my husband now that he's an invalid, but I really find that hard to do. I feel so helpless when I look at him just lying there all the time. It's easier and less painful—and more interesting—to keep on working.

Interviewer A: Don't you remember what you said in your marriage vows—for better or for worse—in sickness and in health? It seems to me that continuing to work is a rather selfish solution to this problem.

Interviewer B: I think I can understand your dilemma. On the one hand, you are certainly committed to your husband. On the other hand, you need to stimulate yourself in other areas so that you have the energy to continue to work with your husband.

Interviewer B neither approves nor disapproves of what this patient is saying, whereas Interviewer A explicitly judges and disapproves of the manner in which the patient is handling the situation. It appears from the patient's point of view that Interviewer A has sided with the husband and has discounted or "written off" the patient. Interviewer B provides an opportunity for the patient to further express and explore the ramifications of this difficult situation, whereas Interviewer A invokes guilt feelings that may eliminate the possibility of further communication with this patient.

A question that health care providers frequently face is how can health professionals overcome personal and cultural biases to deal effectively with an individual who is perceived as unlikeable, worthless, or offensive—for example, a convicted murderer or rapist? George and Christiani (1981) observe that the answer to this question lies partly in the fact that the relationship between health professionals and patients is a helping one. These authors assert that many helpers can respond positively to people who are difficult to like "because the helping relationship allows them to move beyond behaviors, defenses, and facades that others find offensive" (p. 152). In other words, the maintenance of an appropriate professional bearing that demonstrates commitment, understanding, and a nonjudgmental attitude may establish an atmosphere that will allow such patients to discard some of their offensive behaviors, at least for the duration of an interview.

Warmth

According to Goldstein (1980), without the expression of warmth, specific procedures "may be technically correct but therapeutically impotent" (p. 39). Warmth seems to be a key component of effective interactions. The "bedside manner" or interpersonal competence of health professionals is at least as important to their patients as their technical or scientific expertise. The expression of warmth to patients also is important since, as Truax and Carkhuff (1967) observe, most people respond to warmth with warmth and, conversely, to hostility with hostility. In interactions with a hostile or resentful patient, warmth and caring can disarm and diminish the intensity of the patient's angry feelings.

Health professionals can express warmth to patients through specific verbal statements and nonverbal behaviors. Verbally, positive comments about the patient or the relationship, such as "I am concerned about you" or "You're handling this situation very well," express warmth. Ivey and

Simek-Downing (1980, p. 136) describe two kinds of statements that can express warmth—*enhancing* statements and *appreciation-of-differences* statements. Enhancing statements portray some positive aspect or attribute about the patient. Examples of enhancing statements are "You express your ideas well," "You have a very good understanding of your illness," or "You have really done a great job of sticking to this treatment plan since I last saw you." Enhancing statements usually provide positive reinforcement to a patient.

Appreciation-of-differences statements are used primarily when the patient and the interviewer have different opinions about an issue. Examples of appreciation-of-differences statements include "I wouldn't do it that way, but I respect your right to try that out" or "My opinion about it is different, but I can see how you arrived at your conclusion." Such statements support the rights of both parties to retain different ideas or opinions. Explicit disapproval of the patient's point of view is not expressed, but there is no ambiguity concerning the position of either party.

Nonverbally, warmth is communicated through tone of voice, eye contact, facial animation and expressions, gestures, touch, and so on. Johnson (1981) describes some specific nonverbal cues that express warmth or coldness (see Table 2-2). Remember that these behaviors may be interpreted as warm or cold by patients from predominantly western cultures. Patients from other cultures may perceive these nonverbal aspects of warmth and coldness differently.

We should also note that the communication of warmth may have an assertive quality to it. As Egan (1982) has observed, the communication of respect ultimately involves placing demands on people or helping them place demands on themselves (p. 122). On occasion, warmth may be expressed behaviorally by "directiveness, assertiveness, autonomy-enhancing distancing, and even anger" (Goldstein, 1980, p. 45). The presence of warmth allows confrontation to occur between interviewer and patient when necessary and appropriate. We describe effective confrontation in more detail in Chapter 7.

Table 2-2
Nonverbal Cues of Warmth and Coldness

Nonverbal Cue	Warmth	Coldness
Tone of voice	Soft, soothing	Callous, reserved, hard
Facial expression	Smiling, interested	Poker-faced, frowning, disinterested
Posture	Relaxed, leaning toward the other person	Tense, leaning away from the other person
Eye contact	Looking directly into the other person's eyes	Avoiding eye contact
Touching	Touching the other person softly and discreetly	Avoiding all touch
Gestures	Open, welcoming	Closed, as if guarding oneself
Physical proximity	Close	Distant

Adapted from Johnson, 1981.

LEARNING ACTIVITIES

Respect

An important aspect of respect is the capacity to respond to disagreements or differences of opinion in a helpful and nondefensive manner. Four patient situations are described in this learning activity. For each situation, you are to formulate and write an example of an "appreciation-of-differences" statement that could be used as a response (Chapter Objective 2). Situation 1 is completed as an example. See if your statements are similar to those given in the feedback that follows.

1. You request the patient to repeat an extensive series of laboratory tests that were originally performed three months ago. The patient says that he would rather wait for several more months before undergoing the same tests again.

   Appreciation-of-differences response:

   I'm sorry that you don't share the same sense of urgency to repeat the laboratory studies that I do. However, because of the discomfort that is associated with the tests, I can understand your position.

2. You advise a distraught patient to see a psychiatrist for consultation. The patient refuses to do so, explaining that her "emotionally upset state" is only temporary.

   Appreciation-of-differences response:

   _____

   _____

3. You advise a patient requesting teeth restoration that all of her teeth must be removed because they have deteriorated too far to salvage. She refuses to have the extractions performed.

Appreciation-of-differences response:

_____

_____

4. You advise a patient to obtain a second opinion about a rare illness. The patient refuses, stating that he has complete faith in your tentative diagnosis.

Appreciation-of-differences response:

_____

_____

Feedback

2. I don't believe this emotional upset will disappear in a short period of time. But I respect your decision to try to handle it on your own for the time being.
3. I don't feel that it is possible or worthwhile to try to restore your teeth because they are already in such poor shape. However, I can understand your reluctance to have them all removed.
4. I really appreciate your confidence in my capabilities. But because your illness is so unusual, I feel it would be in your best interest to get a second opinion. Also, that would make me feel more comfortable with the diagnosis.

Genuineness

Genuineness refers to the interviewer's ability to be sincere without presenting a facade. According to Egan (1982), "genuine people are at home with themselves and therefore can comfortably be themselves in all their interactions. This means that they do not have to change when they are with different people—that is, they do not constantly have to adopt new roles to be acceptable to others" (p. 127). Many patients are able to relate better to someone who is genuine or "real" because they see that person as human, as someone similar to themselves. This identification process can contribute to the development of rapport and trust in the relationship.

Congruence

There are several aspects to genuineness and several ways in which it can be communicated to patients. One aspect is congruence. Congruence means simply that the interviewer's words, actions, and feelings are consistent. Congruence also implies that interviewers are aware of any discrepancy that exists between their feelings, words, and actions and are careful not to let such discrepancies interfere with the interview or the patient.

Consider the differences in the following examples. Interviewer A, while sitting down, facing the patient, looking at the patient, and pausing for the patient to respond, says "I think that what you're saying about your health is very important. We need to spend some time today talking about it." Interviewer B, after glancing at the clock and the door, taps one foot on the floor and stands up, saying "I think that what you're saying about your health is very important. We need to spend some time today talking about it."

Interviewer A's nonverbal behavior is consistent with the verbal message. The patient is likely to believe that the health professional is genuinely interested in spending the time to discuss the issue. Interviewer B's nonverbal behavior is inconsistent with the verbal message. The nonverbal behavior contradicts the verbal message, and the patient may reasonably assume that the interviewer is insincere or too rushed to discuss the issue. If Interviewer B was aware of this incongruence, he or she might say something like this:

> I think that what you're saying about your health is very important, and we need to spend some time talking about it. However, today is not a good time for me to do this. When can we schedule another appointment to discuss the matter?

The patient will probably respond more positively to the second response because the interviewer is not sending simultaneous conflicting messages. When the patient does return, the interviewer's behavior is more likely to be congruent because of his or her awareness that the earlier time was not an opportune one, and the return visit was scheduled for a specific purpose.

Role Behavior of the Interviewer

Another aspect of genuineness involves the role behavior of the interviewer. Interviewers who do not overemphasize their role are more likely to be perceived as genuine than interviewers who constantly remind the patient of their role, posi-

tion, authority, and status. Too much emphasis on role and status can create distance between the health professional and the patient, and the patient may feel intimidated or resentful. Consider the differences in the following examples:

Nurse A: Mr. Green? I'm the head nurse on this floor. I'm the one who's in charge of what goes on. I just wanted to stop in to introduce myself because if there's anything you need, you should let me know. Being head nurse carries a certain amount of weight around here, and I can get things straightened out in a hurry.

Nurse B: Hello, Mr. Green. I'm the head nurse on this floor. I just wanted to stop in to introduce myself and see if there's anything in particular you need.

In the first example, Nurse A emphasizes his or her role and status first. The patient's needs appear secondary. Nurse B, in contrast, simply states the role to the patient as part of an introduction, emphasizing the desire to meet the patient's needs. The patient will probably be more responsive to sharing concerns with Nurse B than with Nurse A. Nurse B conveys genuine interest in the patient's needs, whereas Nurse A seems more infatuated with authority or control over the patient.

Spontaneity

A third aspect of genuineness is spontaneity. Spontaneity is the capacity to say or express oneself naturally without acting in a contrived manner. It also implies the use of tact without conversational hesitancy (Egan, 1982). Spontaneity does not mean the interviewer must verbalize every passing thought or feeling to the patient, nor does it give interviewers license to say whatever is on their minds. Effective interviewers are spontaneous and assertive without being blunt and aggressive (Egan, 1982). Spontaneity involves the ability to speak freely and easily without "putting your foot in your mouth." Observe the difference in the way two interviewers respond to a patient about his weight:

Interviewer A: Mr. Tysons, I've noticed you've gained a few pounds since your last visit. Can you tell me how your efforts at dieting have been working out?

Interviewer B: Mr. Tysons, you've gained six pounds since I saw you several weeks ago. Shame on you! I guess I know someone who's been cheating on his diet!

Interviewer A expresses concern about the patient's weight gain in an open yet tactful manner. Interviewer B is blunt and depicts disbelief and scornfulness through his or her comments. Mr. Tysons is much more likely to reveal honest and significant information about his weight problems to Interviewer A than to Interviewer B. The bluntness of Interviewer B is likely to strangle, rather than encourage, patient communication.

Genuineness is also communicated by the interviewer's use of appropriate or supporting nonverbal behaviors. Nonverbal behaviors that convey genuineness include eye contact, smiling, and leaning toward the patient while sitting (Seay & Altkreuse, 1979). These three nonverbal behaviors, however, should be used discreetly. For example, direct yet intermittent eye contact is perceived as more indicative of genuineness than is persistent gazing, which patients may interpret as staring. Similarly, continual smiling or leaning forward may be viewed as phony and artificial, rather than as genuine and sincere. (Table 2-1 summarizes the various characteristics of genuineness.)

LEARNING ACTIVITIES

Genuineness

An important aspect of being genuine is sending consistent or congruent verbal and nonverbal messages to a patient. In the learning activity that follows, four health professional verbal statements are given, along with a description of the health professional's corresponding nonverbal behavior. Your task is to decide whether each verbal and nonverbal message is congruent or incongruent (Chapter Objective 3). The first interaction is completed as an example. Check your responses with the ones presented in the feedback following the learning activity.

1. A rehabilitation counselor, speaking in a barely audible voice and with averted eyes, says "I certainly do believe we can help you."

    _____Congruent   ___✓___ Incongruent (the nonverbal cues do not support the verbal message)

2. A home health aide, with a broad smile, facial animation, and direct eye contact, states "I'm so glad it was convenient for me to drop by to see you today. I wanted to see how you were getting along."

    _____Congruent   _____Incongruent

3. While leaning back in his desk chair and glancing at the mail, Dr. Gray says "I'd be glad to talk over this diagnosis with you in more detail. It's important that you understand what it means."

    _____Congruent   _____Incongruent

4. "I really don't have the time today to discuss your alcohol problem. But please ask the receptionist to schedule another appointment in two weeks so we can address that problem," said Dr. Owens as she stood up and offered to shake hands.

_____Congruent   _____ Incongruent

Feedback

2. These messages are consistent; the home health aide's nonverbal behaviors match the feeling or tenor expressed by verbal message.
3. These messages are inconsistent; Dr. Gray's nonverbal behavior contradicts the verbal statement.
4. These messages are consistent; Dr. Owens's nonverbal cues support the verbal message.

Competence

Competence, also referred to as *expertness,* is another factor that enhances the respect component of a helping relationship. Evidence suggests that patients' respect for the interviewer increases in direct proportion to their perception of the interviewer's competence or expertise (Goldstein, 1980). According to Egan (1975), competence refers to a person's belief that the interviewer has the necessary information, skill, and ability to be of help (p. 109). Competence (or the perception of it) is extremely important in the interactions of health professionals with patients for several reasons. First, it enhances the patient's faith and belief in health professionals. This added degree of confidence endows the professionals with an additional degree of authority. Second, competence is related to patient compliance. Patients are more favorably disposed to accept and act on the recommendations of someone whom they perceive as competent or as having particular expertise.

Schmidt and Strong (1970) present some college students' description of an expert helper and an inexpert helper:

The expert shakes the student's hand, aligning the student with himself, and greets him with his first name. He seems interested and relaxed. He has a neat appearance but is not stuffy . . . He talks at the student's level and is not arrogant toward him. The expert assumes a comfortable but attentive sitting position. He focuses his attention on the student and carefully listens to him. His voice is inflective and lively, he changes his facial expressions, and uses hand gestures. He speaks fluently with confidence and sureness. The expert has prepared for the interview. . . . He asks direct and to-the-point questions. His questions are thought-provoking and follow an apparently logical progression. They seem spontaneous and conversational. . . . The expert moves quickly to the root of the problem. . . . He makes recommendations and suggests possible solutions.

The inexpert is awkward, tense, and uneasy. He seems to be afraid of the student. He does not greet the student by name to put him at ease. . . . He is not quite sure of himself or of some of his remarks. He seems too cold, strict and dominating, and too formal in attitude and action. His gestures are stiff and overdone. . . . The inexpert slouches in his chair. He is too casual and relaxed. . . . His voice is flat and without inflection, appearing to show disinterest and boredom. . . . The inexpert comes to the interview cold. He has not cared enough about the student to acquaint himself with the student's records. The inexpert asks vague questions which are trivial and irrelevant and have no common thread or aim. His questioning is abrupt and tactless with poor transitions. He asks too many questions like a quiz session, giving the student the third degree.... The inexpert is slow in getting his point across and is confusing in his discussion of what the student should do.... The inexpert does not get to the core of the problem.... He just doesn't seem to be getting anywhere (p. 117).*

Role

Egan (1975) has defined three variables that contribute to a person's perception of interviewer competence. These three factors are role, reputation, and behavior. *Role* refers to the interviewer's title, position, and credentials. Role can be established very quickly, simply by the way interviewers introduce themselves and by their dress, demeanor, office decor, diplomas, and so on. Several studies, for example, have demonstrated that an individual introduced as "Doctor" is more likely to be perceived as an expert than someone introduced as "Mister" or "Ms." The health professional can establish role expertise without overemphasis, simply by stating his or her role to the patient upon introduction. Such introductions are demonstrated in the following examples.

> Hello, Ms. Baker. I'm Dr. Greenberg. I'm the physician who was called in to have a look at your leg.
>
> Hello, Ms. Baker. I'm Dr. Brown. I'm the dentist who will be examining your teeth.
>
> Hello, Ms. Baker. I'm Miss Simons, the nurse assigned to this part of the ward.
>
> Hello, Ms. Baker. I'm Mrs. Blackburg. I'm the new pharmacist for this clinic.

_____

*From "Expert and Inexpert Counselors," by L. D. Schmidt and S. R. Strong. *Journal of Counseling Psychology,* 1970, *17,* 115–118. Copyright © 1970 by the American Psychological Association. Reprinted by permission of the publisher and the authors.

Role expertise is also defined for patients by the way interviewers dress and by their general demeanor. Interviewers who dress and act in concert with their roles are apt to be perceived as more competent than those who don't. A health professional who dresses in a careless, slovenly, or inappropriate fashion or who acts timid or uncomfortable is not likely to convey much role expertise to the patient.

Patients may also look at nameplates, diplomas, and certificates to establish the role expertness of the interviewer. Consequently, it may be prudent to judiciously display certificates showing board certification, membership in professional societies, service awards, and so on. Such "external trappings" may serve the dual purpose of establishing role capability and enhancing the decor of an office or clinic.

Reputation

Reputation refers to the fact that other people have testified publicly about an interviewer's ability or competence (Egan, 1975). Such testimony may come from friends or other colleagues. In health care, many patients seek to establish the reputation of a health professional before deciding to seek her or his services. They may do so by seeking the opinion of other patients, of other health professionals, or even by noting whether the person in question is associated with a prestigious or well-known practice or institution. Unfortunately, reputation is not always a reliable indicator of the health professional's actual competence. In some instances, a very skilled health care worker may receive "bad press." In other cases, a less skilled health professional may be held in very high esteem by others.

Behavior

The third and most important aspect of competence is a behavioral one—whether professionals actually measure up to the expectations of their roles and reputations by demonstrating the necessary skills and knowledge for helping patients. Implicit in this concept is the condition that health professionals must be able to meet the emotional as well as the physiological needs of their patients. According to Gilbert (1978), the behavioral aspect of competence is established by what the interviewer actually accomplishes with the patient.

Behavioral competence is also related to trustworthiness. Egan (1982) observes that "trust in a helper can evaporate quickly if little or nothing is accomplished" (p. 139). Table 2-3 summarizes guidelines for communicating competence.

Table 2-3
Relationship Enhancers
(Competence, Trustworthiness, and Attractiveness)

Relationship Variable	Definition	Purposes	Guidelines for Use
Competence	A patient's belief that the interviewer has the necessary knowledge and skills to be of assistance.	1. To enhance the patient's belief and faith in the health professional; 2. To increase patient compliance with the interviewer's recommendations.	1. Introduce yourself with your title without overemphasizing your role. 2. Make your dress and demeanor appropriate to your role and setting. 3. Deliver what you promise in terms of helping patients.
Trustworthiness	A patient's belief that the word or promise of a health professional can be relied on.	1. To increase the patient's respect toward the interviewer; 2. To increase the patient's confidence in the health professional and the prescribed treatment regimens.	1. Deliver accurate and reliable information to patients. 2. Be dependable in interactions with patients; deliver what you promise. 3. Maintain confidentiality. 4. Respond to the patient with dynamism and frequency; avoid passivity. 5. Demonstrate sincerity in your motives and intentions.
Interpersonal Attractiveness	A patient's perception of the health professional as similar to and compatible with the patient.	1. To enhance the helping relationship, especially the liking or regard component;	1. Convey attentiveness, friendliness, and understanding to the patient.

Table 2-3 (cont'd)

Relationship Variable	Definition	Purposes	Guidelines for Use
Interpersonal Attractiveness (cont'd)		2. To increase the health professional's influence with the patient.	2. Use appropriate self-disclosure of similar attitudes, opinions, or experiences. 3. Engage in structuring—telling the patient what will happen during the interview.

LEARNING ACTIVITIES

Competence

The following learning activity presents descriptions of eight interviewer behaviors. According to Chapter Objective 4, you are to identify in writing whether the behavior reflects an expert or an inexpert interviewer. The first behavior item is completed as an example. Feedback follows the learning activity.

1. The interviewer greets the patient by name.

   __✓__ Expert _____ Inexpert
   (An expert interviewer always uses the patient's name.)

2. The interviewer asks questions that seem redundant or irrelevant.

   _____ Expert _____ Inexpert

3. The interviewer is formal in both attitude and actions.
   _____ Expert _____ Inexpert

4. The interviewer talks on the patient's level, using language the patient can understand.

   _____ Expert _____ Inexpert

5. The interviewer does not seem acquainted with the background of the patient.

   _____ Expert _____ Inexpert

6. The interviewer changes the subject frequently.

_____ Expert   _____ Inexpert

7. The interviewer speaks fluently and with vocal and facial animation.

_____ Expert   _____ Inexpert

8. The interviewer asks questions that relate directly to the topic or to the patient's expressed concerns.

_____ Expert   _____ Inexpert

Feedback

2. Inexpert
3. Inexpert
4. Expert
5. Inexpert
6. Inexpert
7. Expert
8. Expert

Trustworthiness

Trustworthiness or *credibility* is another interviewer characteristic that enhances the respect component of a helping relationship. The patient's respect for the interviewer is greater if the interviewer is perceived as having a high degree of credibility. Rotter (1971) defines trustworthiness as "an expectancy held by an individual or group that the word, promise, verbal or written statement of another individual or group can be relied on" (p. 444). As Froelich and Bishop (1977) note:

In the professional office the development, or lack, of trust depends on the actuality of what the professional says will or will not happen. If you say, "This will not hurt," whether it does or does not hurt makes a difference in the development of the patient's trust. If you say, "I will see you next Tuesday at 11:00," whether you see that patient at 11:00 or 12:00 makes a difference. Each of these situations leads to the ability of the patient to accurately predict your behavior and learn that what you say can (or cannot) be trusted (p. 71).

Trustworthiness or credibility is critical in health professional/patient interactions. If the patient does not believe in the health professional, this lack of confidence can jeopardize the entire treatment process. Enelow and Swisher (1979) observe that "at the very least, every health care worker must establish himself as a humane and sensitive person whose opinions, skills, and recommendations can be trusted. Sadly, this simple requirement is often neglected, even by health care workers who expect patients to commit their lives and welfare to them, albeit briefly" (p. 89). When health professionals establish a trusting relationship with their patients, "the patients recover quicker, experience less pain, and experience a greater variety of physiological, psychological, and behavioral gains . . ." (Gerrard, Boniface, & Love, 1980, p. 112).

Trustworthiness is communicated in several ways. Like competence, trust in health professionals may be enhanced simply because of a reputation for honesty and the social role (Strong, 1968). Patients are more likely to trust health professionals if they have heard descriptive statements about them affirming their honesty and scrupulousness. For example, a patient may hear other patients or colleagues remark:

> That dentist is just out to make money to pay for that new office and equipment. **Or**, That dentist is really interested in providing quality care and at reasonable prices.

The patient's trust in the dentist would be diminished by overhearing the first statement and increased by the second statement.

Patients also are likely to trust health professionals implicitly because of the status of their role in our society. According to Egan (1975), "In our society, people who have certain roles are usually considered trustworthy until the opposite is demonstrated. Physicians and other medical professionals usually fall into this category, and when exceptions do occur (as when a dentist is convicted of molesting a patient), the scandal is greater because it is unexpected" (p. 111).

During long-term care or interactions, it is especially important to communicate trustworthiness. Egan (1982), Johnson (1981), and Strong (1968) suggest ways in which the interviewer's actions convey trustworthiness and credibility (see Table 2-3). First, be reliable as an information source. Accurate and reliable information will enhance the interviewer's credibility. Second, be dependable. Patients need to believe that the health care worker will "come through" for them. Egan (1982) suggests that one way to establish dependability is to formulate a contract with the patient and live up to its provisions. Such a contract may be explicit or implicit. The essence of dependability can be summarized this way: Don't promise what you can't deliver, and be sure to deliver what you promise. Third, maintain confidentiality of the patient's communications. Nothing will destroy trust more quickly than a patient's discovery that confidential information has been shared inappropriately or without permission. Fourth, respond to the patient with some frequency and dynamism. A patient's level of trust will be decreased if the interviewer is passive, lethargic, or inactive; it will be enhanced by a dynamic, growing, and changing relationship

LEARNING ACTIVITIES

Trustworthiness

This learning activity presents descriptions of eight health professional characteristics. Your task is to determine whether each characteristic is an example of trustworthiness or nontrustworthiness and record your answer in the appropriate answer blank (Chapter Objective 5). The first exercise is completed as an example, and feedback follows the learning activity.

1. The health professional is a respected pharmacist in the community.

   __✓__Trustworthy   _____ Nontrustworthy
   (Trustworthiness is conveyed by the social role and status of a health professional.)

2. The health professional has a reputation for charging excessive fees.

   _____Trustworthy   _____ Nontrustworthy

3. The health professional provides accurate information to patients.

   _____Trustworthy   _____ Nontrustworthy

4. The health professional is late for appointments.

_____Trustworthy _____ Nontrustworthy

5. The health professional provides false reassurance to patients.

_____Trustworthy _____ Nontrustworthy

6. The health professional gives realistic information to patients.

_____Trustworthy _____ Nontrustworthy

7. The health professional appears lethargic.

_____Trustworthy _____ Nontrustworthy

8. The health professional seems curious about the patient's extramarital love affair.

_____Trustworthy _____ Nontrustworthy

Feedback

2. A reputation for seeking personal gain is likely to make the health professional nontrustworthy.
3. The reliability of the information provided suggests trustworthiness.
4. The lack of dependability displayed by this characteristic suggests nontrustworthiness.
5. The lack of reliability is an indicator of nontrustworthiness.
6. The reliability of the information is an indicator suggesting trustworthiness.
7. The passivity of the health professional contributes to an impression of nontrustworthiness.
8. The curiosity of the health professional about the patient's extramarital love affair suggests voyeurism and implies nontrustworthiness.

Finally, demonstrate sincerity in your motives and intentions. Patients view health professionals as more trustworthy if they perceive the professional as working on their behalf and not simply for personal gain. Egan (1982) suggests that helping professionals should "avoid behavior that might indicate the presence of ulterior motives as voyeurism, selfishness, superficial curiosity, personal gain, or deviousness" (p. 137). Evidence of these personality traits may erode trust.

Patients who view the health professional as trustworthy are likely to be cooperative. The failure of a patient to carry out his or her part of a treatment plan may be one of the first indications

of a lack of trust. Froelich and Bishop (1977) suggest that a patient's difficulty in trusting a health professional is a problem of some magnitude and should not be taken lightly (p. 71). They observe that trust is affected by the perceptions of the individuals involved in the relationship. They state:

> Because "believing is seeing," the person who generally trusts others will "see" that he/she can trust what you do and say. Likewise, when a person generally distrusts others, he/she will "see" distrust in what you do and say. You may have to confront such a person with the fact that although he/she did not trust you about a certain matter, in fact you did what you said

you would do. Thus, it may take a very active, aggressive assault on the distrust to establish a trusting relationship (1977, p. 72).

Interpersonal Attractiveness

A patient's perception of the interviewer's interpersonal attractiveness is based on "perceived similarity to, compatibility with and liking for" the interviewer (Strong, 1968, p. 216). Although physical characteristics and general appearance may influence a patient's perception of an interviewer's attractiveness, they are only two aspects of this relationship variable. Role, reputation, and interpersonal behavior are other factors that enhance an interviewer's perceived attractiveness. Social-influence theory contends that if patients perceive the interviewer as attractive, the helping relationship will be strengthened and enhanced and the patient will like and cooperate with the interviewer to a greater extent. Presumably, health care workers will have more influence with patients who feel compatible with and like them.

In addition to physical appearance, role, and reputation, certain behaviors will enhance interpersonal attractiveness (see Table 2-3). These include attentiveness, friendliness, and understanding. Appropriate self-disclosure may also increase perceived attractiveness by communicating shared attitudes, beliefs, and dilemmas to the patient. For example, suppose a female patient states:

> I have the opportunity to go back to work—they have held my old job open for me. But now that my maternity leave is almost over, I feel very, very reluctant to return to work—at least for now. I'd really like to stay home and take care of my baby. It's very important—at least to me, anyway—to enjoy my baby in these early years.

An interviewer may choose to respond by disclosing similar attitudes or opinions about the subject, thereby increasing the perceived similarity between the patient and the health professional. The health care worker, in this situation, may respond by saying:

> I can understand your dilemma. I agree that it is very important for a young child to have a strong bond with the parents. One way, though not the only way to establish that bond, is to be there with the child when she is very young.

One word of caution: If your opinions are significantly different from the patient's regarding a given issue, it is probably better to remain silent than to feign similarity just to promote attractiveness. The facade becomes all too quickly apparent, and patient trust may be irreconcilably eroded.

Another way to enhance interpersonal attractiveness, suggested by Goldstein (1980), is through structuring. Goldstein distinguishes two kinds of structuring: trait structuring and role structuring (p. 21). In *trait structuring*, before the initial interview, a third party describes to the patient particular traits or characteristics of the health professional. Trait structuring is intended to give the patient a "sneak preview" of the new professional and his or her qualifications by setting the stage for the initial interaction. The patient thus has some foreknowledge of the interviewer, and there is an increased chance of compatibility between the patient and the professional. For example, after requesting a specialist for a consultation, a general practitioner may say to a patient:

> I believe you will find Dr. Gibraltar extremely helpful and competent. She will be very interested in your well-being, and, of course, she's had a great many years of experience in working with other patients who have had leukemia.

Some evidence suggests that in trait structuring it is important to emphasize the health professional's warmth and experience (Goldstein, 1980) in contrast to simply mentioning the consultant's name and title.

Role structuring involves either a third party or professionals themselves. Role structuring means clarifying for patients what they can realistically expect to occur during interactions with health professionals. Patients should understand what the health professionals will do (their roles) and what will actually transpire during the interview or examination.

In scheduling appointments for new patients at a public health facility, a receptionist or aide may use role structuring. He or she may tell the patients which health care worker they will see, the background of the health care worker, and the procedures to be followed during the initial visit. Or, alternatively, health professionals at the facility may describe their roles on the health care team so that patients understand their functions and importance. For example, a patient may be told:

> At your first visit you will be seeing Mr. Keen, a medical social worker. He will spend some time talking with you about your health-related concerns and obtaining some background information about you and your family. After that, he will make some recommendations to you about seeing one of our physicians or nurses. Mr. Keen, however, will continue to follow you as long as you use this facility, so there will always be at least one person with whom you will have continuous contact.

Such information reduces apprehension and establishes realistic expectations in prospective patients. It also corrects misconceptions, which in turn contributes to increasing the interviewer's perceived attractiveness.

As Goldstein (1980) observes, if a person experiences surprising or puzzling events during an interview due to misinformation or lack of information, negative feelings may result. In contrast, events that confirm the patient's expectations increase his or her compatibility with the interviewer (pp. 22–23).

LEARNING ACTIVITIES

Interpersonal Attractiveness

An important part of attractiveness is the appropriate use of structuring. The following learning activity describes six patient situations. Your task is to write two examples of trait structuring (Part One) and two examples of role structuring (Part Two) (Chapter Objective 6). The first item in each part is completed for you. See if your responses are similar to those provided in the feedback.

Trait structuring

1. You are preparing to refer a pregnant, diabetic patient to another health professional who specializes in the care of patients with high-risk pregnancy. Write an example of the use of trait structuring with this patient prior to the referral. *Example Response:*

   > I believe you will find Dr. Plante to be very helpful. High-risk obstetricians specialize in the care of patients like you. Dr. Plante has worked with women with high-risk pregnancies for many years.

2. You are going to consult an endocrinologist regarding a patient who has been diagnosed as having Addison's disease. Write an example of the use of trait structuring with this patient prior to the consultation. *Your response:*

   _____

   _____

_____

_____

3. You have suggested the name of a very competent private-duty nurse to the family of a critically ill, comatose patient. Write an example of the use of trait structuring prior to introducing the family to the nurse. *Your response:* _____

_____

_____

_____

Role structuring

1. You are a physician's assistant in a private health care setting. You are about to meet a new patient and obtain the health history. Write an example of the use of role structuring with this patient. *Example response:*

Hello, I'm Mr. Waverly, the assistant to Dr. Gerrard. I'd like to talk to you for about 30 minutes today to try to discover more about how you've been feeling. I'll be asking you a number of questions, and I'll need your help in providing as much information as possible. After I complete the history, I will conduct a physical examination. I will share the information only with Dr. Gerrard. It will help him in making an accurate diagnosis and assessment of your health. Next week, at your second appointment, Dr. Gerrard will have all this information together, and he will talk with you and examine you personally. Do you have any questions at this time?

2. You are a nurse in the VD clinic of a public health facility. You are about to meet a patient for the first time. Write an example of the use of role structuring with this patient. *Your response:* _____

_____

_____

_____

_____

3. You are a technician in a radiology department. A patient is about to undergo an upper gastrointestinal X-ray series for the first time. Write an example of the use of role structuring with this patient. *Your response:*

_____

_____

_____

_____

Feedback

Trait structuring

2. I think you will like Dr. Thomas. He's had a great deal of experience in working with other patients who have Addison's disease, and I think his expertise will be invaluable to you.
3. I have given the name of Mrs. James to you because she is an extremely competent and caring private-duty nurse. I believe she will provide excellent care for your father during this difficult time.

Role structuring

2. I'm Ms. Downs, the nurse from the VD clinic. First, I want you to know that whatever you tell me will be confidential or between us. While you are here, I will first need to obtain some basic information from you like your name, address, and so on. Then I'd like to talk with you about what brought you to this clinic. Do you have any questions?
3. I'm Fred Smith. I'm the X-ray technician in charge of this room. An upper GI series provides your doctors with some X-ray photographs that show how your esophagus, stomach, and upper intestine work and look. In order to provide a better contrast between the intestinal tract and the other organs in your abdomen, I will ask you to drink this chalky-tasting liquid. Then, as you swallow it, I will be able to take the X-rays. Do you have any questions?

Chapter Summary

The basic premise of this chapter is that health professionals, in their interactions with patients, are part of a helping process. Helping is an interactional process that involves four elements: (1) someone seeking help and (2) someone willing to give help who is also (3) capable of or trained to help (4) in a setting that permits help to be given and received.

This chapter described differences between helping, crisis intervention, and psychotherapy. Although all three are methods of responding to persons in need and overlap to some degree, they differ in various dimensions, including the nature of problems presented by patients, the goals of the interaction, the duration of the interaction, and the methods utilized.

This chapter also described two helping models that are applicable to health professionals. The human relations model emphasizes the importance of the helping relationship as characterized by three facilitative conditions: empathy, respect, and genuineness. In the social influence model, the helper attempts to establish an influence base with the patient through his or her competence, trustworthiness, and interpersonal attractiveness. This influence base is used to effect opinion and behavior change on the part of patients.

This chapter also defined and illustrated the use of these six relationship variables in interactions with patients. Empathy was defined as the capacity to communicate understanding to patients. The communication of empathy is an important means of establishing rapport, showing support, demonstrating civility, clarifying patients' problems, and collecting pertinent information. Respect was defined as the ability to view the patient as a person with inherent worth and dignity. Respect consists of commitment, understanding, a nonjudgmental attitude, and warmth. Respect communicates the health professional's interest in and acceptance of the patient. Genuineness was defined as the ability to be oneself without presenting a facade—being real rather than phony. Genuineness can reduce the emotional distance experienced by patients and may promote trust and rapport.

Competence was defined as the interviewer's capacity to utilize special knowledge and skills to help patients. If patients perceive the health professional as competent, they are more likely to have confidence in diagnostic procedures and to comply with treatment. Trustworthiness was defined as the ability of health professionals to deliver what they promise. Trustworthiness involves both reliability and dependability. The patient's respect for and confidence in the health professional may increase if the patient views the health care provider as trustworthy. Interpersonal attractiveness was defined as the ability of the health professional to establish a compatible working relationship with patients. Health professionals are likely to have greater influence with patients if patients like them and perceive some degree of similarity between themselves and the health care workers.

Although we discussed these six relationship conditions separately, in practice they are interrelated. For example, a health professional whom patients view as empathic is also likely to be regarded as genuine, competent, trustworthy, and attractive. The presence of one of these conditions enhances the overall quality of the relationship. Likewise, the absence of any of the conditions tends to erode the influence of the others.

Suggested Readings _____

Bernstein, L., & Bernstein, R. *Interviewing: A guide for health professionals.* New York: Appleton-Century-Crofts, 1980. Chapter 1, "The Relationship between the Health Professional and the Patient," focuses on the nature of the interaction between health professionals and patients.

Egan, G. *The skilled helper.* Monterey, Calif.: Brooks/Cole, 1975. Chapter 4, "Helper Response and Client Self-Exploration," gives an excellent discussion of the relationship variables reflected in both the human relations and social influence helping models.

Egan, G. *The skilled helper* (2nd ed.). Monterey, Calif.: Brooks/Cole, 1982. Chapter 5, "Problem Exploration and Clarification," describes important behavioral components of respect and genuineness.

Froelich, R. E., & Bishop, F. M. *Clinical interviewing skills.* St. Louis, Mo.: Mosby, 1977. Chapter 9, "The Cooperative Patient," describes a number of factors that lead to trust and cooperation in the health professional/patient relationship.

Gerrard, B., Boniface, W., & Love, B. *Interpersonal skills for health professionals.* Reston, Va.: Reston Publishing Company, 1980. Chapter 4, "Developing Facilitation Skills," discusses the importance of trust and warmth in health professional/patient interactions. A variety of skill-building exercises are also presented in this chapter.

Goldstein, A. P. Relationship enhancement methods. In F. H. Kanfer & A. P. Goldstein (Eds.), *Helping people change.* New York: Pergamon Press, 1980. This chapter describes a number of ways to enhance a helping relationship with special emphasis on helper expertness, attractiveness, empathy, and warmth.

Leigh, H., & Reiser, M. F. *The patient: Biological, psychological, and social dimensions of medical practice.* New York: Plenum, 1980, Chapter 1, "Illness and Help-Seeking Behavior," defines help-seeking behavior and identifies a number of factors that influence whether or not a person decides to seek health care.

The Health Care Interview: Stages and Special Problems____

Objectives

Following completion of this chapter, you will be able to:

1. Demonstrate 10 out of 12 steps associated with beginning a health care interview, given a role-play patient situation.

2. Demonstrate 8 out of 10 steps associated with managing a health care interview, given a role-play patient situation.

3. Demonstrate 6 out of 8 steps associated with terminating a health care interview, given a role-play patient situation.

4. Identify your beliefs and values about a particular health care issue, given five hypothetical patient case reports.

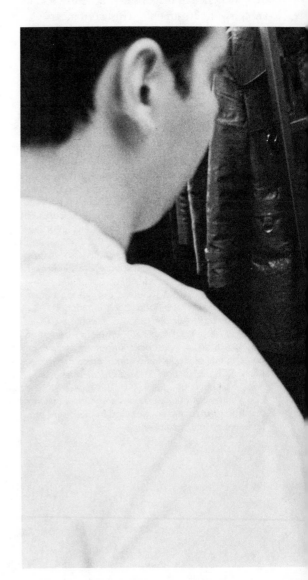

3

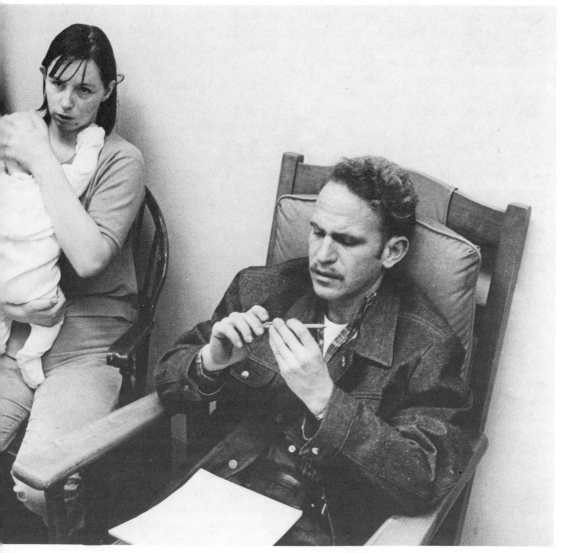

Beginning interviewers are especially apprehensive at the thought of interviewing an actual patient for an extended time period. They worry about such things as "How should I introduce myself to the patient?", "What will we talk about?", "What if the patient cries?", and "How will I terminate this interview in order to be on time for my next patient?" Interviews with patients always flow more smoothly if the interviewer has a plan or framework for conducting the interview. Although all of the skills presented in the remaining chapters of this book are used in patient interviewing, this chapter specifically attempts to place these skills in a conceptual framework and to identify where they may be used in the sequence of a typical patient interview. This information should help health care interviewers to understand the sequence of events in a typical interview and also to fit the skills described in the remaining chapters into a proper framework.

This chapter also describes a variety of particular problem areas unique to health care interviewing. They include the "trap" of jargon, adequate role taking, appropriate emotional objectivity with patients, and value conflicts. If not well understood or properly handled, these traps have the potential to cause interviewers to lose temporary control of their own feelings, to interfere with delivery of appropriate professional patient care, and to thwart the conditions necessary for an effective helping relationship.

Typical Sequence of a Patient Interview

Every patient interview has three parts: a beginning, a middle, and an end. These three phases of an interview are referred to as: (1) beginning the interview; (2) managing the interview; and (3) terminating the interview. The time spent on any one of these phases varies with the type of interview being conducted. For example, the health professional may spend less time on the opening and closing phases of a telephone interview than of a face-to-face interview. This may also be the case during an in-patient interview with a hospitalized patient or a follow-up contact with a known patient. In an initial interview with an out-patient, the health professional is likely to schedule sufficient time for all three aspects of the interview. An effective initial interview is critical because it "sets the stage" for all future interactions with that patient (Froelich, Bishop, & Dworkin, 1976, p. 15).

The style of the interview also will vary, depending on the formality or informality of the setting and the interviewer's own interactional style. Each interview with a patient, however, can be distinguished by these three phases, regardless of the length or the level of formality. In each phase the health professional and the patient have certain goals, purposes, and tasks to be accomplished.

Beginning the Interview

The three purposes of the opening phase of a health care interview, as depicted in Figure 3-1, are *building rapport with the patient, establishing the interview structure,* and *clarifying expectations.* These tasks are generally accomplished by an introduction and an explanation of the interview structure to the patient.

Building Rapport

Getting acquainted is the primary task at the outset of a health care interview. An adequate introduction is required to establish rapport, particularly with a new patient. With established or known patients, rapport must be re-established with each successive interaction. The initial introduction should be brief and concise. The health professional needs simply to address the patient by name, reveal his or her own name, and describe his or her role to the patient. The interviewer might say something like "Hello, Mrs. Jones" (greeting patient by name). "I'm Miss Brewer" (reveals own name). "I'm one of the physical therapists, and I'm going to be working with you during your stay here" (brief description of professional role).

Interviewers may also reinforce their name and role to the patient by wearing a nametag. However, the introduction is more personalized when the interviewers recite both names. Many adult patients expect a certain level of formality, and for that reason the interviewer may want to ask the patient how he or she prefers to be addressed. Young children almost always feel more comfortable if called by their first name. The oral greeting and introduction should be supplemented with appropriate nonverbal behavior, such as smiling and maintaining eye contact with the patient. It is also perfectly acceptable for interviewers to shake hands with patients as long as the handshake is an action that is comfortable for the interviewer (Froelich & Bishop, 1977).

With many patients, this simple and short introduction will suffice, and the interviewer can move on to establishing the interview structure and clarifying patient expectations. For some patients, however, discussion of expectations may be premature without additional "social amenities." Patients who seem apprehensive or uneasy may "let their guard down" after the interviewer has taken a few more moments to discuss a non-health-related topic with them. Elder (1978) recommends that health professionals attempt to learn something about patients before talking to them. They can then use such knowledge at this point in the interaction to help allay patients' fears or distrust.

The use of such additional social amenities recognizes the role of the patient's emotions in seeking health care assistance from a stranger. Froelich, Bishop, and Dworkin (1976) note that "the most universal reaction to a new situation or new people at a time when you are asking for help, feeling a little helpless, and needing to depend on someone else whom you don't yet know is anxiety" (p. 15). These authors also point out that some patients may feel trapped or intruded upon by having to interrupt their daily routines for a medical visit, whereas others may equate the need for health care with a loss of youth or wholeness. If the patient's anxiety or irritation persists beyond the opening phase of the interview, the health professional should respond to it by acknowledging its presence and encouraging the patient to discuss the apprehension or irritation in more depth.

Establishing the Interview Structure

Once rapport is established and introductions are made, the interviewer should explain the inter-

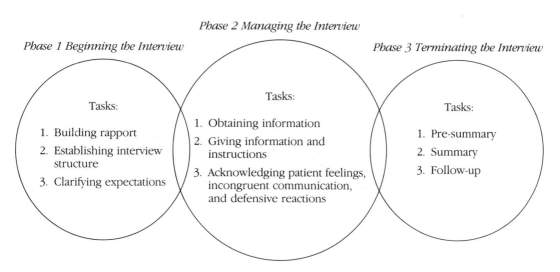

Phase 2 Managing the Interview

Phase 1 Beginning the Interview

Phase 3 Terminating the Interview

Tasks:

1. Building rapport
2. Establishing interview structure
3. Clarifying expectations

Tasks:

1. Obtaining information
2. Giving information and instructions
3. Acknowledging patient feelings, incongruent communication, and defensive reactions

Tasks:

1. Pre-summary
2. Summary
3. Follow-up

Figure 3-1
Three Phases and Corresponding Tasks of a Health Care Interview

view and role structure to the patient. As discussed in Chapter 2, role structuring reduces patient apprehension and misconceptions about the interview process. One simple way to role structure is to briefly describe the purpose or agenda of the interview to the patient and to note the time available for the session. Specifying the amount of time available at the outset facilitates a smoother ending to the interview and helps the patient focus on necessary topics rather than on unrelated ones. It is also important to obtain the patient's agreement to the agenda or to the proposed interview. Typically, these three activities can be accomplished in one sentence, as illustrated in the following examples:

> Mrs. Jones, we have about 30 minutes available to talk today. Since I haven't seen you for about three months, I'd like you to tell me how you've been doing. I'd also like to examine you to determine if we need to do more lab work at this time, OK?

> Mrs. Brown, since this is the first time I've seen you, I'd like to spend some time obtaining the health history of your child and your family. Then I'll examine your baby. This will take about 45 minutes. All right?

> Hello, Mr. Green. I just wanted to stop by for a few minutes to see how you have been feeling since yesterday. Are you having a good or not-so-good day?

> Miss Friend, I'd like to talk to you about any problems you've had during the last six months with your teeth or mouth and then examine your teeth. This will take about 45 minutes or so, OK?

Once the patient has agreed to the interview and its expressed purpose, the health professional must be certain that the atmosphere is conducive to accomplishing the stated tasks. He or she must not only ensure a certain amount of privacy and comfort but also assure patients that the interview content is confidential. If there are limits to the confidentiality of the communication, patients also have a right to know these limits. For example, a general statement of confidentiality might go something like this: "What you tell me is confi-

dential. Nothing in your records will be revealed without your permission." If there is an exception to this policy, such as particular information that the health care worker is required by law to reveal, the patient should be so advised. For example, the interviewer might say "If you have a venereal disease, I am required to report the disease to the State Health Department."

After this brief role structuring, it is useful to elicit the patient's reason or rationale for the visit or the interview. For example, an interviewer might use an open-ended question (see also Chapter 7) and ask "What do you hope to accomplish today?" or "What are your reasons for being here?" The interviewer could also ask "What would you like to discuss?" or "What problems have you been having?" The content of the question can be adapted to the setting and the patient. Regardless of the specific questions asked, it is most important to allow patients to state their goals for the interaction and to give them enough time to respond to questions with minimal interviewer interruptions (Hillman, Goodell, Grundy, McArthur, & Moller, 1981).

Clarifying Expectations

Patients and health care personnel have expectations concerning each other's role and behavior. Usually these expectations are implicit and surface only when they are not met or are in conflict. To reduce such conflict or frustration, it is important that both patients and health care workers share their expectations explicitly with another and do so early in the interview process. If such expectations are shared explicitly, both the health professional and the patient are made aware of the "ground rules" at the outset; the probability of either party having frustrated expectations is decreased. As Leigh and Reiser (1980) note, "covert differences in expectations can, of course, lead to difficulties in the doctor-patient relationship and interfere with the treatment process. Clearly, problems of this nature can be prevented and/or corrected by effective and open *communication*" (p. 25).

Patients develop expectations based on their cultural-ethnic affiliations and on their past experiences with medical care and health care settings. These include expectations about what the health professional will do, how the patient should behave, and how the health care worker should behave as a professional. These expectations can have great impact on the health professional's effectiveness with the patient. For example, patients with positive expectations are more likely to seek health care when needed. Patients who have negative expectations may delay seeking care or may use the negative expectation to undermine the health professional's efforts, thereby creating a "self-fulfilling prophecy." A health professional can obtain information about the patient's expectations by asking open-ended questions such as:

What experience have you had with nurses (or physicians, dentists, physical therapists, and so on)? What was the experience like for you?

How long have you waited before seeking care or treatment for these symptoms?

In what ways do you hope I can help you?

What are your expectations of me?

How do you believe this will benefit you?

What do you want me to be able to do for you?

Depending on the patient's response, the interviewer can capitalize on the positive expectancies and challenge the negative ones. At this point the interviewer can discuss unrealistic expectations or "false hopes" the patient may secretly harbor.

Expectations in the health care process are not one-sided, however, but mutual. The health professional also holds certain expectations about the patient, based on previous experience with certain types of patients and illnesses, his or her cultural-ethnic affiliation, personal style of communication, and, perhaps most of all, societal expectations of appropriate sick-role behavior. Leigh and Reiser (1980) explain the sick role as follows: "Society assigns specific expectations to the ill person by virtue of his being ill. These expectations comprise what is known as the sick

role" (p. 16). Parsons (1951), a sociologist, has formulated four elements of the sick role. These elements include two rights and two responsibilities or obligations:

Two Rights
1. Patients are exempted from carrying out their normal, social role responsibilities (that is, a homemaker is excused from washing, cooking, and child care, or a laborer is excused from strenuous exertion).
2. Society recognizes that sick persons cannot be expected to get well simply by "pulling themselves together."

Two Responsibilities
3. Patients are in a situation that requires care or help, but patients also must exhibit a desire to get well.
4. Patients are obliged to seek technically competent health care.

Based on this sick-role concept, most health professionals share three expectations for patient behavior: (1) patients will cooperate with professionals in order to help themselves achieve wellness; (2) patients will trust professionals and be candid and frank with them; and (3) patients will voluntarily disclose important and necessary information to professionals. Additionally, some health professionals harbor additional expectations of patients, including the assumption that patients will recognize and accept their authority, be willing to surrender some autonomy, and exhibit evidence of "suffering." Such suffering should be physical in nature.

Patients who do not conform to one or more of these expectations may be labeled by health care personnel as "bad" patients, with various consequences. The patient may be suspected of malingering or be denied continued hospitalization (Leigh & Reiser, 1980, p. 17). Health professionals who hold such beliefs about patients may need to re-examine their expectations in order to enhance the quality of care they give patients.

Health professionals' expectations may influence their behavior with patients in a number of other ways as well. For example, those who expect patients automatically to disclose important personal information "may fail to inquire into personal situations and matters that may be relevant . . ." (Leigh & Reiser, 1980, p. 24). Or if health professionals expect their patients to present evidence of physical suffering, there is a tendency to assume that the presenting symptoms always reflect physical illness or disease rather than destructive emotions, personality traits, or lifestyles.

Health professionals can avoid conflicts between their expectations and those of their patients first by understanding their own expectations and then by understanding the determinants of the patient's sick-role performance (Leigh & Reiser, 1980). The latter may include the realization that the "problem patient" is often someone who is not intentionally a "bad" patient but whose adjustment to the sick role is unusually difficult (Leigh & Reiser, 1980).

Health professionals can share their expectations with patients and their roles by simply describing these to the patient as illustrated below:

> Mrs. James, I will do my best to help this gum condition improve. However, this is not something I can do without your help. I will need your fullest cooperation in following any recommendations I might make regarding the care of your gums and taking the prescribed medicine regularly. . . .
>
> Mr. Caddell, I'd like very much to find out why you've been bothered by so much pain. However, I need your help. I hope you will be frank with me and will feel comfortable in answering any questions I may need to ask, even those that may seem a bit personal to you.

If, during continuing care, patients display by their actions a failure to meet the basic expectations of the health professional, the interviewer may decide that confrontation or referral is warranted (see Chapter 7). After establishing the interview structure and clarifying expectations, the health professional can proceed beyond this phase of the interview to the middle portion, or the "heart" of the interview. We refer to this phase as *managing the interview*.

Managing the Interview

The middle phase, managing the interview, takes up most of the interview time; it is during this phase that most of the work or the agenda is accomplished. The health professional needs to actively direct this phase in order to ensure that desired objectives are met.

As depicted in Figure 3-1, this phase has three general functions—obtaining relevant patient information, giving information and instructions to the patient, and recognizing and responding to patient feelings and to indirect and incongruent patient communication. The proportion of time spent on any one of these functions varies according to the time allotted for the interview, the patient's reasons or rationale for the interview, the type of interview, and other factors. More than one interview may be required in order to accomplish all of the objectives.

Obtaining Information

The purpose of obtaining information is to identify the patient's problems and their parameters. Before seeking information, the interviewer should explain the purpose of his or her request. Such an explanation enhances the patient's trust and cooperation with the interviewer. The interviewer may say something like "I'm going to be asking you some questions now. These may seem like a lot of questions to you, but your answers will help me identify particular problems you are having, OK?" Health professionals who fail to explain why they are requesting information communicate disrespect and lack of concern for their patients.

The health professional now requests information about both medical and psychosocial aspects of the patient's problems. The particular health problems to be identified depend on the interviewer's specialty area. For example, a dentist might request information primarily about medical problems related to the teeth, gums, and mouth, whereas a nurse might request information about a patient's emotional and physical condition following surgery. In general, all health professionals regardless of their orientation need to be concerned with both medical and psychosocial problems, since both are relevant parameters of health and illness. Chapter 4 discusses specific ways to obtain information about patients' physical, environmental, and psychological problem areas. The astute health professional will also determine whether any problems the patient reveals appear to be crisis situations—that is, with the potential to arouse severe emotional consequences if not handled immediately.

Next the health professional will take a health history from the patient if one is not already available or if the existing history is obsolete or incomplete. The content of the history depends partly on the expertise and specialty interests of the interviewer. But, as Chapter 8 illustrates, most health professionals obtain information about the patient's primary complaint, history of the presenting problem or "present illness," past medical or health history, family history, social history, and a review of many physiological systems.

By this time the interviewer has probably reviewed a rather thorough list of questions about potential or existing problem areas. It is important to remember that any time an interviewer requests information from a patient, the patient needs time to respond before another question is introduced. Finally, when the interviewer is satisfied that all the necessary and pertinent questions have been asked, he or she should give the patient a chance to express any additional opinions, concerns, or queries that were not previously mentioned. The interviewer can ask the patient questions similar to the following:

What else do you think might be wrong?

What other areas are of concern to you?

Is there anything else we have not covered that you believe is important or should be mentioned?

Following the receipt of all the verbal historical and diagnostic information, the health professional may conduct a physical examination of the patient or use other diagnostic procedures to add to the assessment of the problems. When all the relevant diagnostic information has been obtained,

the interviewer should be in a position to make a diagnosis and to inform and instruct the patient about the diagnosis and possible treatment alternatives.

Giving Information and Instructions

As far as patients are concerned, the giving of information and instructions is the most sensitive and critical part of the interaction. As Leigh and Reiser (1980) note, patients expect health professionals to communicate diagnostic findings and treatment plans. Much evidence suggests that there is a higher level of dissatisfaction among patients about the amount of information provided to them by health care workers than about any other aspect of their health care (Cartwright, 1964; Duff & Hollingshead, 1968; Waitzkin & Stoeckle, 1972). Either underestimating or overestimating the extent to which patients comprehend their illness can lead to poor communication and inadequate information giving (Leigh & Reiser, 1980).

Generally, health professionals need to inform patients about the nature of the illness, the diagnosis, and specific treatment options, with their relative benefits and risks. This information is the minimum amount that satisfies the requirements of "informed consent" (see Chapter 14). Once the patient chooses a specific treatment, the health professional is responsible for explaining the treatment procedure and outlining specific instructions and recommendations. Patient education is a critical component of a health care plan. Jargon should be avoided if possible, and if technical terms are required, definitions in lay language must be provided to ensure patient comprehension. The interviewer also should solicit the patient's emotional reaction to the information presented, since it is likely to have some emotional impact. Chapter 9 discusses specific guidelines for giving information and instructions to patients.

During this second phase of the interview, patient reactions to the interview, to the health care worker, and to the health care setting are most likely to become evident. These reactions often take the form of emotional outbursts, incongruent communication, or defensive reactions. Thus, another important part of managing the interview effectively involves acknowledging patient feelings, incongruent communication patterns, and defensive reactions.

Acknowledging Patient Feelings, Incongruent Communication, and Defensive Reactions

In Chapter 2 we noted that patients seek medical help to relieve symptoms and/or distress. Such help-seeking behavior implies that patients may need interpersonal support and relief from emotional distress as well as medical intervention and relief from physical discomfort. Consequently, it is appropriate for health professionals to indicate their awareness and understanding of patient feelings and emotions as they are expressed—overtly or covertly—during the interaction. This acknowledgement conveys empathy and communicates the health professional's interest in the patient as a person and not just a "case" with a collection of signs and symptoms.

Patients may also *unconsciously* express significant emotions, conflicts, or concerns by incongruent or indirect communication. Some patients may reveal conflict through inconsistent or incongruent communication, whereas others may reveal anxiety or hidden concerns by using defense mechanisms or other reactions such as inappropriate humor, questions, and topic changes. Communication between patient and professional and the reliability of the information obtained are usually enhanced when consistent patterns of incongruent or indirect communication are acknowledged and discussed. Chapters 5, 6, 7, 10, and 11 present guidelines for responding to patients' feelings, defensive reactions, and incongruent communication.

Terminating the Interview

Many health professionals have no difficulty initiating or managing an interview, yet find it very awkward to close or terminate an interview

smoothly and efficiently. The termination can be particularly troublesome if the patient desires additional time and the health professional has another appointment scheduled. Effective terminations, like effective beginnings, can be achieved using a plan of action and plenty of practice. There are three parts to an interview closing, as depicted in Figure 3-1: (1) pre-summary; (2) summary; and (3) follow-up. The objective of the termination phase is to review and synthesize what has been accomplished in the interview.

Pre-summary

Some health professionals attempt to "shut down" the interview by making a summary statement or giving exit cues at the last possible moment. This plan often backfires because it does not allow the patient adequate time to prepare and assimilate the fact that the interview is almost over. This error can be avoided by engaging in a *pre-summary*, which simply gives the patient a warning or a signal that the time is almost up and allows for any additional patient input. The pre-summary should be started about ten minutes prior to the designated termination time. The interviewer can say something like "Miss Peabody, I just noted that we have about ten minutes left. Is there anything else you want to discuss before we review what we talked about today?" This kind of statement has three effects. First, it informs the patient of the amount of time left in the interview. Second, it gives the patient one final opportunity to disclose any problems that have been overlooked or avoided. It is not uncommon for patients to deliberately avoid mentioning some problem areas, especially highly emotional or distressing ones, until near the end of the interview. Third, it helps the patient understand that the end of an interview is not synonymous with rejection. As Hein (1980) observes, an abrupt closing "that causes interruption of the patient's line of thought or cuts off his critical problem-solving efforts may contribute to the patient's feelings of rejection" (p. 75).

Summary

Once the pre-summary is completed and any additional topics discussed, the interviewer can comfortably and appropriately terminate the interview with a summary statement. The summary statement should provide appropriate support and reassurance to the patient and at the same time highlight the content of the interview in a brief and concise fashion. The summary statement is also useful for clarifying misunderstandings or differing perceptions and for determining the agenda for subsequent interviews. A good summary statement contains two parts: (1) a review of what has been learned and done during the interview; and (2) instructions for what the patient is supposed to do following the interview. The summary statement is not the time for either the interviewer or the patient to introduce new information. As Froelich, Bishop, and Dworkin (1976) note, a summary statement "should contain no new information but should review in a positive manner the interaction with the patient . . ." (p. 60). If the patient attempts to discuss a new topic, the interviewer can respond by saying something like "I can see you have something important to bring up, yet we don't have the time today. Let's see when we can get together again." The summary statement also "should contain your specific instructions and encourage the patient to accept responsibility" for his or her share of the planned treatment regimen (Froelich et al., 1976, p. 61).

After making the summary statement, the interviewer should confirm the accuracy of the statement with the patient. The entire process is accomplished in several sentences, as illustrated in the following example:

> Miss Geary, today we confirmed that you are indeed two months pregnant, and we reviewed the prenatal care you will need. Also, we discussed some ways for you to take care of yourself and the baby during the pregnancy. I want you to schedule another appointment in four weeks. At the time of the next visit we will schedule sonography, which, as I mentioned, will give us information about the size of the baby's head and the position of the placenta. Is this your understanding also?

The patient also can participate in the summary by being asked to review the most significant areas covered during the interview.

Follow-up

An important part of the termination phase is the scheduling of a follow-up. The interviewer can accomplish this objective by expressing appreciation to the patient for the present interview and then instructing or inviting the patient to return for a follow-up visit. Hillman et al. (1981) assert that a health professional "should never end an interview without expressing appreciation for the patient's cooperation and your sincere wish for his or her future welfare" (p. 14). The follow-up statement may go something like this:

> Mr. Kramer, I want to thank you for being so patient today and for answering all of my questions so completely. I appreciate your cooperation. I would like to see you again in three months.

Or

> It's not necessary to have another checkup until two years from now, unless something comes up before then that concerns you.

After making the follow-up statement, interviewers should prepare to leave the interview by giving exit cues. Exit cues include standing up, shaking the patient's hand, saying goodbye, turning away, and walking toward the door. Many interviewers fail to terminate an interview punctually simply because their nonverbal behaviors are inconsistent with their verbal statements, leaving patients either confused or believing that the interviewer really does have more time available. Patients are not likely to try to manipulate health professionals into hearing "just one more problem" if health professionals demonstrate by both words and actions their intentions to leave at the designated time.

In addition to the skills involved in beginning, managing, and terminating a health care interview, there are certain situations in a health care interview that are troublesome enough to warrant specific mention. These include the "trap" of the indiscriminate use of jargon, inadequate role assumption, lack of emotional objectivity, and value conflicts with patients. We discuss these problems in the next section.

LEARNING ACTIVITIES

Beginning a Health Care Interview

According to Objective 1, you will be able to demonstrate at least 10 out of 12 steps associated with beginning a health care interview using a role-play patient. This learning activity can be conducted in triads, with one person taking the part of a selected patient role (described below), a second person assuming the role of the interviewer, and a third person being the observer. The observer can use the Interview Rating Checklist for Beginning an Interview (page 57) as a guide for providing feedback. If you do not have an observer, interviewers can audiotape the interview and assess their own performance using the checklist as a guide. Change roles twice so that each person has an opportunity to be the patient, the interviewer, and the observer. For purposes of this activity, assume that the scenario depicts the interviewer's initial contact with the patient. Each interview should last approximately 15 minutes. Remember the three tasks to be accomplished during the beginning phase of the interview: (1) building rapport; (2) establishing the interview structure; and (3) clarifying expectations.

Patient roles

1. You are an eight-year-old child. This is your first visit to a dentist or a hygienist, and you are nervous and unsure about what to expect. You are there only because your grandmother, with whom you are staying for the summer, "made" you come in for teeth cleaning and a checkup. You expect the process to be painful and uncomfortable.

2. You are a middle-aged woman who has scheduled a general physical checkup because you have been feeling tired and run down for several months. Although this is your first visit to this particular clinic, you have had numerous other contacts with health professionals and clinics previously. You seem to hold all health professionals in very high regard and are a very cooperative and pleasant patient.

3. You are an elderly man who is being admitted to a nursing home. It is part of the nursing home admission procedure to give new residents a general physical examination and health assessment. You are somewhat forgetful and repeatedly confuse the present interviewer with another one you knew and disliked. Consequently, you are not very pleased to be here and are not too compliant.

4. You are a young woman who has been admitted to the hospital for observation and tests after coming to the emergency room for severe headaches that have persisted for more than a year. Although this is the first time you have been hospitalized, you have heard a lot of "war stories" about hospital errors from your friends. Consequently, you are highly suspicious of all health care personnel, their procedures, and their motives.

Interview rating checklist: Beginning an interview

Instructions: Determine which of the following behaviors for beginning the interview were demonstrated by the interviewer during the role-play. Use the Yes/No blanks following each item to record your observations.

Building Rapport

1. Did the interviewer greet the patient by name?

_____ Yes   _____ No

2. Did the interviewer greet the patient with appropriate supporting non-verbal behaviors such as direct eye contact, smiling, handshaking, and so on?

_____ Yes   _____ No

3. Did the interviewer introduce himself or herself to the patient by name?

_____ Yes   _____ No

4. Did the interviewer briefly describe his or her role to the patient?

_____ Yes   _____ No

5. Did the interviewer engage in any "social amenities" to reduce patient apprehension?

_____ Yes   _____ No

Establishing the Interview Structure

6. Did the interviewer state the purpose of the interview to the patient?

_____ Yes   _____ No

7. Did the interviewer note the amount of time available for the interview?

_____ Yes   _____ No

8. Did the interviewer obtain the patient's agreement to the interview?

_____ Yes   _____ No

9. Did the interviewer note the confidentiality of the information obtained during the interview?

_____ Yes   _____ No

10. Did the interviewer obtain the patient's rationale or reasons for the interview?

_____ Yes   _____ No

Clarifying Expectations

11. Did the interviewer elicit the patient's expectations of the health care worker and of the interview?

_____ Yes   _____ No

12. Did the interviewer describe his or her expectations for the patient?

_____ Yes   _____ No

Observer Comments: _____

_____

_____

Managing a Health Care Interview

According to Objective 2, you will be able to demonstrate 8 out of 10 steps associated with the procedure for managing a health care interview given a role-play situation. This learning activity can be conducted in triads, with one person assuming the role of a patient, another the role of an interviewer, and a third as the observer. The observer can use the Interview Rating Checklist for Managing an Interview as a guide for providing feedback. The role-play patients should assume the same roles they used for the previous role-play on beginning an interview.

Each interview should last approximately 20 minutes. Remember the three tasks to be accomplished during the middle phase of a health care interview: (1) obtaining relevant patient information; (2) giving information and instructions to patients; and (3) recognizing and responding to patient feelings and to indirect and incongruent communication.

Interview rating checklist: Managing an interview

Instructions: Determine which of the following behaviors for managing the interview were demonstrated by the interviewer during the role-play. Use the Yes/No blanks following each item to record your observations.

Obtaining Relevant Patient Information

1. Did the interviewer explain the purpose of any information sought from the patient?

   _____ Yes   _____ No

2. Did the interviewer obtain information about both medical and psychosocial problems of the patient?

   _____ Yes   _____ No

3. Did the interviewer identify whether any of the patient's problems were crisis situations that needed to be handled immediately?

   _____ Yes   _____ No

Giving Information and Instructions to the Patient

4. Did the interviewer provide information to the patient about the nature of the illness and/or the diagnosis?

   _____ Yes   _____ No

5. Did the interviewer give information to the patient about any treatment procedures used?

   _____ Yes   _____ No

6. Did the interviewer outline specific instructions and/or recommendations for the patient to follow?

   _____ Yes   _____ No

7. Did the interviewer avoid the use of jargon or explain to the patient any technical terms used?

————— Yes   ————— No

*Recognizing and Responding to Patient's Feelings
and Indirect Communication*

8. Did the interviewer elicit the patient's emotional reactions to any information given to the patient?

————— Yes   ————— No

9. Was the interviewer supportive and nonjudgmental in responding to the patient's feelings and emotions?

————— Yes   ————— No

10. Did the interviewer acknowledge the presence of any indirect or incongruent patterns of patient communication (if present)?

————— Yes   ————— No

Observer comments ————————————————————————————————

——

——

Terminating a Health Care Interview

According to Objective 3, you will be able to demonstrate six out of the eight steps associated with the procedure for terminating a health care interview using a role-play situation. This learning activity also can be conducted in triads, with one person assuming the role of a patient, another the role of an interviewer, and a third as the observer. The observer can use the Interview Rating Checklist for Terminating an Interview as a guide for providing feedback. The role-play patients may wish to assume the same roles they used for the first role-play on beginning an interview. Each interview should last approximately ten minutes. Remember the three tasks to be accomplished during the closing phase of the interview: (1) pre-summary; (2) summary; and (3) follow-up.

Interview rating checklist: Terminating an interview

Instructions: Determine which of the following behaviors for terminating the interview were demonstrated by the interviewer. Use the Yes/No blanks following each item to record your observations.

Pre-summary

1. Did the interviewer give the patient a cue about the time limits of the interview?

————— Yes   ————— No

2. Did the interviewer elicit additional patient concerns?

————— Yes   ————— No

Summary

3. Did the interviewer review what was learned during the interview with the patient?

_____ Yes _____ No

4. Did the interviewer provide instructions to the patient for any actions or events to be carried out following the interview?

_____ Yes _____ No

5. Did the interviewer avoid introducing any new information during the summary?

_____ Yes _____ No

Follow-up

6. Did the interviewer express appreciation to the patient for completing the present interview?

_____ Yes _____ No

7. Did the interviewer instruct or invite the patient to return for a follow-up visit?

_____ Yes _____ No

Observer comments: _____

_____

_____

Some Specific Interviewing Problems

Although a variety of potential problems exist for health care interviewers, there are several that create sufficient difficulty to warrant special attention. These include giving information and explaining health care procedures without the excessive use of jargon, remaining emotionally objective while interacting with patients, and dealing with patients who have different values or who are from different cultural and socioeconomic backgrounds.

The "Trap" of Jargon

Health care personnel are sometimes at a loss to explain diagnoses, illnesses, and health care pro-cedures to patients in language that the patient can understand and that is still descriptive enough to be accurate. Frequently interviewers are unaware of lapsing into the use of medical jargon while giving information to patients. And at the same time they fail to observe how little the patient comprehends their explanation. According to Froelich et al. (1976), "when professional jargon is used, the patient may feel put down, misunderstand what you say, and be very confused. We are so accustomed to jargon that we are not aware of its use until we notice a patient's confusion. . . . When the patient fails to follow our plans for treatment, our first reaction is that the patient is just being difficult. It is more productive to explore his/her misunderstandings. Excessive jargon contributes to misunderstandings" (p. 59).

The best rule of thumb for this problem is, whenever possible, to translate medical terminology into nontechnical language. In making such a translation, the interviewer must be careful to retain accuracy and precision so that the information is still descriptive and concrete. Leigh and Reiser (1980) observe that "in translating medical jargon to lay terms, specificity is very often lost. . . ." Patients are likely to have their *"own fantasies and ideas"* about what they are being told (p. 28). After giving information to patients, health professionals should ask them what they understood from the explanation provided (Leigh & Reiser, 1980).

Health care workers also can contribute to patients' confusion and apprehension by using jargon while talking with another health professional in the presence of the patient. For example, a head nurse may say something to another nurse about the patient's diagnosis or condition while the patient is present and "all ears." This situation is potentially dangerous. Patients are likely to hear and understand only a portion of what they hear and thus may resort to their own fantasies and interpretations, which may be distorted and inaccurate.

Health care personnel must also remember that a patient's interpretation and understanding of language is likely to be affected by that patient's cultural background. For example, the concept of time varies greatly among different cultures. If an interviewer says "I'll see you at 11:00 A.M.," one patient might interpret that to mean she is to be there at 11:00 A.M. sharp, and another might believe the interviewer doesn't intend for her to be there until 11:30 or so.

Adequate Role Assumption and Emotional Objectivity

Beginning interviewers report considerable difficulty in assuming an adequately professional role and in gauging the appropriate emotional distance to assume with patients. Beginning interviewers may evidence inadequate role assumption by becoming easily flustered when introducing themselves or while responding to patient questions. Such discomfort takes the form of excessively long introductions or explanations about their beginner or student status or apparent ambiguity in explaining their roles to patients. The best introduction is always concise and focuses on the patient, rather than on the health professional, as depicted in the following examples:

> Hello, Mr. Bernard. I'm Miss White, a student nurse on this floor. How are you feeling today?
>
> Hello, Mrs. Petronis. I'm Dr. Dennison, a third-year medical student assigned to this floor. What kind of a day are you having?
>
> Hello, Darla. I'm Mr. Shaw. I'm a student dentist in this pediatric dental clinic, and I am working under the supervision of Dr. Breen. He and I will be examining your teeth today. What kinds of problems have you been having with your teeth since your last checkup?

Some health professionals also have difficulty determining the appropriate amount of personal/emotional objectivity for interactions with patients. Feeling insecure about this issue, such interviewers may become either excessively aloof or excessively involved with their patients. This problem is not uncommon among beginning interviewers, especially. Even experienced health professionals sometimes begin to lose objectivity by developing strong emotional feelings about a patient or even overidentifying with a patient. A health professional may develop intense positive feelings for a patient, such as tenderness or protectiveness, or strong negative feelings, such as contempt or dislike. Health professionals need to be aware of such feelings, although it is generally not helpful to express them to the patient (Reiser & Schroder, 1980, p. 101).

Occasionally, health professionals find themselves so emotionally involved with patients that *countertransference* occurs. Countertransference refers to the development of a strong, emotional reaction to a patient. For instance, a health professional may be treating a young, female adult who is dying from cervical cancer. The health professional may become very attached to this patient, to the point of overidentifying with her and feeling very protective of her. These feelings may reduce the interviewer's objectivity and ultimately interfere with the ability to provide the patient with professional care. In another instance, a male health professional who was recently divorced may find himself very attracted to or repelled by a particular female patient who reminds him of his former wife. Countertransference can be a significant problem if the health professional begins to treat the patient as if she were his wife and has difficulty in emotionally separating the two as distinct and different persons.

Astute interviewers realize there are certain kinds of patients who consistently elicit strong positive or negative feelings in them. This awareness can help them manage their feelings instead of allowing their feelings to control them. Transference and countertransference are not unusual phenomena. Many health professionals find themselves developing certain emotional reactions to patients. However, they need to be constantly vigilant for occasions when such reactions occur so that their judgment and professional care of patients is not adversely affected. Reiser and Schroder (1980) observe that a clue to transference and countertransference is a sudden eruption of strong emotions that seem inappropriate in timing or intensity, given the context in which they arise (p. 150).

One very difficult problem in the area of objectivity involves the use of touch with patients. Interviewers wonder if they should sit on a patient's bed or hold a patient's hand if the patient is crying. The difficulty with any form of body contact is that it may have a significant and often unconscious meaning to a patient, which may be very different from the meaning the interviewer intended to convey (Reiser & Schroder, 1980, p. 101). Froelich and Bishop (1977) note that the interviewer's "best intentioned touch may be misinterpreted" (p. 21). To assist interviewers in understanding their (sender) intentions and possible patient (receiver) interpretations about body contact, Table 3-1 depicts a *touch spectrum* adapted from Froelich and Bishop (1977). Froelich and Bishop recommend that if an interviewer feels some sort of touch is appropriate, but is uncertain of the patient's expectations, he or she should follow the rule: "When there is hesitation, no manipulation." In other words,

Table 3-1
Touch Spectrum

Feeling	Response
Avoidance	Withdrawal
Affection	Handshake
	Arm on or around shoulder
	Hug
Sensuality	Massage or stroking
Sexuality	Skin-to-skin intimate touch
	Kissing
	Sexual intercourse

interviewers should clarify their intentions with the patient before actually engaging in any form of touch. For example, the interviewer might say "I would like to comfort you; may I put my hand on your shoulder?" or "Is it OK with you if I put my hand on your shoulder?" (Froelich & Bishop, 1977, p. 21).

Values

Values are those things a person prizes, cherishes, and affirms (Raths & Simon, 1966). Values differ from attitudes because they represent ways in which people invest themselves. Values cause a person to act (or refrain from acting) in a repeated, consistent way. Values are related to lifestyle and give weight to positive or negative courses of action (Egan, 1975; 1982). According to Elder (1978), our values are stored in our brain like "thousands of recordings" and form the "shoulds, oughts, and musts" of our personal style (p. 11). Most of us learned our values as children from our parents or from teachers, peers, and the influence of mass media. Elder (1978) observes that some people accept values wholeheartedly from authority figures, whereas others store and assume values only after a careful, independent assessment of their merit.

In interactions with patients, it is impossible to be "value free." Values permeate every interaction. Health professionals cannot be "scrupulously neutral" in their interactions with patients

(Corey, Corey, & Callanan, 1979, p. 85). Okun (1982) asserts that "in recent years, we have recognized that in any interpersonal relationship, whether or not it is a helping relationship, values are transmitted either covertly or overtly between the participants" (p. 229). Interviewers may unintentionally influence a patient to embrace their values in subtle ways, by what they pay attention to and by nonverbal cues of approval and disapproval (Corey et al., 1979, p. 98). If patients feel they need the interviewer's approval, they may act in ways they think will please the interviewer instead of making choices independently according to their own value system.

Values that are especially likely to affect patient interactions include health professionals' "attitudes and feelings about kinds of people, what is 'good' or 'bad,' what is acceptable or unacceptable..." (Okun, 1982, p. 229). Corey, Corey, and Callanan (1979) and Elder (1978) have identified some situations in which the values or ideologies of interviewers are likely to affect their behavior toward patients. These areas are age, health and self-care, death and dying, sexuality, and cultural-socio-economic factors.

Age. Many health professionals find it difficult to work with patients who are either much younger or much older than they. Health professionals may have internalized stereotypical values about the elderly, such as "they are too helpless to be allowed to do anything for themselves" or "they are in a process of disengagement and don't really want contact with other people anyway." Elder (1978) asserts that often health professionals go out of their way to avoid older patients in order not to feel their pain. She states that "most elderly people are not afraid of death. More often than not they fear loneliness, dependency, and incapacitation in the years that precede dying" (p. 164). Unfortunately, some health professionals may contribute to this fear by avoiding contact with elderly patients as much as possible.

Death and dying. The issues associated with death and dying in the health care field are too numerous to list separately. One issue that often poses a values dilemma for health professionals is under what conditions, if any, a patient has the right to refuse necessary medical treatment and, ultimately, the "right to die." Health professionals are confronted with these difficult situations daily when treating persons being maintained on a respirator, when badly deformed infants are born, when terminally ill persons are in severe pain, when elderly persons are steadily deteriorating, or when very disturbed people have attempted suicide. Although health professionals may be legally obligated to do everything possible to prolong life, their actual feelings about a particular patient situation may conflict wih their legal responsibilities. Sometimes in such situations the values dilemma of the health professional is exacerbated because of the conflicting wishes of the patient's family.

Another issue posed by death and dying is the predominant value held by health professionals and health care settings that death is an indication of a health care failure. Health professionals may identify so strongly with saving lives that they are unable to confront death objectively. Health professionals who are unable to recognize their own limitations may be especially vulnerable in this situation. As a consequence, "people at the end of the road, such as the aged and the terminally ill, are avoided" (Elder, 1978, p. 165). Even patients who are comatose or unconscious are likely to be avoided because in their condition they may seem more representative of death than of life. Health professionals may respond by treating such patients as if they were dead or at least as "persona non grata." Yet, as Elder (1978) observes, evidence suggests that unconscious patients can hear. She recommends treating them as thinking, feeling human beings (p. 166).

Health and self-care. Presumably most health professionals have strong values that favor wellness over illness and self-care behaviors over self-injurious behaviors. Occasionally these values may create a conflict between health professionals who are strongly committed to wellness and patients who seem to prefer illness. Health professionals may come to believe that patients have no right to choose illness over wellness and may needlessly argue, berate, or object to caring for such a patient. Other health professionals may be so personally and professionally committed to particular self-care behaviors, such as daily exercise or non-smoking, that they have considerable difficulty treating smokers or nonexercisers with objectivity, respect, and concern.

Other health professionals may become so invested in particular medical procedures that they have difficulty tolerating patients who do not agree to such procedures. For example, a health professional who believes strongly that all pregnant women over age 35 should undergo prenatal tests for genetic defects may not treat a dissenting patient with much respect and may strongly encourage her to undergo a procedure against her will. This example illustrates the *misuse* of the social influence base of helping. Social influence is ethical only if the patient's values are respected.

According to Egan (1982), interviewers may encourage patients to re-examine their values, but they should not influence patients to adopt actions or procedures that are inconsistent with their values (p. 217). Okun (1982) also contributes to understanding this issue. She observes that people "who have strong ideologies are often dismayed by the philosophy that they should not impose their values" on patients (p. 233). She notes that imposition of values does not result in "independence" but rather "submission to or withdrawal from" the interviewer (p. 233).

Sexuality. Sexuality cannot be avoided in dealing with patients, no matter how uncomfortable health professionals may be in dealing with this issue. In working with patients, health professionals may discover they have particular values or prejudices about patients who engage in unusual sexual practices or patients who have different sexual preferences, such as homosexuality. Transvestism, premarital sex, extramarital sex, and group sex are other areas in which health professional values may conflict with those of patients.

Value dilemmas in the area of sexuality show up in a number of ways. For example, if a female health professional is insecure about her own sexuality and relationships with men, she may feel very uncomfortable working with a patient who has identified herself as a lesbian. The health professional may go out of her way to avoid this patient or, if physical avoidance is not possible, to avoid discussing this issue with the patient. Okun (1982) believes that when "helpers are uneasy about their values in any one of these areas, they may deliberately and subtly avoid these areas . . ." (p. 231).

Health professionals can create a major barrier to an effective helping relationship by being intolerant of different sexual preferences or practices. For example, a very religious health care worker may communicate strong anger, disapproval, and scorn to a patient with venereal disease or to a patient who has openly discussed his or her numerous extramarital affairs. Strong disapproval is likely to interfere with the creation of empathic conditions necessary for an effective helping relationship.

Being accepting of a patient does not mean an interviewer must condone all of the patient's behavior. It does mean that interviewers "can tolerate differences, ambiguity, and uncertainty" and "can accept that what is right or good for one person may not be right or good for another" (Okun, 1982, p. 231). Practically speaking, there may be times when any health professional has difficulty tolerating or accepting the behavior or principles of a patient. A values conflict between professional and patient poses a real problem if the values clash to such an extent that the interviewer's ability to function in a helpful manner is jeopardized (Corey et al., 1979). If a health professional cannot offer a minimum of respect and empathy, he or she should consider referring the patient to another health care worker, or, if that is not possible, limit the relationship to discussion of particular topics (Okun, 1982). In such dilemmas the health professional should probably try to sort out her or his own values and feelings about the conflict by talking with a colleague or a supervisor.

LEARNING ACTIVITIES

Personal Values

The following learning activity presents descriptions of five hypothetical patient case reports. Your task is to read each report and then examine your values on each of the issues represented by the case (Chapter Objective 4). We suggest you use the following five questions, adapted from Corey, Corey, and Callanan (1979) as a guideline for this process. There is no feedback provided for this learning activity because there are no right or wrong answers. You may wish to write your reactions down or discuss them in a small group of colleagues or with an instructor.

Questions

1. What is my position on this particular issue?

2. Where (how) did I develop my views?

3. To what extent have I challenged or questioned my values about this issue?

4. In this particular situation would I be likely to impose my values on the patient or communicate disapproval of the patient's values?

5. Could I work with this person effectively?

A second way to use this learning activity is to role play the cases with one or two other people. One person should assume the role of the patient, and another should take the role of the interviewer. A third person can provide feedback and indicate to what extent the interviewer avoided imposing his or her values on the patient or avoided communicating disapproval to the patient.

Patient Cases

1. Mr. Grimes is a male patient in his 30s. He informs you that he has been having some sexual problems and his wife asked him to come in to determine if something was physically wrong. Finally, he discloses that, although his wife believes he is impotent, he is gay and has been having an affair with another married man for the last year.

2. Mrs. Beaulieu is a middle-aged woman who is married and has three children still living at home. She is terminally ill with cancer of the pancreas and has begged you for a week to give her an overdose of pills to put an end to her excruciating pain. She states she believes she has a right to die in peace before she totally disintegrates in front of her family members.

3. Sarah Young is a 16-year-old patient who says she has engaged in sexual relationships with a number of older men for several years. She has never used any birth control method because she never believed she would

get pregnant. Now she is pregnant and wants an abortion. She is also not sure whether the father of her unborn child is her current boyfriend or her own father.

4. Mrs. Worth is a 40-year-old widow who is pregnant for the second time. Although her first child, who is 10 years old, was normal, there is a history of Down's syndrome in her family. Mrs. Young states that despite her history and her age, she is strongly opposed to having an amniocentesis performed to determine if any chromosomal abnormalities exist in the fetus. She states that she sees no reason to submit to the procedure because her religious beliefs would not permit her to consider abortion.

5. Jose Martinez is a six-year-old boy who has acute leukemia. His parents have refused to sign any consent forms for medically oriented treatment, stating that medical intervention is in opposition to their cultural and religious beliefs. They believe God will save their child "if he and they have been good enough to deserve another chance for his life."

Cultural and socioeconomic factors. There is no doubt that cultural and socioeconomic factors significantly affect health professional/patient interactions. Trust, respect, and cooperation may vary inversely with the amount of social distance between the patient and the interviewer (Simmons, 1958). Although many health professionals prefer to work with patients of cultural and ethnic backgrounds similar to their own, such choices are not always available. Health care personnel need to learn to work effectively with patients from a variety of cultural and ethnic backgrounds. The ability to do so can, to some extent, be enhanced if the health professional understands how different cultural-socioeconomic factors influence a patient's help-seeking behavior, type of illness, and response to health care workers.

Individuals who are white, urban, educated, and middle- or upper-class Americans "whose definitions of health and illness are most congruent with those of the health professional ... are also most likely to fulfill the patient role in a way that meets the expectations of the clinician ..." (Enelow & Swisher, 1979, p. 27). In contrast, Clark (1970) has reported that Mexican-Americans in the Santa Clara Valley of California are likely to resist the sick role for fear that family and friends will lose respect for them and consider them inferior. They make every effort to continue normal daily activities despite signs of illness or poor health.

Cultural and socioeconomic factors influence what constitutes an illness, when and if to seek medical help, what to report about the illness, and how to report it (Koos, 1967). For example, cultural and socioeconomic factors may affect the patient's perception and report of pain (Zborowski, 1969). According to Bernstein and Bernstein (1980), "the health professional needs to be aware of the influence of ethnicity when patients report symptoms, especially where diagnoses and treatment are to a large extent based on what the patient tells the [health professional]. Important diagnostic leads might be overlooked" (p. 154).

Socioeconomic class and social mobility also affect the type of disorders likely to occur in patients. Disorders that have been significantly correlated with socioeconomic status include hypertension, peptic ulcers, breast cancer, and coronary artery disease (Graham, 1963). Neurosis, peptic ulcers, and proneness to infectious diseases appear to be connected with upward mobility (Susser & Watson, 1971).

A health professional may find it especially troublesome to work with a patient who identifies with a religious group whose values system clashes with medical treatment modalities. Religious affiliations can affect a patient's decision to seek health care assistance, to accept or reject certain medical procedures, and to trust or distrust health care workers. For example, many members of the Christian Science faith are reluctant to seek medical help for illness. Jehovah's Witness members usually refuse to accept blood transfusions.

Because values affect all relationships with patients, health professionals need to be aware of their values and to know how their values may influence their interactions with patients. Interviewers aware of their values are "less likely to impose them covertly on others" (Okun, 1982, p. 229). Elder (1978) suggests that awareness of values can assist health professionals to handle difficult situations effectively. She states: "If you are conscious of how you feel you are more likely to be able to handle the situation or choose not to handle it in ways that will not have unpleasant future consequences for you. It is dangerous for your feelings to take you by surprise because then they control you. You may say and do things you don't really want to do" (Elder, 1978, p. 164).

Chapter Summary

This chapter presented the typical sequence of a health care interview. Most health care interviews have three distinct phases: beginning the interview, managing the interview, and terminating the interview. During the opening phase of the interview, the health professional attempts to build rapport with the patient, explain the interview structure to the patient, and clarify both patient and interviewer expectations. The middle phase of the interview is devoted to obtaining relevant patient information, giving information and instructions to patients, and acknowledging significant or persistent patient emotions, incongruent communication, or defensive reactions. Terminating an interview effectively involves use of a pre-summary, a summary, and a follow-up statement.

Also discussed in this chapter were some specific problem situations encountered during interviews with patients. These problem situations include: how to explain and give information to patients that is specific and precise without excessive use of jargon; how to assume an adequate professional role with patients; how to achieve a balance of emotional objectivity in relationships with patients, and how to relate to patients from different cultural-socioeconomic backgrounds or with different value systems. Interviewers were encouraged to become aware of their own values in order not to subtly impose them on patients or communicate disapproval to patients with different backgrounds and belief systems.

Suggested Readings _____

Bernstein, L., & Bernstein, R. *Interviewing: A guide for health professionals.* New York: Appleton-Century-Crofts, 1980. Chapter 11, "Social Distance and Patient Care," describes some variations in cultural and socioeconomic background of patients and possible effects on interactions with health professionals.

Corey, G., Corey, M., & Callanan, P. *Professional and ethical issues in counseling and psychotherapy.* Monterey, Calif.: Brooks/Cole, 1979. Chapter 5, "Values and the Therapeutic Process," describes a number of important ways in which values of professionals affect the helping process.

Elder, J. *Transactional analysis in health care.* Menlo Park, Calif.: Addison-Wesley, 1978. Chapter 13, "Conflicts, Alternatives, and Reasonable Expectations," discusses ways in which health professionals may hold values that conflict with the needs of patients.

Enelow, A. J., & Swisher, S. N. *Interviewing and patient care.* New York: Oxford University Press, 1979. Chapter 2, "The Nature of Medical Information and the

Social Context of the Interview," describes ways in which the social context and role of the patient and health professional affect the interaction.

Froelich, R. E., & Bishop, F. M. *Clinical interviewing skills.* St. Louis, Mo.: Mosby, 1977. Chapter 6, "Closing the Interview," illustrates a variety of ways a health professional can terminate a health care interview effectively.

Froelich, R. E., Bishop, F. M., & Dworkin, S. F. *Communication in the dental office.* St. Louis, Mo.: Mosby, 1976. Chapter 2, "Initial Contact with the Dental Office," depicts a number of possible expectations and emotional reactions of new patients prior to their initial contact with a dental health professional.

Hillman, R. S., Goodell, B. W., Grundy, S. M., McArthur, J. R., & Moller, J. H. *Clinical skills: Interviewing, history taking, and physical diagnosis.* New York: McGraw-Hill, 1981. Chapter 1, "Medical Interviewing," describes some techniques for opening and closing a health care interview.

Leigh, H., & Reiser, M. *The patient: Biological, psychological, and social dimensions of medical practice.* New York: Plenum, 1980. Chapter 2, "The Sick Role," and Chapter 3, "Expectations in the Consulting Room," describe a number of patient/health professional expectations and various implications of those expectations for health care practice.

Okun, B. *Effective helping: Interviewing and counseling techniques.* Monterey, Calif.: Brooks/Cole, 1982. Chapter 9, "Issues Affecting Helping," discusses the impact of the helper's values on interactions with others. Specific types of values conflict are described and illustrated.

Reiser, D. E., & Schroder, A. K. *Patient interviewing: The human dimension.* Baltimore: Williams and Wilkins, 1980. Chapter 5, "Before the Interview," and Chapter 7, "After the Interview," discuss some parameters of the health professional's role behavior and some effects of transference and countertransference.

Focusing the Health Care Interview

Objectives

After completing this chapter, you will be able to do the following:

1. Identify accurately three focus areas (physical, psychological, environmental) using a written patient case.

2. Identify accurately two interview tasks (assessment and transition) from a written dialogue of a health professional/patient interview.

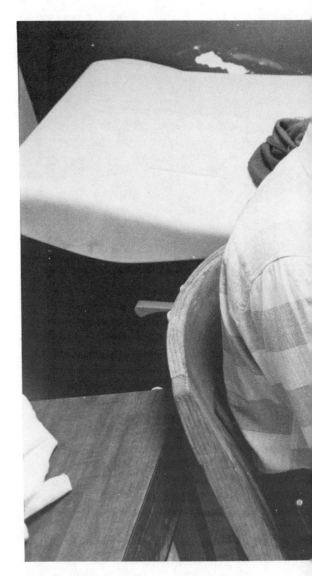

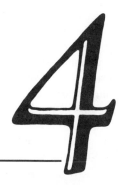

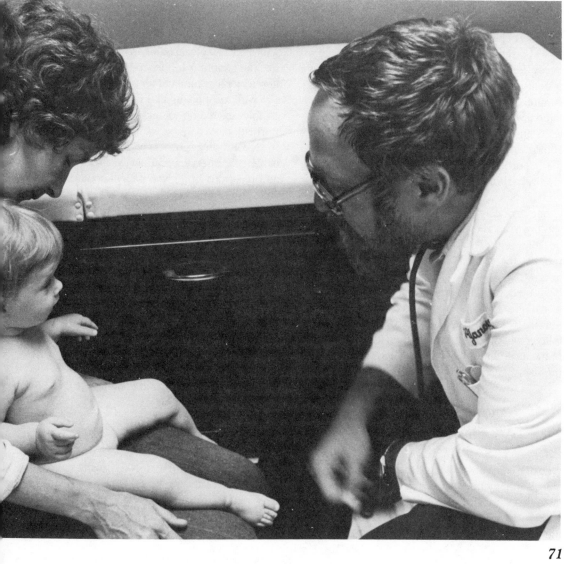

Interviews with patients are conducted for three purposes. The first purpose is to establish an atmosphere of trust and openness in which patients can communicate easily about themselves and their health. The second purpose is to obtain specific information about the nature and duration of the patient's symptoms and the patient's experience with the illness. The third purpose is to provide an opportunity for the health professional to make observations of and about the patient. Stated another way, a successful health care interview has three goals: (1) to establish a positive professional/patient relationship; (2) to elicit information about the patient's condition; and (3) to observe the patient's behavior (Sheppe & Stevenson, 1963).

In order to attain these three goals, it is necessary for the health professional to scrutinize patients and their problems in terms of varying parameters. For example, an effective health care interviewer will inquire not only about the physical signs of illness but also about possible psychological and environmental aspects as well. Further, in order to achieve all the desired goals in a relatively short period of time, the professional must develop a certain adeptness at shifting focus—either obviously or imperceptibly—from one perspective to another. Likewise, the professional must be able—either subtly or overtly—to direct or redirect the patient's focus into other areas of interest.

To effect such shifts in emphasis the professional must use a variety of effective communication tools during the interview. The chapter that follows will first describe and then illustrate some of the techniques that can be effective in facilitating such a change in emphasis.

Integrating a Physical and Psychological Focus in the Interview

One of the major challenges facing health professionals in patient interviewing is achieving a balance in focus. The verbal behavior of the interviewer sets the stage or establishes the focus for the interview (Cormier & Cormier, 1979). For example, if a nurse addresses her questions and remarks to a patient's recent physiological (organic) *symptoms* of hypertension, the comments will reflect the nurse's physical focus and will implicitly direct the patient to think and reply in terms of physiological symptoms.

On the other hand, if a social worker interviews the same patient and restricts the discussion to the patient's *feelings* about hypertension and recent stressful events in the patient's life, the comments will suggest a psychological focus and encourage the patient to discuss his or her psychological reactions to the illness.

There are two reasons why it is important for the health professional to be aware of the various focus areas emphasized in any patient interview. First, the patient is influenced by the focus of the interviewer's comments and questions and typically will respond in like fashion to that focus, possibly excluding other potentially pertinent information.

Second, an awareness of different focus areas enables the interviewer to analyze specific assets and limitations in a given patient contact. Often, after an interview, a clinician may complain that "the interview didn't go anywhere—the patient just rambled on and on." A focus analysis of this interview may reveal that the session lacked direction because the clinician constantly shifted or allowed the patient to shift from one focus to another. As Engel and Morgan (1973) note, the health professional is responsible for subtly directing the course of an interview. These authors suggest that "far from being merely a passive listener, [the health professional] indicates to the patient by his responses and questions the need for certain organization and content" (p. 38).

Specific Areas of Focus in a Health Care Interview

Three general areas of focus will usually suffice to obtain most of the pertinent information. These areas are depicted in Figure 4-1. Note the three focus areas: (1) physical; (2) psychological; and (3) environmental. Although these areas are discussed separately in this section, in actual practice they are integrated, as depicted in Figure 4-1 and in the case illustration found on pp. 75–76. Achieving the proper balance among all three focus areas is critical. An interviewer who focuses only on physical symptoms to the exclusion of psychological and environmental factors may help a patient recover from disease but may fail to assist the same patient in discovering ways to maintain health and prevent recurrence of disease.

Physical Focus

The physical focus is concerned primarily with bodily states—that is, condition of a patient's tissues, organs, and organ systems (Leigh & Reiser, 1980, p. 202). Important information regarding a patient's physical state includes early signs of current illness, possible contributing factors to illness, previous diagnosis and treatments, predis-

position to disease, and so on. The physical focus typically involves discussion of symptoms, physical signs of disease, laboratory tests, medication, procedures such as surgery or radiation therapy, and examination of the patient.

A major purpose of the physical focus is to obtain sufficient information to make an accurate diagnosis of the current illness. Such information also forms the basis of many decisions about proposed health care treatments. Another reason for obtaining information about previous and current signs of illness is to establish a pattern of illness or to monitor the cause of a complaint. Frequently such a pattern will reveal a very apparent, new diagnosis from what was previously a perplexing collection of signs and symptoms.

An additional reason for the physical focus is to provide the patient with specific information about his or her illness and the options for pallia-

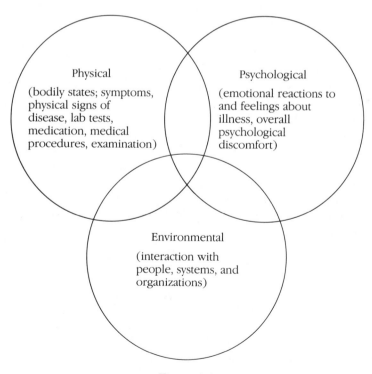

Figure 4-1
Areas of Verbal Focus in a Patient Interview

tion or cure. The health professional should share with the patient the rationale, strategy, and meaning of a proposed diagnostic procedure or treatment regimen to alleviate patient anxiety and to encourage patient compliance and confidence.

We should note that the physical state of the patient is most often the underlying basis of the patient's illness and the primary reason for which most patients seek health care services (Leigh & Reiser, 1980). There is, however, increasing evidence that some patients, under the guise of physical complaints, seek health care services for psychological distress (Anstett & Collins, 1982).

Psychological Focus

A psychological focus is reflected in any interview content that deals with emotional reactions and psychological distress. This distress may be the factor that prompted the patient to seek health care, or it may be a reaction to physical illness or to proposed treatment procedures. Psychological interventions are aimed at exploring and modifying the patient's reactions to and feelings about the illness and also at alleviating pain, anxiety, and overall psychological discomfort. The psychological status of patients is usually assessed in an interview by listening to their verbal accounts and observing their behavior during the interaction (Enelow & Swisher, 1979, p. 16).

Almost every illness and/or medical procedure elicits an emotional reaction in the patient. The type and intensity of the reaction depends on the nature and course of the illness, the type of medical procedure or treatment, and the patient's style of coping with stressful situations. During illness, habitual ways of dealing with stress often become exaggerated (Leigh & Reiser, 1980).

The most pervasive emotional reactions to illness are fear, anxiety, and depression. Since many patients are reticent about discussing feelings, they may present evidence of their emotional distress in terms of somatic complaints (Anstett & Collins, 1982). For example, a patient who is feeling very anxious may reveal such physical complaints as muscle tension, headaches, and stomach upset, yet fail to disclose associated feelings of fear and tension.

Emotional reactions such as anxiety and depression can also indicate the presence of a physical illness even before it is diagnosed. Anxiety and depression, for example, may be associated with particular metabolic disorders such as hyper- and hypothyroidism. According to Verwoerdt (1972), vague feelings of depression may be symptomatic of physical disease with widespread systemic effects such as cancer of the pancreas. An astute interviewer can determine when somatic complaints represent legitimate signs of illness or when they are disguising emotional/psychological distress.

If emotional reactions and psychological distress are ignored, they may sap the patient's strength and consume energy that could be used to combat illness, to promote recovery, or to achieve wellness. Strong emotional reactions, over the course of time and illness, can become even more intense if ignored or taken lightly. For example, a patient who has a rather temporary and mild depressive reaction may start to harbor thoughts of suicide as the depressive state increases in intensity. In contrast to the role that "negative" emotions may have in contributing to and exacerbating illness, "positive" emotions such as joy, happiness, and satisfaction may promote a more rapid and thorough recovery or may prevent an illness from becoming more serious or prolonged.

As Leigh and Reiser (1980) note, health professionals who understand the psychological meaning of their work with patients can "wittingly, judiciously and deliberately utilize the psychotherapeutic potential inherent in the relationship to promote healing and to maximize the beneficial effects of medical treatment" (p. 292). In addition to the use of a therapeutically oriented relationship, the health professional also can focus on psychological issues in health care by using systematic and effective communication responses, such as attentiveness, good listening habits, clarification, and so on. We discuss use of such responses in Chapters 5 and 6.

Environmental Focus

An environmental focus is reflected in any discussion about the patient's interaction with persons, systems, or organizations to which he or she belongs. These may include health care setting, work setting, family setting, educational setting, community/social setting, and cultural setting. These settings are important variables in health and illness and may influence how patients perceive their symptoms as well as their decision to seek appropriate health care (Enelow & Swisher, 1979, p. 17).

Environmental factors may precipitate disease or promote wellness. For example, in the case of Frank Boyce presented after this section, it is possible to identify how Frank's work setting may have contributed to his diagnosed illness of essential hypertension. Frank reported he had a sedentary job and had to endure a doubling of work responsibilities because of a recent hiring freeze. Effects of work settings on illness are evident in the increased incidence of respiratory disease in coal miners. Persons who work constantly under frequent deadlines may be more susceptible to heart disease (depending on other circumstances as well).

In an example of the effects of a community setting and illness, an increase in tooth decay is reported in children who live in communities with nonfluoridated water and who do not receive fluoride supplements. A cultural setting may influence a young mother's decision to bottle feed rather than breast feed, even though the latter option may be better for the infant. Cultural settings also influence what patients regard as an illness as well as the way they describe or report it (Enelow & Swisher, 1979, p. 21).

Finally, family settings can affect health and illness in various ways. For example, some research has found that an identified patient with a psychosomatic illness may be resorting to illness to act out the conflicts of the family system (Minuchin, Rosman, & Baker, 1978). In another study of 200 families who had a hospitalized family member, there was evidence that the illness was linked to unsatisfactory family relationships in almost half of the families studied (Duff & Hollingshead, 1968). Also, "significant others" in the patient's family and social settings may be reacting to physical symptoms in a way that maintains or exacerbates these complaints. Focusing on environmental factors

during the interview can assist patients in determining whether environmental settings are affecting their health and whether any modification in these settings might bring about a change in the patient's condition.

The following case study illustrates the use of these three focus areas in a patient case report. Read the case carefully and note how the patient interview integrates various focus areas. Specific focus areas are underlined, with the corresponding focus area noted in parentheses.

Case Example:
Identifying Focus Areas _____

Frank Boyce is a 60-year-old black male who reluctantly presented to the office for a routine physical examination.

The history of present illness revealed little except fatigue and some episodes of "lightheadedness" not associated with nausea, vomiting, or vertigo (physical focus). His symptoms were ill defined and generally did not seem to be of concern to him. His wife had scheduled the office visit.

Social history indicated that he was a two-pack-a-day cigarette smoker, rarely engaged in any physical exercise, was employed in a sedentary job as a packing supervisor in a chemical research center, and had endured a doubling of his job responsibilities during the past two years because of a hiring freeze (environmental focus). In addition, it became apparent that he was very apprehensive about his impending retirement in two years after 39 years with the same company (psychological focus).

The review of systems was noncontributory except that he added salt to his food before he tasted it (physical focus).

On physical examination, he was a well-developed 20-pound-overweight black male who appeared somewhat older than his stated age. Pulse was 108, and blood pressure was 160/100 sitting (physical focus).

Examinations of the retina revealed blood vessel changes usually seen with moderate high blood pressure. Cardiac evaluation revealed a grade II/VI systolic murmur at the left sternal border and a S-4 gallop. The remainder of the physical exam was within normal limits (physical focus).

Mr. Boyce was advised of his tendency for high blood pressure and requested to return two weeks later for recheck. Meanwhile, because he had evidence of eye and cardiac abnormalities, a chest X-ray, electrocardiogram, serum electrolytes, BUN, and blood count were obtained (physical focus). The results of all the studies were within normal limits except for a mild left ventricular strain pattern on the electrocardiogram.

By the time of his second visit two weeks later, several intervening blood pressures had been obtained, which ranged from 150–175 systolic to 94–110 diastolic. He was advised that he probably had "essential hypertension" and that a complete treatment program would include diet with weight loss, cessation of cigarette smoking, decreased use of table salt, and medication (environmental and physical focus). The rationale for each of these therapeutic modalities was explained to him (physical and psychological focus). He was started on hydrochlorothiazide, 50 mg each morning, and requested to return in two weeks.

Two weeks later, his blood pressure was unchanged, despite the fact that he had lost three pounds and, except for smoking, claimed almost 100% compliance with the treatment regimen. The treatment program was again reviewed, and he was started on alphamethyldopa, 250 mg morning and night, in addition to the hydrochlorothiazide.

After four weeks he had lost five pounds and repeated blood pressures were in the acceptable range of 140/90. By now he had begun to confide in the health professional that his major concerns were related to stresses on the job and the fact that in two years he will be forced into retirement and is concerned about boredom and lack of substantial savings (psychological focus). He also expressed concern over the fact that he felt his medication had rendered him impotent (psychological focus).

He was counseled by the health professional regarding the availability of alternate medication regimens in the event that the impotence persisted and was reassured that the side effects usually diminish with the passage of time (physical and psychological focus). The health professional also praised the positive changes in lifestyle that Mr. Boyce had effected in losing the five pounds and encouraged him to seriously begin thinking about diminishing his cigarette smoking (environmental focus). The remainder of the visit focused on techniques for stress reduction and ways to reduce the excessive work load (psychological and environmental focus). When seen again one month later, he had attained a normal blood pressure of 136/88 and had continued to lose weight slowly.

Further follow-up visits will continue to re-emphasize the elements of the comprehensive treatment program and explore concrete methods of stress reduction and retirement planning.

LEARNING ACTIVITIES

Identifying Focus Areas

Chapter Objective 1: Identify accurately three focus areas (physical, psychological, environmental) from a hypothetical written case. In the following case study, focus areas reflected in the health professional's verbal communication are underlined and numbered. Indicate by underlining which of the three focus areas—physical, psychological, or environmental—is the *predominant* one of the communication. (Occasionally two focus areas may be equally represented.) The first one has been completed as an example. The correct responses (feedback) are provided following the learning activity.

The case of Mary X

A 24-year-old white female graduate student presented to the Emergency Room with a 48-hour history of fever, chills, and very sore throat (1) (example) Physical/psych./environ. Further history revealed that for the preceding six weeks she had suffered from malaise, lassitude, easy fatigability, generalized aches and pains, and some abdominal tenderness. (2) Physical/psych./environ. Past medical history, family history, and social history were noncontributory except that as a graduate student, she had been studying for her comprehensive examinations and complained that because of her low energy level, she was unable to study efficiently. (3) Physical/psych./environ. In addition, she was concerned because one of her closest friends with similar complaints had recently been diagnosed as having acute leukemia. (4) Physical/psych./environ.

On physical examination, the temperature was 39 degrees Centigrade, the pulse 104 beats per minute, and respirations 24 per minute. She appeared to be quite ill. Examination of the head, eyes, ears, nose, and throat were within normal limits except for bilateral inflammation of the tympanic membranes, marked inflammation of the pharynx, and gross enlargement of the tonsils. Both tonsils were covered with exudate. The remainder of the examination was unremarkable except for numerous small (less than one centimeter in diameter), nontender lymph nodes in the anterior and posterior cervical chains, both axillae, and the inguinal regions. A spleen tip was felt. (5) Physical/psych./environ.

Laboratory evaluation on the Gram strain of a throat swab revealed numerous pus cells and occasional Gram positive organisms in pairs and chains resembling streptococci. The blood count revealed 9600 white blood cells with 45% lymphocytes and several atypical lymphocytes. A mono-spot test was positive. (6) Physical/psych./environ. A throat culture was obtained and sent to the bacteriology laboratory.

A diagnosis of probable mononucleosis with an accompanying streptococcal sore throat was explained to the patient. Penicillin VK, 250 mg, four times daily was prescribed and she was requested to telephone in 48 hours to verify the presence of the strep infection and the need to continue the penicillin. In addition, she was told to use regular aspirin, 10 grains every four to six hours as required for relief of the fever and muscle aches until she called the office to verify the need for antibiotics. She was also told that she could resume her regular routine as soon as she felt well enough, but that she should avoid vigorous exercise, which might traumatize her enlarged spleen. (7) Physical/psych./environ.

To aid in her recovery, it was suggested that she should plan for extra sleep and rest and consume a well-rounded diet for the duration of her illness. The importance of a good fluid intake in the presence of fever was emphasized. (8) Physical/psych./environ. It was emphasized that the symptoms from the very sore throat could be expected to resolve over the following three or four days and that the malaise could persist for a period of several weeks or even months, but that the disease usually followed a benign course. (9) Physical/psych./environ. Ways to manage her difficult study/teaching schedule to provide additional time for rest were discussed. (10) Physical/ psych./environ. Finally, a return appointment was scheduled within the week to ensure the correctness of the diagnosis, a positive response to treatment, and additional reassurance. (11) Physical/psych./environ.

Feedback

Determine if your answers are similar to the following:

2. Physical—focus on symptoms

3. Environmental—focus on the patient's work/study setting

4. Psychological—focus on patient's feelings of concern about illness

5. Physical—focus on physical signs

6. Physical—focus on objective laboratory findings related to the physical findings of the disease process

7. Physical—focus on objective treatment protocols related to physical finding of the disease process

8. Environmental—focus on the patient's personal health care setting—sleep, diet

9. Physical; psychological—focus on symptoms and on benign course of the disease to relieve patient's anxiety

10. Environmental—focus on managing the patient's work/study setting

11. Physical; psychological—focus on response to treatment and evaluation of patient's psychologic response to plan

Transitions in Focus: ART

The goals of the interview are best achieved when the clinician deals with and weaves all three focus areas into the interview. It is difficult to conduct a relaxed and yet efficient interview in which there is a balance among physical, psychological, and environmental content. Reiser and Schroder (1980) have described one useful way of achieving this balance during patient interviews. They suggest that the clinician should constantly be engaged in three tasks during an interview: (1) assessment; (2) ranking; and (3) transitions. To aid in remembering these tasks, the authors suggest the acronym ART.

Assessment

The *assessment* is that phase of the interview (perhaps only a few minutes in duration) during which the professional is "maximally open-minded, receptive and non-directive" (Reiser & Schroder, 1980, p. 195). One goal of the assessment phase is to elicit as many associations about the patient's concerns as possible. A second goal is to elicit information and elaboration regarding these concerns. Reiser and Schroder (1980) note that "the key to accuracy during the assessment phase of the medical interview lies in one's ability to maintain a relaxed receptiveness" (p. 195). Interviewing skills that typically may be used during the assessment phase include verbal and non-verbal attentiveness, listening, and the use of open-ended questions. These skills will be discussed in more detail in subsequent chapters.

An illustration depicting a dentist engaged in the assessment phase of a patient interview is shown in the following example:

Dentist: Good morning, Mrs. Smith. What brings you here today?

Patient: Well, I have had a very sore tooth for the last three weeks. The pain is almost constant.

Dentist: Almost constant? Do you notice any time it seems to get better or worse?

Patient: It always seems worse at night. I've been taking aspirin then and that helps some.

Dentist: What about temperature—does it seem more sensitive with either hot or cold food and drink?

Ranking

The second part of the strategy proposed by Reiser and Schroder is *ranking*—that is, arranging topics in order of importance, or establishing the priority in which the various areas of focus will be considered.

Even though topics may be discussed in any chosen sequence, the health professional is wise to consider the physical focus before the others. Many patients, although aware that psychological and environmental factors have some bearing on their health, may be "put off" or confused if too much consideration is given to the nonphysical sphere at the outset. Patients must be confident that their somatic complaints will receive a thorough evaluation before they will accept consideration of psychological and environmental concerns. It is almost always wise to evaluate the physical focus thoroughly in order to determine if physical problems or disease exists and then shift into the psychological and environmental areas. Further, convincing patients that their problems are other than physical in origin is often facil-

itated if the professional can present a patient with a list of "positive negatives"—meaning that a number of considerations and diagnoses have been ruled out. Notice the progression in the following example of a health professional talking to Mrs. Jackson, who has complained of chronic headaches:

> Mrs. Jackson, I have the results from the laboratory tests you took to try to determine a possible cause of your headaches. I'm delighted to report that all the tests are within the normal range. I'm sure you'll be relieved to know that there is no evidence to suggest the presence of an illness or condition such as a brain tumor, aneurysm, or hypertension that could be causing these headaches. However, since you have mentioned that the headaches are still occurring just as frequently, I'd like to spend some time talking with you about some other factors that could be causing the headaches. For example, can you think of anything in your environment such as loud noises or noxious fumes in your house or neighborhood that might be related to your headaches? How about people in your life who give you a headache? Or do you notice whether the headaches seem to start or get worse when you're thinking about certain problems or during particular stressful situations?

Ranking is primarily a covert process or something that the interviewer does automatically and almost instinctively. It is based on the interviewer's experiences, hunches or intuition, and style and on the purpose of the interview and the urgency for discussion of any specific problem areas.

Transitions

In contrast to the covert process of ranking, the third task proposed by Reiser and Schroder (1980)—*transitions*—is a more overt or conscious action on the part of the health professional. Transitions occur in an interview whenever the health professional shifts from one focus to another. It is important for such shifts in focus to occur smoothly but deliberately. To ensure that smooth transitions occur, it is good practice to inform the patient when and why the focus is changing. As Reiser and Schroder note:

> Effecting transitions is fairly simple, if one remembers to do it. . . . Not only is this one of the easier techniques of medical interviewing, it is also one of the most frequently overlooked. It is essential to remember that the patient cannot read your mind. . . . Therefore, make sure that you *share* your thinking aloud with the patient (pp. 197–198).

Verbalizing transitions involves some of the skills presented in following chapters, including confronting, reflecting, and instructing. The following example depicts a nurse shifting the focus of an interview from the physical to the psychological. Note how the nurse effects this transition by telling the patient this shift is occurring.

Nurse: What kinds of problems have been bothering you lately?

Patient: Well, I've been very frustrated with my new baby. He cries all the time and doesn't hardly sleep at all. I think he might be sick.

Nurse: Have you noticed anything else about him that makes you think that he might be ill?

Patient: Well, he doesn't eat that much. And he seems to have a runny nose constantly.

Nurse: All right. I'll look at him in a few minutes. Right now I'd like to shift gears a little and ask you how you're coping with all this? You appear a bit frazzled to me. Is your concern about your baby upsetting you?

During an actual interview, because assessment and transitions are overt, it is possible to determine exactly when and how the health professional engages in assessment and transitions. In contrast, because ranking is a covert process, it is not obvious but implicit. However, each time the clinician makes a transition from one focus area to another, ranking occurs. The clinician has, in

his or her own mind, established priorities for the topics and has selected the next one for discussion by making the transition to it. Covert ranking also occurs during assessment. The questions the professional asks reflect the selection of priorities and decisions regarding the interview content and focus.

The following interview dialogue illustrates how a health professional engages in assessment, ranking, and transition in a coordinated fashion during an interview. In this example, each remark of the health professional that reflects assessment or transition is underlined and the corresponding task noted in parentheses. Note what the interviewer says that indicates he or she is engaged in assessment or transition. Also, note that these tasks are not necessarily conducted in any specific order or sequence. In the example, for instance, the interviewer moves back and forth between assessment and transition. (Ranking is not noted, since it is a covert activity and is implicit in each response.)

Interview Example: Transitions in Focus

Health Professional: Hello, I'm Dr. Elmore. I'm on the staff here, and I'd like to talk to you about the health problems that caused you to come here. I will be asking you a lot of questions. I will appreciate your help in answering them as accurately as possible because that will give both of us a better picture of what is going on. Do you have any questions at this time, Mr. Boyce?

Patient: No, I guess not. I don't know how helpful I'll be because I'm not too sure why I'm here, but I'll try.

Health Professional: That's fine. Now you just said you weren't exactly sure about why you were here. Have you not been having some health problems? [assessment]

Patient: Well, my wife suggested I come in. She has noticed that during the last few months I seem to get easily upset as she puts it. She thought that might indicate a problem. Since I haven't had a health check-up for several years, I thought maybe I should come in.

Health Professional: OK, so your wife is concerned about your becoming upset recently. How have you been feeling in the last few months, Mr. Boyce? [assessment]

Patient: Pretty good. I've been a little tired, but other than that, good. I've had a great many more responsibilities at work in the last two years so that probably explains the fatigue.

Health Professional: How often do you feel fatigued? [assessment]

Patient: Well, not all the time, but maybe several days out of a week. I mean I just don't seem to have any "get up and go."

Health Professional: Will you tell me about your sleep patterns—how much do you usually sleep each night? [assessment]

Patient: Well, I usually sleep about seven hours—from about midnight to 7 A.M. I don't usually have any trouble going to sleep though occasionally I'll wake up once or twice.

Health Professional: Does this waking up during the night happen often or only sometimes? [assessment]

Patient: Oh, maybe two or three times a week.

Health Professional: Can you think of any other problems that sometimes bother you?

Patient: Well, not anything that I can think of right now.

Health Professional: You did mention you don't do much exercise. Is your weight about right, or too high or too low? [assessment]

Patient: Well, I'm not fat, but I could stand to lose about 15 or 20 pounds. I don't seem to be able to lose it, though, with all the rich food I eat.

Health Professional: Could you describe your diet to me? [assessment]

Patient: Well, my wife likes to cook and a lot of my meetings are over large lunches or dinners.

Health Professional: Do you eat a lot of fried foods? [assessment]

Patient: Yes, I love fried foods.

Health Professional: What about your use of salt? [assessment]

Patient: Oh, I always salt everything. I guess it's just a habit.

Health Professional: Mr. Boyce, I'd like to shift the topic here and inquire about another problem that you mentioned earlier. You said that the responsibilities on your job had changed significantly and that you often felt overburdened with your work. Can you tell me more about your job and those extra responsibilities? [transition] What's been happening there? [assessment]

Patient: Well, I'm due to retire in two years. That's sort of a worry to me. But I'm employed now—have been for 39 years— as a packing supervisor in a chemical research center. Due to a hiring freeze two years ago, my job responsibilities have now doubled. I'm just constantly busy and on the go now. I do enjoy it, but there's almost never a free moment.

Health Professional: I'm getting a picture that you're up at 7 every morning, working all day and perhaps some evenings, too, with little time for personal relaxation. Is that an accurate description of your daily routine now? [assessment]

Patient: Yes, pretty much. Many evenings I stay late at work. Some weekends I go in on account of my job, too. It doesn't allow for much free time.

Health Professional: What do you usually do with your free time? [assessment]

Patient: Oh, sit and read, watch TV or do something with my wife.

Health Professional: How often do you engage in any regular exercise of any kind? [assessment]

Patient: Not very often. I just don't seem to have the time for it.

Health Professional: OK, I see. Now you mentioned a few minutes ago you were worried about your retirement that's coming up. Let's get back to that. [transition] Could you tell me more about your concern there? [assessment]

Patient: Well, I've always worked hard. I guess to some degree I've been married to my job. It's hard for me to imagine life without work. I'm sort of afraid I might get bored or just waste away doing nothing.

Health Professional: So in a sense you are caught between two extremes. Right now you're overworking with almost no free time, yet you see retirement as no work and too much free time.

Patient: Yup. That's about it.

Health Professional: It sounds as if you've been under some stress with all your job responsibilities—is that true? [assessment]

Patient: Yes, to some degree.

LEARNING ACTIVITIES

Transitions in Focus

Chapter Objective 2: Identify accurately two interview tasks—assessment and transitions—using a written dialogue of a health professional/patient interview. In the following dialogue, specific health professional verbal communications are underlined and numbered. For each numbered communication, identify whether it is an example of assessment or transition by checking the blank indicating the correct choice. Provide a reason for your selection. The first one is given as an example. The feedback that follows the learning activity gives the correct answers.

Health Professional: Hello, I'm Ms. McGloughlin. I'm on the staff here, and I'd like to spend some time asking you some questions about yourself and your health. All right?

Patient: OK, sure, go ahead.

Health Professional: What sort of problems bring you here today?

1. __✓__ assessment _____ transition
(An open-ended lead to elicit description of patient's health problems.)

Patient: Well, the most recent thing happened about four days ago. It started with a sore throat and a fever. I felt so tired I went to bed. I tried to get up after two days, but any time I walked around my knees hurt. It seems like I've gotten worse. My fever is up to 103°, and my throat is very sore. When I was a child I had tonsilitis several times, and I've got exams coming up, so I thought I'd better get in here and get some medicine for my throat.

Health Professional: You said these symptoms are the most recent thing that has happened to you. How have you been feeling generally?

    2. _____ assessment   _____ transition

Patient: Well, fairly good until about the last four or six weeks, I guess.

Health Professional: What happened then?

    3. _____ assessment   _____ transition

Patient: Well, sort of the same symptoms. I had a fever, sore throat, and headache then, too. But I went to bed for a couple of days, and then these symptoms seemed to get better after that. But I've had this awful feeling of fatigue and no energy—like I have to push myself to do simple little things.

Health Professional: I see.

Patient: I guess when these symptoms started again a few days ago, it sort of jolted me. I'm sure it's all due to my studying, but I'm a little worried because it's not usual for me to be feeling so "blah."

Health Professional: Ms. Jones, I want to follow up on these symptoms in a few minutes. Right now, though, I'd like to change topics here and ask you to tell me more about your studying responsibilities and how you typically spend your time.

    4. _____ assessment   _____ transition

Patient: Well, I don't know if the last couple of months are typical of the year, but the last few months I've spent almost all of my free time studying. This is usually at night. During the day I'm busy taking classes and teaching. I'm in a graduate program, and I have comprehensive exams coming up in six weeks. So I've been staying up rather late at night. I can't flunk them or else I'm out of the program. It's highly competitive.

Health Professional: But at least for the last few months you've been burning the candle at both ends, so to speak?

    5. _____ assessment   _____ transition

Patient: Yes, and I've got six more weeks to go. The way I'm feeling, I wonder if I can make it. What can you give me to help?

Health Professional: OK, let's go back and discuss your symptoms again.

    6. _____ assessment _____ transition

Health Professional: You mentioned recurring fever, sore throat, and headache. Where do you feel the pain when you have a headache?

    7. _____ assessment _____ transition

Patient: Mostly in front of my head, around my eyes, I guess.

Health Professional: What about the muscular aches—do you notice they are more predominant in a particular part of your body?

    8. _____ assessment _____ transition

Patient: Well, I hadn't thought about it, but I guess so. It's been uncomfortable, especially around my knees when I walk or move around.

Health Professional: Anything else that you've noticed that doesn't seem to feel right?

    9. _____ assessment _____ transition

Patient: No, not really. Of course when my throat is sore it feels very swollen all around my neck.

Health Professional: OK, I'm going to check that out in a minute. I'm also going to get a throat swab, and I'd like you to have some blood work done right after we're finished.

Patient: Do you think something is really wrong? I mean, do I have some severe illness?

Health Professional: Well, probably nothing life-threatening if that's what you mean by severe. You seem a little anxious about the severity of your illness—are you?

    10. _____ assessment _____ transition

Patient: Well, in a way. You see I had a friend who had similar symptoms and she was recently found to have leukemia. I guess that made me think that you never know when something like that could happen.

Health Professional: How do you believe this applies to you and what you're feeling now?

    11. _____ assessment _____ transition

Patient: I guess I got a little concerned that I had similar symptoms and also that I've been feeling blah for six weeks or so, which isn't usual for me. But then I've been getting very little rest, and I've been under some stress with these exams coming up.

Health Professional: Your concern about your illness is understandable, as sometimes it's easy to assume that when someone close to us has a certain illness, we have the potential for it, too. Of course, there are many factors that influence why one person develops leukemia and another person does not. My hunch is that you may have something like strep throat. After I examine you, I'll talk to you again and tell you what's going on. I'd like to shift the focus though and go back to something you said earlier. You mentioned you were under some stress from your exams and that the next six weeks are going to be difficult.

12. _____ assessment _____ transition

Health Professional: You seem to feel pretty overwhelmed with the task facing you.

Patient: Yes, because I feel like I still have so much studying left to do, and it's so important for me to do well on these exams. Yet at this point I'm so worn out I don't feel like I have the stamina to really put forth much effort. I do feel pretty discouraged about all of this.

Health Professional: I'd like to talk a little while about this. What options do you have so that the next six weeks are not going to just wear you down further and perhaps aggravate your condition?

13. _____ assessment _____ transition

Feedback

Check to see if your responses and rationale are similar:

2. Assessment—another open-ended lead to elicit description of her recent health

3. Assessment—open-ended lead to elicit information from patient

4. Transition—shift in focus from physical (symptoms) to environmental (studying responsibilities)

5. Assessment—question to clarify and assess patient's recent time management and lifestyle

6. Transition—shift in focus from environmental (studying) to physical (symptoms)

7. Assessment—open-ended lead to elicit clarification and refinement from the patient concerning her headaches

8. Assessment—open-ended lead to elicit patient information and description

9. Assessment—open-ended lead to elicit description of other problems or symptoms

10. Assessment—clarifying lead to determine intensity of patient's feelings of anxiety about illness

11. Assessment—open-ended lead to elicit patient discussion of concerns about having severe illness

12. Transition—shift in focus from physical (discussion of possible illness, diagnosis) to psychological (patient's feelings of being overwhelmed) focus

13. Assessment—open-ended lead to elicit patient discussion of possible alternatives to manage stress

Chapter Summary

An effective interviewer directs the course of a patient interview smoothly and efficiently. Maintaining direction and balance in an interview assures that important information in all relevant areas of the patient's life is obtained. This chapter discussed the importance of a multiple focus in patient interviewing that includes inquiry and discussion of physical, psychological, and environmental parameters of illness. A physical focus means any treatment, intervention, or discussion directed at determining and alleviating the etiologic or symptomatic cause of a disease. A psychological focus refers to interview content that deals with behavior related to the patient's illness and the patient's psychological reactions to the illness. An environmental focus is reflected in interview content that examines the patient's interaction with various settings (such as cultural, family, and work).

It is difficult to conduct an efficient yet relaxed interview in which there is a balance among physical, psychological, and environmental content. Achieving this balance can be facilitated by completing three specific tasks during an interview: assessment, ranking, and making transitions. Assessment is that phase where the interviewer is receptive and nondirective and seeks to elicit as much information about patient concerns as possible. Ranking is a covert task in which the interviewer ranks or arranges topics in order of importance or priority. Transitions occur whenever the health professional shifts from one focus area to another. To ensure that such transitions occur smoothly, it is wise to inform the patient when and why the focus is changing. By engaging in these three interview tasks, the clinician can explore and direct patient discussion of physical, psychological, and environmental parameters of health problems.

Suggested Readings _____

Anstett, R., & Collins, M. The psychological significance of somatic complaints. *The Journal of Family Practice,* 1982, *14,* 253–259. This article discusses ways in which somatic complaints and psychological distress of patients are often related. The authors provide a valuable chart depicting a list of commonly presented somatic complaints that may be psychological rather than physical in origin.

Enelow, A. J., & Swisher, S. N. *Interviewing and patient care.* New York/Oxford: Oxford University Press, 1979. Chapter 2, "The Nature of Medical Information and the Social Context of the Interview," discusses four classes of information or focus areas explored in a medical interview: biological, psychological, social, and cultural.

Leigh, H., & Reiser, M. *The patient: Biological, psychological and social dimensions of medical practice.* New York: Plenum, 1980. Chapters 9–12 on patient assessment provide particularly useful descriptions of obtaining relevant patient information in the interview.

Reiser, D. E., & Schroder, A. K. *Patient interviewing: The human dimension.* Baltimore: Williams and Wilkins, 1980. Chapter 9, "Obtaining the Medical History," discusses the role of assessments, ranking, and transitions (ART) in patient interviewing.

Listening to Patients

Objectives

After completing this chapter, you will be able to do the following:

1. Identify in writing pauses the interviewer should allow to continue and those that the interviewer could interrupt.

2. Demonstrate at least 13 out of 16 behaviors associated with nonverbal, psychological, and verbal attentiveness, given a simulated patient interview.

3. Identify in writing the major ideas presented in selected patient messages.

4. Identify in writing the cognitive and affective components of selected patient messages.

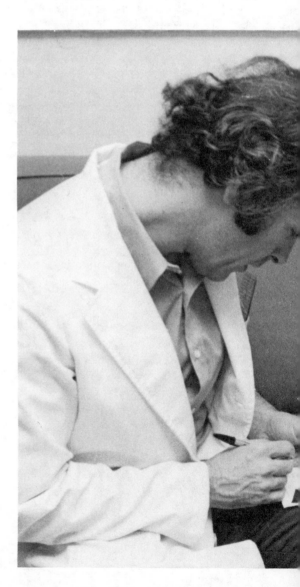

5

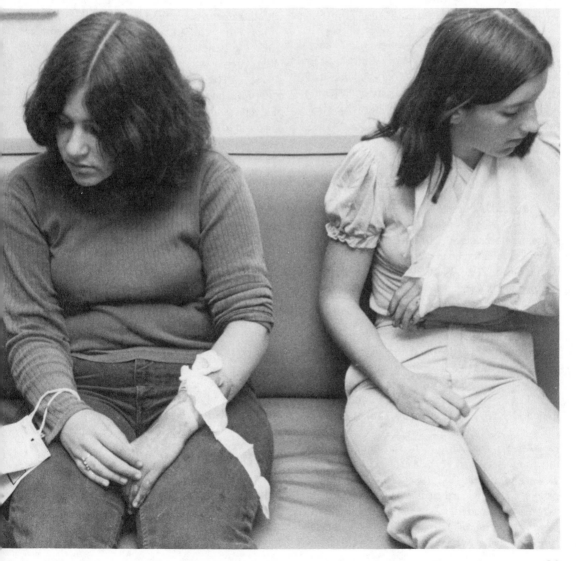

Communication is ever two-way. Listening is the other half of talking. Listening well is no less important than speaking well and it is probably more difficult. Could you listen to a 45-minute discourse without once allowing your thoughts to wander? Good listening is an art that demands the concentration of all your mental facilities. In general, people in the western world talk better than they listen (Potter, 1965, p. 6).

Most health professionals today are aware of the importance of listening to patients, yet patients frequently complain that the attending professional is too busy to do so. Too often, instead of being willing to listen, the interviewer feels compelled to explain (Burton, 1977). Unfortunately when the professionals do most of the talking, they do not learn anything about the patient. Listening and attentiveness are primary conditions for effective interviewing.

Benefits of Listening and Attentiveness

Listening and being attentive toward patients have several positive effects in a patient interview. Bernstein and Bernstein (1980) note that attentive listening "creates a climate in which the patient can communicate" (p. 19). Attentiveness can contribute to a patient's sense of security, which can result in greater expression and openness.

Listening also communicates the professional's interest and respect for the patient. It lets patients know that they and their concerns are important. If the patient perceives a lack of interest or respect, communication may be impeded, resulting in "a perfunctory and uninformative interview" (Engel & Morgan, 1973, p. 31).

A third beneficial effect of listening is that it establishes a base of influence or authority with the patient (Egan, 1975). It enhances the interviewer's credibility and trustworthiness with the patient, may increase the patient's confidence, and may make the patient more receptive to the interviewer's suggestions and explanations. In health care, compliance with medication or with a treat-

ment regimen may increase. Egan (1975) suggests that attentiveness also implies a reciprocal response from the patient. As he notes, "If I am with you fully, invest myself in you, and work with you, all of this demands a response on your part" (p. 64).

A fourth benefit of attentiveness is reinforcement. Much research documents the fact that showing attention is a powerful reinforcer in all human interactions (Hackney, Ivey, & Oetting, 1970; Ivey & Authier, 1978). Attentiveness can make patients feel as if they and their communication are worthwhile and valued. People converse most with those who pay attention to them!

Health professionals also should remember that these benefits of listening apply not only to interactions with patients and their families but also to everyday relationships with subordinates, colleagues, and supervisors. Nothing enhances job motivation and performance more than paying close attention to the communication of other persons.

Behavioral Expressions of Attentiveness

There are three ways in which listening and attentiveness can be expressed: nonverbally, psychologically, and verbally. All three channels of attentiveness are important. Failure to listen in one way may negate the effects of other expressions of attentiveness. Each expression of attentiveness supports the others.

Nonverbal Attentiveness

It is important that health professionals appear to be listening to patients. Patients often determine whether interviewers are attentive to them by observing the interviewer's nonverbal behavior. In fact, even if a clinician *states* "Go ahead and talk—I'm listening to you," the patient may not believe this verbal message if the interviewer is looking away, leaning back in the chair, or generally appearing disinterested. Even the interviewer's personal demeanor and appearance may discourage the patient from talking, as in the case of an interviewer who is dressed sloppily or has poor personal hygiene. Mehrabian (1968) reported that a major part of human communication is expressed nonverbally rather than verbally.

Whereas verbal communication is intermittent, nonverbal communication is constant. When verbal and nonverbal messages are in contradiction, the patient will usually believe the nonverbal message (Gazda, Asbury, Balzer, Childers, & Walters, 1977). Actions speak louder than words. Consequently, it is important for health care providers to be aware of the degree to which they nonverbally express attention to patients.

A variety of nonverbal behaviors communicate attentiveness (see Table 5-1). First, if possible, the health professional should sit rather than stand while talking with the patient. This has the psychological effect of communicating with the patient literally "on the same level." It may be particularly important when talking with children or people who are of short stature. Standing up to talk with

patients while they are seated usually exaggerates the distance the patient already feels and inhibits communication.

Second, the health professional should face the patient directly. Sitting sideways or at an angle may impose a barrier that inhibits communication. Leaning forward slightly, particularly while the patient is talking, communicates receptiveness to the patient's ideas. At the same time it is important for the health professional to maintain a comfortable body posture that appears relaxed rather than tense.

Another important aspect of nonverbal attentiveness relates to the physical distance between the interviewer and the patient. A distance of three to four feet seems to generate ease, comfort, and verbal expression on the part of the patient. Too little distance (two feet) or extreme distance (seven to nine feet) between interviewer and patient may produce anxiety and inhibit patient communication (Knight & Bair, 1976; Stone & Morden, 1976).

Table 5-1
Types of Attentiveness and Example Behaviors

Type	Behaviors
Nonverbal attentiveness	1. Sitting down to talk 2. Facing patient directly 3. Leaning forward 4. Distance of three to four feet between interviewer and patient 5. Maintaining eye contact 6. Relaxed body posture 7. Head nodding 8. Smiling 9. Animated facial expression
Psychological attentiveness	1. Freedom from internal distractions 2. Freedom from external interruptions 3. Psychological privacy
Verbal attentiveness	1. No interrupting 2. Use of one-word verbal encouragers 3. "Tracking"—staying on topic 4. Silence—refraining from overtalking

A third aspect of nonverbal attentiveness involves eye contact. Maintaining consistent eye contact indicates a desire for the patient to talk and a willingness to listen. Constantly shifting eye contact, looking away, or looking down suggests avoidance of the patient or a desire to terminate the interview and tends to change the focus or topic of the interview.

Other ways of communicating nonverbal attentiveness include head nodding, smiling, and animated facial expression. All three of these actions can be reinforcing to the patient. However, these behaviors must fit the context of the situation and must not be exaggerated. There is nothing more distracting than conversing with someone who smiles or nods continuously.

It is important to keep in mind that attentive behaviors, while generally useful, need to reflect both the situation and the individual patient. "High" levels of attention may be too intense for some patients, especially during an initial contact. Nonverbal attentiveness particularly should be adapted to the situation because such behaviors vary across cultures (Ivey & Simek-Downing, 1980). The guidelines presented here for effective nonverbal actions are most applicable to white, middle-class patients from western cultures. For example, several training programs in helping skills for Eskimo and some Oriental cultures do not advocate maintaining eye contact when engaging in a helping interaction. According to Ivey and Simek-Downing (1980):

> In-depth analysis of native American tribes of the Southwest, black rural or inner city populations, Chicano, and other racial or ethnic groups reveals different patterns of nonverbal communication for each culture. The important generalization from this information is that one cannot depend on one's own cultural awareness of nonverbal communication to provide support for understanding another group or culture (pp. 112–113).*

*This and all other quotes from this source are from *Counseling and psychotherapy: Skills, theories, and practice* by A. Ivey and L. Simek-Downing. Copyright 1980 by Prentice-Hall. Reprinted by permission of the publisher.

Table 5-2 contrasts typical nonverbal communication patterns for middle-class culture in the United States with patterns from selected other cultures.

Psychological Attentiveness

Helping interactions demand an intensity of presence, "being there" with the other person in addition to showing an appearance of interest (Egan, 1975). This is referred to as psychological attentiveness or presence. Although it is impossible to teach psychological presence or intensity of presence, there are several components of psychological attentiveness that can be incorporated into helping styles (see Table 5-1). Environmental conditions are then created in which psychological attentiveness is more likely to occur.

The first condition is freedom from internal (personal) or covert distractions. Egan (1975) suggests that attention is facilitated by "getting rid of whatever might distract you from attending" (p. 64). For many people, this means eliminating thoughts about the previous patient, dispelling lingering concerns over a conflict with a spouse or colleague, refusing to be preoccupied with a future task or meeting, or stopping a daydream about anticipated weekend plans. It means, simply, to concentrate on patients while working with them.

A second condition is freedom from external or environmental distractions, such as interruptions from a team member, telephone calls, a "beeper," and so on. Allowing an interview to be interrupted not only communicates disinterest and lack of respect for the client but also breaks the flow and continuity of the session. Bernstein and Bernstein (1980) note that "glancing at mail and taking telephone calls will show the patient that you are very busy and much in demand, but they also will demonstrate that you may be too busy to be interested..." (p. 21).

A rare exception to this condition is the medical or personal emergency. Even then, it is the health professional's responsibility to re-establish contact with the patient as soon as possible. According to Bernstein and Bernstein (1980), health professionals "should indicate their regret for the interruption, acknowledge that the patient must have felt 'put off,' and reschedule the interview for the earliest possible time, preferably when uninterrupted attention can be given" (p. 22).

A third condition for psychological attentiveness involves creating privacy during the session. Conducting an interview in a public setting may reduce the level of the patient's self-disclosure. Unfortunately, geographic privacy is not always easy to secure in some medical settings. However, if psychological privacy can be created and the patient is assured that the interview will not be overheard, then the disclosure level may not be affected. As Bernstein and Bernstein (1980) note, "psychologic privacy does not necessarily demand geographic privacy" (p. 22). Psychological privacy can be created by moving to a corner of a room, draw-

Table 5-2
Nonverbal Communication Patterns of Middle-Class Culture in the United States and Selected Other Cultures*

Nonverbal Dimension	U.S. Middle-Class Pattern	Contrasting Example from Another Culture
Eye contact	When listening to a person, direct eye contact is appropriate. When talking, eye contact is often less frequent.	Some blacks in the U.S. may have patterns directly opposite and demonstrate more eye contact when talking and less when listening.
Body language	Slight forward trunk lean facing the person. Handshake a general sign of welcome.	Certain Eskimo and Inuit groups in the Arctic sit side by side when working on personal issues. A male giving a female a firm handshake may be seen as giving a sexual invitation.
Vocal tone and speech rate	A varied vocal tone is favored, with some emotionality shown. Speech rate is moderate.	Many Hispanic groups have a more extensive and expressive vocal tone and may consider U.S. middle-class styles unemotional and "flat." Speech rate is faster among many Hispanic groups.
Physical space	Conversation distance is ordinary "arm's length" or more for comfort.	Common in Arab and Middle Eastern cultures is a six- to 12-inch conversational distance, a point at which the middle-class U.S. individual is uncomfortable.
Time	Highly structured, linear view of time. Generally "on time" for appointments.	Several South American countries operate on a more casual view of time and do not assume that specified, previously agreed-on times for meetings will necessarily hold.

Note: This table is intended to provide an overview of some key cultural nonverbal patterns in middle-class U.S.A., and to provide an example from another culture to illustrate some major differences. Further study of other cultural patterns is highly recommended. It is also critical to remember that individuals within a single cultural group vary extensively.

*From *Counseling and psychotherapy: Skills, theories, and practice* by A. E. Ivey and L. Simek-Downing, Copyright 1980, p. 113. Reprinted by permission of Prentice-Hall, Inc.

ing a curtain between two beds, speaking in a low-ered voice, and eliminating interruptions.

Verbal Attentiveness

Nonverbal attentiveness is supported by verbal attention—that is, what is said to patients that demonstrates an interest in them. There are different ways of expressing verbal attention (see Table 5-1).

One way to show verbal attentiveness is to allow patients to complete sentences. Cutting off a patient's communication by interrupting may seem punitive and discourage full expression. According to Gordon (1969), interruptions are not always verbal expressions; they include any behavior that distracts the patient or interferes with the patient's ability to continue with the interview at a particular pace.

A second way to demonstrate attentiveness is through the occasional use of one-word or short "verbal encouragers" such as "Mm-hmm," "I see," "go on," and so forth. When used selectively, these short phrases can have a powerful effect in gaining trust and encouraging expression.

A third aspect of verbal attention is called *tracking* (Minuchin, 1974, p. 127). An interviewer engages in tracking by following the content and actions expressed in the patient's communication. Minuchin likens an interviewer's use of tracking to "a needle tracking grooves in a record" (1974, p. 127). The interviewer is nonintrusive and leads by following, accepting, and encouraging a patient's communication rather than initiating or changing topics (Minuchin, 1974, p. 127).

There are a variety of ways in which tracking can be used effectively—it is not restricted to just one type of response. It may be a statement or a question and may take the form of any number of different verbal responses such as a clarification, paraphrase, reflection of feeling, and open-ended question (these responses are discussed in Chapters 6 and 7). The critical element in tracking is to maintain the focus on the topics expressed by the patient.

Finally, it is necessary to refrain from excessive talking in order to give the patient an opportunity to talk. Silence is an important ingredient of verbal attentiveness. Interviewers' judicious use of silence indicates that they are willing to listen and to give patients time to talk. Silence does not mean that nothing is happening. On the contrary, it gives both the patient and the interviewer time to collect their thoughts and provides the interviewer with the opportunity to observe the patient unobtrusively (Hein, 1980, p. 50).

Silence is sometimes most difficult to achieve in an interview. Many professionals find it hard to refrain from talking because of their own anxiety. According to Lewis (1978), "to many persons, silence is frightening and something to be avoided" (p. 36). Lewis (1978) also believes that some professionals are uncomfortable with silence because when pauses occur, they feel they are not doing enough for the patient. The skill of using silence effectively in an interview thus involves the ability to be comfortable with moments of silence and also the sensitivity to discriminate when to remain silent and when to talk. Because of the extreme difficulty of the effective use of silence, we present some guidelines for it in the following section.

Patient-induced versus interviewer-induced silence.

Silence and pauses may be understood best in the context in which they occur. For example, in an initial interview, silence in patients often means they are having difficulty "getting started." In subsequent contacts, their silence may mean they are using the time to think, to search for words, or to assimilate information. According to Enelow and Adler (1979), "this kind of thoughtful silence is rarely accompanied by signs of increased tension" (p. 43).

Hackney and Cormier (1979) point out the difference between patient-induced and interviewer-induced silence. In patient-induced silence the patient talks, then stops and pauses. The pause may represent avoidance or embarrassment of a certain topic or the patient's need to catch up on the progress of the moment, especially if the interviewer has covered a lot of ground (Hackney & Cormier, 1979, p. 41). In interviewer-induced silence, the interviewer assumes the responsibility for the moment and responds with silence, and the silence may occur for several reasons. For example, some interviewers may pause because they are at a loss for words. Others may misuse silence as a way of withholding. Interviewer-induced silence is most appropriate when used deliberately for specific purposes, such as reducing the interviewer's activity, transferring responsibility for talking to the patient, and so on.

We suggest the following guidelines for deciding whether to continue a pause or to interrupt it.

Permitting a pause to continue. It is generally useful to allow the pause to continue when the patient is trying to remember or to clarify thoughts, is deciding whether to say more or to elaborate, is feeling overcome with emotion, or is needing to assimilate information. The time they require to accomplish these tasks varies among patients. As Hein (1980) points out, older people may require longer silences because their physical and mental processes have slowed down with age (p. 51). It is also useful to let a pause continue in order to regulate the pace of the interview. Silence can call attention to the patient's activity and slow down the pace of the interview and can help focus attention on what is happening. A final reason for allowing a silence to continue is to shift the responsibility for talking from the health professional to the patient. As Hackney and Cormier (1979) note, silence may indicate that the interviewer does not want to select or direct the topic at this time.

Interrupting a pause. In contrast, there are occasions during an interview when it is more appropriate to interrupt a silence than to allow it to go on. The duration of a therapeutic silence is approximately 10 to 15 seconds; prolonged silence can cause discomfort, anxiety, or resentment and should be interrupted. Silences should also be interrupted with patients who are severely depressed and say very little. Finally, excessive silence is often inappropriate with a patient who displays distrust by being passive, avoiding topics or questions, and so on. According to Sierra-Franco (1978), "with such a patient, any silence will generally widen the distance between you. If you are silent, he will tend to interpret your silence as disinterest and lack of concern for him" (p. 251).*
Remember, these guidelines are just that. Each interview will require you to judge the appropriateness of silence at any given moment.

---

*This and all other quotes from this source are from *Therapeutic communication in nursing,* by M. Sierra-Franco. Copyright © 1978 by McGraw-Hill. Used with the permission of the McGraw-Hill Book Company.

LEARNING ACTIVITIES

Using Silence

In the following learning activity we present eight descriptions of various types of pauses in an interview. Chapter Objective 1 asks you to identify whether each is an indication for allowing the silence to continue or for interrupting it. Indicate your answer in the blank provided. The first one is completed as an example. The correct responses (feedback) follow the learning activity.

1. The patient seems to be trying to remember something.

   __✓__ Continue   _____ Interrupt

2. The patient is trying to clarify her or his thoughts or feelings.

_____ Continue   _____ Interrupt

3. The patient seems to have difficulty in starting to talk.

_____ Continue   _____ Interrupt

4. The patient seems to need time to think about what has been covered so far in the interview.

_____ Continue   _____ Interrupt

5. The duration of the pause becomes prolonged (over 20 seconds).

_____ Continue   _____ Interrupt

6. The patient seems depressed and has said very little in the interview.

_____ Continue   _____ Interrupt

7. The patient is overcome with emotion such as crying.

_____ Continue   _____ Interrupt

8. The patient seems distrustful and behaves passively in the interaction.

_____ Continue   _____ Interrupt

Feedback

2. Continue—the patient needs the pause to focus and to reduce the ambiguity being experienced.
3. Interrupt—the pause is not helping the patient "get started" and a comment by the interviewer may have a better result.
4. Continue—the pause helps the patient assimilate the information received in the interview.
5. Interrupt—very prolonged pauses often are nontherapeutic and increase the patient's discomfort.
6. Interrupt—the patient's feelings of depression and accompanying lack of verbal interaction will not be helped by pauses. An interviewer comment may be more helpful in this case.
7. Continue—the pause is useful here to allow the patient to experience the emotion and to get control of it.
8. Interrupt—prolonged silence in this case probably will only increase the lack of trust felt by the patient. Interviewer comments may help to put the patient at ease.

Attentiveness

According to Chapter Objective 2, you will be able to conduct a 15-minute role-play interview with a patient in which you demonstrate at least 13 out of 16 various behaviors associated with nonverbal, psychological, and verbal attentiveness. Here is how to implement this exercise.

If possible, conduct this activity in triads: One person takes the part of the interviewer, one person assumes the patient role, and the third person serves as observer. (If no observer is available, try to videotape your interview for feedback via playback.)

The patient should describe a health-related concern to the interviewer. The interviewer's task is to demonstrate attentiveness—not to solve the problem. The observer's task is to observe the interaction and to provide feedback, using the Checklist of Nonverbal, Psychological, and Verbal Attentiveness.

After the 15-minute interview, discuss the interaction; then trade roles. Each person should have the opportunity to be interviewer, patient, and observer one time.

Checklist of nonverbal, psychological, and verbal attentiveness

Instructions to observer: Determine whether the interviewer did or did not demonstrate the desired behaviors listed in the right column. Check yes or no in the left column to indicate your judgment.

Nonverbal Attentiveness

	Yes	No	
1.	____	____	Sat down to talk with patient
2.	____	____	Faced patient directly
3.	____	____	Leaned forward slightly in chair
4.	____	____	Maintained distance of three to four feet between interviewer and patient
5.	____	____	Maintained eye contact without staring
6.	____	____	Body appeared relaxed
7.	____	____	Used occasional head nods
8.	____	____	Demonstrated intermittent smiling
9.	____	____	Responded with facial animation and alertness

Psychological Attentiveness

10.	____	____	Appeared to be "with" the patient and not preoccupied with other things
11.	____	____	Refrained from being interrupted by calls, beeper, etc.
12.	____	____	Created psychological privacy

Verbal Attentiveness

13.	____	____	Did not interrupt patient
14.	____	____	Used one-word verbal encouragers

15. _____ _____   Demonstrated "tracking" responses; stayed on topics introduced by patient

16. _____ _____   Allowed pauses to give patient time to think—refrained from overtalking

Comments: _____

_____

_____

_____

Receiving and Processing Messages

Good listening includes both receiving and processing messages. *Receiving* a message suggests receptivity not only to the words but also to the nuances of the expression, not only to what is said but also to what remains unsaid. *Processing* involves interpretation of the message.

Complete processing of a message implies that the interviewer is objective about the message and does not selectively screen out parts of the message that may be bothersome, disturbing, or offensive. With experience, an objective interviewer learns to recognize particular patient phrases and behaviors that may provoke negative, subjective feelings toward the patient. For example, a female health care interviewer may realize she feels defensive whenever a male patient refers to his wife as "my old lady." Awareness of this dynamic can be useful so that the interviewer does not "tune out" important parts of the patient's message that are offensive to her. Identifying the feelings and the psychological reactions evoked by patient interactions may give the interviewer certain clues about the nature of the patient. According to Froelich and Bishop (1977), "recognition of types of patients who consistently evoke a specific feeling is useful in planning the management of your patient and his/her illness. For example, a patient who creates anger may be the type of patient who

will not carry through with a treatment program of self-medication. The patient who elicits amiable feelings may be the type of patient who overdoes everything and takes more medication than prescribed" (pp. 54–55). Being aware of personal reactions to patients and colleagues can encourage the constructive use of feelings rather than inhibiting communication through ignorant, thoughtless, or impulsive responses. Processing also involves retention. During effective listening interviewers attend so carefully that they can recall quotations, sounds, and expressions long after the conversation has ended.

Listening receptivity can be heightened by improving skills in attentiveness and concentration. To ensure that you will process and recall messages accurately, learn to listen in certain ways. For example, most interviewers usually hear and remember the objective or obvious part of the message (sometimes referred to as the *cognitive* portion of a message) much more easily than the underlying or subjective part of a message (referred to as the *affective* part of a message). Sometimes it is difficult to remember the entire message, and, in responding, the most important part is omitted.

Recalling Messages

One of the first steps in listening is to hear and remember an entire message communicated by a sender. According to Long and Prophit (1981), "most people not only don't hear much of what is said to them but also hear things that are not said. When asked to repeat the content of a message, they usually leave out one or several of the main points and often add content of their own" (p. 40). As these authors point out, a skilled listener who hears both the objective (cognitive) and subjective (affective) communication can then direct the interview to the best advantage by focusing her or his response on the appropriate portion of the message. An interviewer who hears only a portion of the message, however, has much more limited options. Long and Prophit (1981) recommend trying to "remember the whole message in the patient's own words . . ." (p. 40).

As an example, consider the following patient message. The patient, a 75-year-old woman, has just made the following statement prior to her scheduled hip replacement surgery:

> I just hope I made the right decision. I'm sure the surgery will help the pain in the long run but right now I'm just remembering the problems of all the other surgery I've had before. I feel pretty apprehensive about this one, especially at my age.

In this example, the patient communicated four different ideas: (1) I hope this is the right decision; (2) The surgery will help in the long run; (3) I'm remembering problems from previous surgery; and (4) I'm apprehensive, especially now that I'm older. It is the professional's task to learn to recall all the major points communicated by a patient without deleting or omitting important ones and without distorting the meaning. The following exercise will provide an opportunity to practice this skill.

○

═══════════════════ *LEARNING ACTIVITIES* ═══════════════════

Recalling Messages   Chapter Objective 3: To identify in writing the major ideas presented in selected patient messages.

Listed below are four patient messages. Read one message carefully. Without looking at the message again, try to remember exactly what the patient said. Then respond to the questions after each message in writing. The first one is completed as an example. The answers can be found in the feedback section following the learning activity.

1. A 37-year-old woman who has just given birth to her first child:

   Oh, I'm so relieved everything went all right. I know I thought my age might be a factor, that I might be too old for this sort of thing. Now I'm just overjoyed to have a healthy, normal baby.

   Can you recall this patient's message almost word for word—in her words not yours? (Select which blank by marking a √).

   __√__ yes   _____ no

   How many points do you recall? Three—(1) relief that everything went OK; (2) concern about her age; (3) joy to have a normal, healthy baby.

2. A 75-year-old man who is having difficulty tolerating arthritic pain:

   I don't think I can stand this much longer. Can't you give me something for the pain? Why did this have to happen to me?

Were you able to recall the patient's message in his own words?

_____ yes   _____ no

How many different points did he make? What were they?

_____

_____

3. A 15-year-old boy with acute leukemia:

I just wish I didn't feel so down on everything. What's the use—I'm probably going to die soon anyway. What do I have left to live for?

Do you remember the message as expressed in his words?

_____ yes   _____ no

How many different parts of the message do you remember?

_____

_____

4. A 40-year-old businessman with hypertension:

This clinic has got to be one of the most inefficient places I've visited. You have to wait forever before anyone sees you. Then it's another hour before they are ready to take you for your lab work. Why it takes up one of my mornings just to come here for a checkup.

What did this patient say—can you remember his words, not yours?

_____ yes   _____ no

What were the different points he expressed?

_____

_____

Feedback

Patient 2: The three parts to his message were: (1) I can't stand this much longer; (2) I want something for the pain; and (3) Why did this happen to me?

Patient 3: There were four parts to this message: (1) Wish I didn't feel so down; (2) What's the use? (3) I'm going to die soon anyway; (4) What do I have left to live for?

Patient 4: His message had four ideas: (1) This clinic is inefficient; (2) You have to wait forever before being seen; (3) It's another wait before you get your lab work done; (4) It takes a morning just to get a checkup here.

If you had difficulty recalling these various points, try to determine what the problem is and how to correct it. People who have trouble remembering parts of a message or who distort the message by adding their own ideas may not be focusing their attention solely on the patient. Try to remove noise and external distractions to improve your attentiveness. Recall also takes practice. Apply these skills to other situations. For example, focus and concentrate on remembering names of new persons you meet. With practice, your skills in remembering messages accurately will improve dramatically.

Two Parts of Messages: Cognitive and Affective

In responding to any patient message, the health professional must choose which part of the message is the most important and deserving of response. As we mentioned earlier, patient messages may contain an objective or cognitive component and a subjective or affective component. The *cognitive* component includes thoughts and ideas about situations, events, people, or things (Hackney & Cormier, 1979, p. 65) and answers the question "What happened?" The *affective* component refers to the emotions or feelings of the patient and answers the question "How does the patient feel about what happened?" (Hackney & Cormier, 1979; Long & Prophit, 1981). Notice the cognitive and affective portions of the following patient message:

I wish I didn't get so many colds and sore throats. I've always thought I was in pretty good health overall. Most of the time I feel good and pleased about the way my life is going. I try to take care of myself—take vitamins, eat the right foods, take Geritol, sleep regularly, etc. Still I seem to get four or five of these colds or sore throats each year—it's frustrating.

The cognitive component, or "What happened?", refers to the events—trying to take care of herself and yet having frequent colds and sore throats each year. The affective component, or "How is she feeling about what happened?", has two parts:

1. Feeling good and feeling pleased about life;

2. Feeling frustrated about the frequent colds and sore throats.

(Now do the learning activities on pages 102–103.)

Implied Parts of a Message

Not all patient messages contain both cognitive and affective components that are easily recognized. Some messages may have only cognitive content, as when a patient says "I think the nurses here provide good care." Other messages may contain only the affective portion. For example, a patient may state "I feel pretty good today." In both of these examples the other component was omitted from the message and must be discovered through direct inquiry or inference.

Typically patients are more likely to reveal cognitive content and omit the affective part of the message, because they feel uncomfortable discussing their feelings, particularly to someone they hardly know. For example, patients often talk quite directly about a situation and their perception of it but may only imply what their feelings are about the situation. A patient may say something like "This car accident sure was a lousy thing. I've been thinking about why it happened to me." The patient describes the situation (car accident) but leaves the affect or emotions unstated. In such instances, the patient's nonverbal behavior may give important clues about the unstated or implied feelings. In the example above, the patient might be feeling upset, angry, depressed, or confused.

○

┌─────────────────── *LEARNING ACTIVITIES* ───────────────────┐

Identifying Cognitive and Affective Components of Messages

For each of the following patient messages, identify in writing the cognitive and affective parts of the message (Chapter Objective 4). The first one is completed as an example. Feedback follows the learning activity.

1. An elderly woman who was in an automobile accident:

   I think I'm a lucky person—alive after that collision with the bus. That darn bus driver—here I was driving along in the proper lane, within the speed limit, and he crossed over into my lane. I'm just worried now about how long it's going to take me to get over all these bumps and bruises.

   Cognitive component: The event of a car-bus accident resulting in minor injuries.
   Affective component: Feeling worried.

2. A 40-year-old man:

   I know both myself and my wife really want to have a child. But trying so long like this without having it happen is so discouraging. I've tried everything I know to do—have sex a lot, wear loose underwear, etc. Lately I've been thinking maybe I'm just too old.

   Cognitive: _____

   _____

   Affective: _____

   _____

3. A six-year-old girl:

   I can't help crying. I don't want to go to the hospital and have my tonsils out. Hospitals are for sick people and I'm not sick. Besides that, it might hurt really bad and I'm scared.

   Cognitive: _____

   _____

   Affective: _____

   _____

4. A 19-year-old male student with diabetes:

I'd like to make it through college and graduate with all my friends. Now I'm thinking that's not too realistic. My energy level has been pretty low. Consequently I've had to drop two classes. I'm sleepy during study time. It gets pretty frustrating at times.

Cognitive: _____

_____

Affective: _____

_____

5. A colleague who is upset about having to work on a ward that is exceptionally short-staffed:

I'm getting more and more frustrated with trying to do my job well on this floor. There just aren't enough of us to go around, and the patients suffer as a result.

Cognitive: _____

_____

Affective: _____

_____

Feedback

Patient 2
Cognitive: Wanting to have a child and trying various things to make it happen.
Affective: Feeling discouraged.

Patient 3
Cognitive: Having to go to the hospital for a tonsillectomy.
Affective: Feeling scared.

Patient 4
Cognitive: Low energy level and not keeping up with friends in college.
Affective: Feeling frustrated.

Colleague 5
Cognitive: Trying to do job well. Aren't enough staff members to go around. Patient care suffers.
Affective: Feeling more and more frustrated.

When an affective message is implied but not directly stated, the health professional may want to clarify the patient's feelings and moods concerning the situation. The omitted part of a message is not unimportant and should not be ignored. In fact, in some cases, the patient may omit the part of the message that is most significant because it is also the most difficult to talk about or share with someone else. The health professional must use discretion in deciding which part(s) of the message—stated or implied—should be emphasized in responding.

Responding to Patient Messages Selectively

Up to this point, we have emphasized two different skills in learning to process patient messages. The first skill involves remembering the entire patient message without distorting it or adding new content. The second involves discriminating which parts of the message are present or omitted. There is also a third important skill—deciding what part or parts of the message should be emphasized in responding.

It is impossible to be attentive to everything a patient says and does in an interview. Interviewers are continually faced with the decision to respond to or ignore certain parts of a patient communication; in other words, attention becomes selective. Some subjects are chosen for discussion and others are ignored.

It is important to consider what the concept of selective attention implies in actual practice. As Jessop (1979) indicates, selective attention "does not imply that you are not listening to the person or that you are unaware of what is going on. Selective attention is purposive. You are attending to all that is going on in the interview (process), but you are not reinforcing or attending to some parts of what is being said . . . (content)" (p. 32).

Studies of interviewing typescripts have shown that listeners do not discriminate very well between multiple patient messages. When there are two or more parts to a message, interviews tend to make responses that either are nonspecific or include both messages (Tyson & Kramer, 1981). And as we stated earlier, an implied or omitted idea may be more significant than something the patient states directly. There are no hard and fast rules to dictate when to respond to which part of a message. These are decisions that become easier with interviewing experience. However, it is important to be aware of patterns of selective attention. Such patterns usually reveal more about the interviewer than the patient. For example, as mentioned in Chapter 4, the clinician who continually focuses on physical symptoms may feel uncomfortable discussing other topics. Or the interviewer who usually talks about abstract problems or situations may be reluctant to discuss more personal topics that directly involve the patient. Clinicians who continually focus either on other people (typically not present at the interview) or on only physical problems may find their sessions are not personalized. To personalize an interview, it is necessary to focus on the patient rather than on some other person or problem (Ivey & Simek-Downing, 1980, p. 72).

Chapter Summary

Listening and paying attention to patients can, over time, bring enormous benefits to a health professional/patient interaction. Patients will talk more freely about themselves and will participate more actively in an interview when they sense they are the professional's sole concern at that time. Listening and attentiveness are communicated to patients by psychological presence, nonverbal behaviors, and selected verbal responses. Silence is an important ingredient in listening to patients. Some pauses are necessary for patients to assimilate information or to clarify their thoughts. Silence may not be helpful when the patient is having difficulty talking for one reason or another.

Attentiveness to patients is selective; the interviewer observes all parts of the patient's behavior but responds verbally and nonverbally only to particular portions of it. As a set of skills, effective listening can be learned with practice and applied to interactions with both patients and colleagues. It involves recalling verbal and nonverbal mes-sages, discriminating between various parts of a message, and detecting certain parts of a message that are implied or omitted.

Suggested Readings _____

Bernstein, L., & Bernstein, R. *Interviewing: A guide for health professionals.* New York: Appleton-Century-Crofts, 1980. Chapter 2, "An Overview of Interviewing Techniques," discusses the role of attentiveness in effective interviewing.

Enelow, A. J., & Swisher, S. N. *Interviewing and patient care.* New York/Oxford: Oxford University Press, 1979. Chapter 3, "Basic Interviewing," contributed by Enelow and Adler, has a very useful discussion of the role of silence in a medical interview.

Hackney, H., & Cormier, L. S. *Counseling strategies and objectives.* Englewood Cliffs, N.J.: Prentice-Hall, 1979. Chapter 5, "Using Silence," discusses a number of valuable strategies an interviewer can use to handle silence effectively.

Hein, E. C. *Communication in nursing practice.* Boston: Little, Brown, 1980. Chapter 6, "Communication Skills in the Nursing Interview," and Chapter 15, "Listening," offer useful suggestions for silence and attentiveness in patient interactions.

Ivey, A., & Simek-Downing, L. *Counseling and psychotherapy: Skills, theories, and practice.* Englewood Cliffs, N.J.: Prentice-Hall, 1980. Chapter 3, "The Skills of Intentional Counseling: Attending and Influencing," presents an overview of behaviors associated with attentiveness in the helping process. The role of selective attention in interviewing also is discussed.

Long, L., & Prophit, Sister Penny. *Understanding/responding: A communication manual for nurses.* Monterey, Calif.: Wadsworth, 1981. Chapter 2, "Nonverbal Methods for Facilitating Communication," discusses various nonverbal components of attentiveness and their effects on patient interaction.

Responses That Communicate Understanding

Objectives

After completing this chapter, you will be able to do the following:

1. Write examples of clarifying responses for selected patient messages.

2. Write examples of paraphrase responses for selected patient messages.

3. Write examples of accurate reflection of feeling responses for selected patient messages.

4. Write examples of summarization responses for selected patient messages.

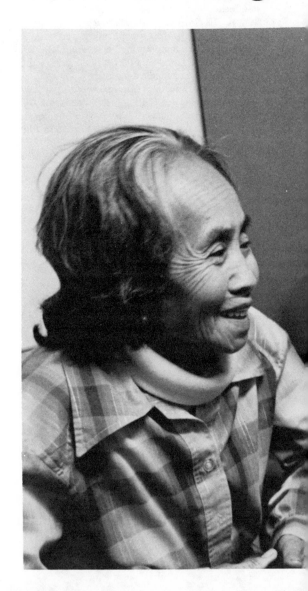

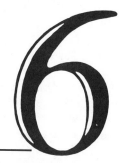

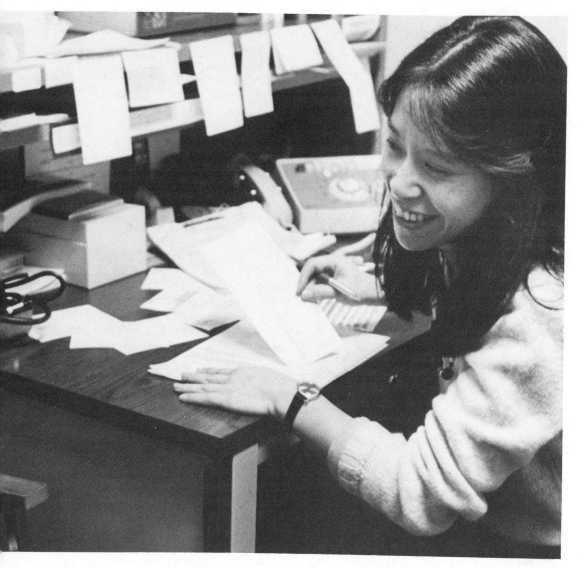

Understanding refers to the ability to perceive the patient's point of view and to communicate that perception back to the patient. Patients interact more easily with someone who they feel understands them. Many health care providers want to understand their patients, yet certain obstacles may inhibit effective comprehension of patient messages. The more common obstacles include judgmental attitude, the tendency to respond to missing information with frequent questions, and the tendency to propose instant solutions to complex patient problems. These barriers to effective understanding can be removed with practice and experience and with the use of tools that aid in understanding patient messages and communicating that understanding to patients. In this chapter we present four such tools for communicating understanding to patients—clarification, paraphrase, reflection of feeling, and summarization.

Request for Clarification

As Hackney and Cormier (1979) note, sometimes patient messages sound cryptic or confused and you are left wondering just what the person was attempting to communicate (p. 51). Communication that may be particularly confusing includes inclusive terms ("they" and "them"), ambiguous phrases ("you know"), and words with double meaning ("stoned," "trip") (Hein, 1980, p. 35). When what a patient means is unclear, it is useful to ask for clarification. Otherwise you may collect inaccurate information and fail to check out distorted assumptions. A clarification asks the patient to elaborate on "a vague, ambiguous, or implied statement" made previously in the interview (Hein, 1980, p. 56). The request for clarification is usually expressed as a question, asking the patient to rephrase the communication (see Table 6-1). It may begin with phrases like "Do you mean that . . ." or "Are you saying that . . ." or "Could you try to describe that . . ." in an attempt to encourage the client to restate the previous communication. The clarification can pertain either to the cognitive or to the affective part of the message. Consider the following examples of the request for clarification.

Patient: I just feel sick all over. My mouth hurts. My lips are jabbing me, my stomach is in knots, my head feels like it's bursting, my back is sore, and my hands are shaking.

Health Professional: <u>Could you try to describe that sequence of events for me again?</u> I'm not sure I followed you. [clarification of cognitive part of message]

Health Professional: How have you been feeling lately?

Patient: Terrible, like the whole world is caving in on me.

Health Professional: I'm not sure I know what you mean by that feeling—the world is caving in on you. <u>Could you clarify that feeling for me?</u> [clarification of affective part of message]

Now do the clarification learning activity on pages 110–111.

Paraphrase

A paraphrase is an encapsulated repetition of the patient's primary words and thoughts (Cormier & Cormier, 1979; Ivey & Simek-Downing, 1980). Paraphrasing involves selective attention to the cognitive or objective part of a message—with the patient's key words and ideas translated into other words. An effective paraphrase thus does more than simply "parrot back" what the patient has said. "The goal should be to rephrase what has been said in such a way that it will lead to further discussion or to increased understanding of the topic" (Jessop, 1979, p. 63). Consider the following interchange.

Patient: I know I should give up smoking and get more exercise. What I'm doing now isn't helping my old heart.

Health Professional: You know you should give up smoking and get more exercise in order to help your heart.

In this example, the interviewer merely "parroted" the patient's words. The likely outcome of such a response is that the patient may merely say "Yes" or "I agree" and not elaborate or that the patient may feel belittled or ridiculed by the interviewer. A more effective paraphrase would be "You are aware that making some lifestyle changes will be better for your heart." This response encourages the patient to keep talking and to expand on particular lifestyle changes that would be beneficial.

The paraphrase has several purposes. First, it tells patients what you have understood them to say. It gives them the opportunity to validate the accuracy of your perceptions. Second, an astute

Table 6-1
Definitions and Intended Purposes of Understanding Responses

Response	Definition	Intended Purposes
Clarification	A question asking the patient to rephrase or restate a previous message	1. To clear up confusion or ambiguity—to avoid misunderstanding 2. To confirm the accuracy of what you heard the patient say
Paraphrase	A statement rephrasing the cognitive part of a patient message	1. To encourage patient elaboration on the cognitive part of the message 2. To let patient know that you have understood or heard the message 3. To help the patient focus on a specific situation, idea, or action 4. To highlight content when attention on affect would be premature or inappropriate
Reflection of feeling	A statement rephrasing the affective part or emotional tone of a patient message	1. To clarify patient feelings in a particular situation or interview contact 2. To help patient feel understood—to establish the interviewer's interpersonal as well as technical competence 3. To encourage the patient to express her or his feelings about a situation 4. To help the patient learn to manage feelings, especially negative ones 5. To reflect negative feelings directed toward the health care provider or setting in order to avoid an emotional conflict
Summarization	A collection of several paraphrase or reflection responses that condenses patient messages or an interview or series of interviews	1. To tie together multiple elements of patient messages 2. To identify a theme or pattern of patient communication 3. To interrupt excessive rambling and bring back a particular focus to the interview 4. To help regulate the pace of an interview 5. To review progress and suggest areas for discussion in future interviews

○

═══════════ *LEARNING ACTIVITIES* ═══════════

Clarification

In this learning activity, we present four patient messages. Read each message carefully, then verbalize or write a request for clarification (Chapter Objective 1). Your request for clarification should be directed to the part of the message that is confusing or misleading or requires additional explanation in order for you to understand the patient. The first example is completed for you. Feedback follows the learning activity.

1. *A teenage girl:* You know it's hard to have much of an appetite when you're feeling the way I feel right now.

   Clarification: Could you tell me exactly how you're feeling today? [clarification of affective component]
   Could you describe what your typical appetite is? [clarification of cognitive component]

2. *A middle-aged man:* It's hard for me to understand why I'm having so many problems with my teeth—it's pretty confusing. For years I've been taking care of them so well—brushing them, using floss—you know, the whole bit.

   Clarification: _____

   _____

3. *An elderly man:* I don't know why I have to have this therapy. I think it's a waste of time.

   Clarification: _____

   _____

4. *A young woman:* I just feel so down. I keep thinking what's the use? And then I can't stop crying.

   Clarification: _____

   _____

Feedback

Here are some examples of various clarifications used to respond to these patient messages. Determine if your responses are similar.

Patient 2
a. Could you describe for me the specific problems you've been having with your teeth? [clarification of cognitive component]

b. Can you explain more about what you mean by saying "it's pretty confusing"? [clarification of affective component]

Patient 3

a. Are you saying that you feel irritated about having to have this therapy? [clarification of affective component]
b. Could you try to describe in what ways you believe it will be a waste of your time? [clarification of cognitive component]

Patient 4

a. Could you try to clarify what feeling down is like for you? [clarification of affective component]
b. Are you saying that there's something specific causing you to feel this way or just things in general? [clarification of (unstated) cognitive component]

---

paraphrase encourages patients to talk further and in greater depth. Another purpose of the paraphrase is to draw the patient's attention to a specific situation or event, idea or cognition, or action or behavior. The patient can then focus on selected portions of the message more clearly. For example, the paraphrase may highlight the cognitive portion of the message when attention to the affective part of the message would be premature or inappropriate for the goals of the interview. (Table 6-1 summarizes the purposes of the paraphrase.) The paraphrase is not suitable for restating the affective part of a message; the appropriate response to affect, *reflection of feeling,* is discussed in the next section.

Here are some examples of paraphrasing the cognitive part of a selected message:

Patient, a 19-year-old male student with diabetes: I'd like to make it through college and graduate with all my friends. Now I'm thinking that's not too realistic. My energy level has been pretty low. Consequently, I've had to drop two classes and I'm sleeping through study time. It gets pretty frustrating at times.

Paraphrase of cognition: With the drop in your energy level, you're aware that it may not be feasible to move through college at the same rate as your friends. **Or** It's very important to you to be able to finish college at the same time your friends do.

Patient, a 40-year-old woman: Having to get all these tests and scans done is a real pain. I don't think these tests will show anything, so what's the point? It seems like all I do in my free time anymore is come to the hospital for another test.

Paraphrase of cognition: It's hard to see the value in these tests since you don't think the results will show much. **Or** Having to take the time to have the tests done is a bother.

The following three-step sequence shows an easy way to formulate paraphrase responses. First, listen to and recall the entire patient message by restating it in your own mind. Second, identify the nonaffective parts of the message—that is, the parts of the message that describe an event, situation, thoughts, ideas, or people (cognitive). Third, select the most important part of the message for emphasis and restate this component in fresh words. Try out this three-step sequence in the following learning activity.

○

═══════════════ *LEARNING ACTIVITIES* ═══════════════

Paraphrase

Four patient messages are presented below. Read each message carefully and recall it by restating it. Identify the nonaffective parts of the message and translate these parts into your own words. You may want to try out several different paraphrase responses for each patient message (Objective 2). The first one is completed as an example. Feedback follows.

1. *A teenage girl:* You know it's hard to have much of an appetite when you're feeling the way I feel right now.

   Paraphrase: Food doesn't have much appeal to you now. **Or** You don't feel like eating that much right now.

2. *A middle-aged man:* It's hard for me to understand why I'm having so many problems with my teeth—it's pretty confusing. For years I've been taking care of them so well—brushing them, using floss—you know, the whole bit.

   Paraphrase: _____

   _____

3. *An elderly man:* I don't know why I have to have this therapy. I think it's a waste of time.

   Paraphrase: _____

   _____

4. *A young woman:* I just feel so down. I keep thinking what's the use and then I can't stop crying.

   Paraphrase: _____

   _____

Feedback

Determine if your paraphrase responses are similar to the ones presented here.

Patient 2
a. It seems like suddenly you're having a lot of unexpected teeth problems.
b. You've been taking care of your teeth for a long time.

Patient 3

a. The purpose of this therapy is unclear to you.

b. You believe this therapy won't have any useful results.

Patient 4

a. You think that nothing seems to matter.

b. You don't feel as if you have control over your crying.

Several precautions must be taken to use the paraphrase response effectively. First, it should not be overused. Its use should be confined to one of the specific purposes described above. Second, paraphrasing is most appropriate when it relates directly to the expressed goals of the interview. Jessop (1979) explains this as follows:

> When the goals relate to completion of specific concrete tasks such as teaching the client self care skills, more emphasis will probably be placed on using paraphrasing. On the other hand, discussion of implications and adjustment to chronic illness will likely necessitate increased use of reflection of feeling (p. 69).

The following section discusses the definition and use of the *reflection of feeling* response.

Reflection of Feeling

Whereas paraphrase involves rephrasing the non-affective or cognitive parts of a message, the reflection of feeling response rephrases the affective or emotional tone of the message. According to Jessop (1979), "reflection of feeling consists of verbalizing the client's *present feeling states* as they are observed in the interview" (p. 54). A reflection has more impact when it focuses on present rather than past feelings.

There are several purposes for using reflection of feeling in a patient interaction (summarized in Table 6-1). First, use of reflection can help clarify what the patient is or is not feeling about a certain situation. For example, in an initial interview a patient may talk very little and with great difficulty. The health professional may interpret this as resistance or lack of cooperation. The patient's underlying emotional tone, however, may be one of apprehension. With additional interactions, the patient's feelings may change from apprehension to calm, and the patient's ensuing behavior also changes. Reflecting the patient's feelings helps to ensure that the patient's real feelings are not misinterpreted.

A second important purpose of reflection of feeling, if it is used effectively and accurately, is to help patients feel understood. Increasingly patients look for health professionals who show not only technical competence but also interpersonal competence. Patients tend to relate best to people who understand them and to communicate most freely with people they believe will understand them. As Buggs (1975) notes, "understanding never makes feelings worse; it only gives them permission to be revealed" (p. 193).

A third important reason for using reflection is that it encourages patients to express their own feelings about a particular situation or event. Many patients will not express feelings without some encouragement for doing so. Some patients have never learned to talk about their feelings; others are fearful of the interviewer's reaction if they do so. This point is emphasized by Long and Prophit (1981) who state that "feelings are the least likely thing to be declared by the speaker and the most likely thing to be ignored by the listener" (p. 82). Although identification and expression of feelings do not have intrinsic value, this process does help to discover the ideas, attitudes, and thoughts that underlie or are attached to the feelings. In other words, encouraging patients to express feelings is not an end in itself but a means of helping patients and clinicians understand the nuances and scope of the problem.

The emotional atmosphere surrounding an illness may play a pivotal role in recovery from that illness. Recognition of the importance of this aspect of health care and provision of a proper setting to discuss the patient's emotions are important parts of effective patient/professional interactions. As Sierra-Franco (1978) states,

> Many health professionals are also becoming more and more aware that a patient's emotions are often the most important factor in his physical status. As a destructive factor, emotions may cause physical symptoms, set off a physical disease, and prevent or delay recovery. As a constructive factor, they may assist in maintaining health, speed recovery, and even help to effect so-called miraculous cures (p. 245).

Chronic anger, for example, has been found to correlate significantly with the onset of heart disease (Thoresen, Telch, & Eagleston, 1981; Williams, Haney, Lee, Hong Kong, Blumenthal, & Whalen, 1980).

Although emotional expression is not a substitute for medical treatment, negative emotions such as fear and anger can exacerbate an illness while positive emotions such as happiness, affection, calmness, and humor can diminish the effects of illness and contribute to improvement. Norman Cousins' description of his recovery from a crippling and supposedly irreversible disease (ankylosing spondylitis) in his book *Anatomy of an Illness* (1979) vividly illustrates this fact. According to Cousins (1979), "we know so little about fear, rage, frustration, the negative emotions, and how they affect the body. If negative emotions exert a downward pull, it seems inescapable that positive emotions exert an upward force . . ." (p. 1).

Reflection of feeling can assist the patient not only in identifying and expressing feelings but also in learning to manage or deal with them. Such learning is especially critical in the case of negative emotions such as dependency, anger, or fear. These emotions, if very intense, often make a patient feel helpless or unable to act on his or her own behalf (Sierra-Franco, 1978). As this author explains,

> When a patient is experiencing emotions such as anger or fear, he is generally unable or unwilling to take, or even consider, positive actions to help himself. These emotions block communication, and when they are very strong, a patient may not even be able to hear or think about any information or other evidence that you might expect to be reassuring (p. 326).

For example, a dentist may explain the process of a root canal to a new patient, or a radiologist may explain the process of radiation therapy to a cancer patient, and assume the patient "heard" and understood the explanation and will carry out instructions. However, if the patient's fear or apprehension about the ensuing procedure was very strong, he or she may not have heard a word the clinician said. Strong negative emotions may interfere with a patient's understanding of a particular procedure or treatment and can reduce confidence in a prescribed medical regimen. In such cases, using reflection to identify and deal with feelings is critical to heighten patient participation in and compliance with a prescribed treatment plan.

Reflection also can be used very effectively with a patient who expresses negative feelings about the health professional, the health care setting, or the lack of progress of treatment. Unfortunately in these instances, it is all too easy to get "trapped," to take the negative remarks personally, and to respond defensively rather than with understanding. Using reflection in the event of a disagreement with a patient "lessens the possibility of an emotional conflict, which often arises simply because two people are trying to make themselves heard and neither is trying to listen" (Long & Prophit, 1981, p. 59). In this situation the use of reflection demonstrates to patients that they have been heard, and the intensity of their emotions is usually reduced. At this point an opinion probably can be offered with more likelihood for success than before. However, as Long and Prophit (1981) note, "you should avoid giving an opinion on specific patients' feelings and confine your remarks to external matters and events" (p. 59).

Steps in Reflecting Feelings

Reflecting feelings can be a difficult skill to use, but once understood, it can be learned quickly. The first step in acquiring this skill is to learn to identify the patient's feelings or the emotional tone of a message. This process involves listening for the presence of feeling or *affect words* in the patient's messages and also by observing or "reading" the patient's nonverbal behavior and the way the message is expressed. Feelings can be positive, negative, or ambivalent. Positive feelings include happiness, love, affection, caring, humor, energy, enthusiasm, calmness, and so on. Negative emotions include fear, apprehension, tension, sadness, confusion, dependence, anger, irritation, resentment, and so on. Ambivalent feelings are expressed as two conflicting emotions; for example, a patient may feel both happy and apprehensive about discovering she is pregnant for the first time. According to Bernstein and Bernstein (1980), "in the course of interviews, and frequently within a single interview, feelings are likely to change from negative to ambivalent to positive" (p. 87). For example, a woman who discovers she is pregnant may initially express apprehension, followed by happiness. As the interview or interviews ensue, and she gains more confidence in her ability to handle her pregnancy and more information about the process, the apprehension may dissipate and be replaced by elation.

The patient's positive feelings are more likely to emerge when negative feelings have been consistently recognized and reflected, although the first expression of any positive feelings may sound highly tentative and even ambivalent (Bernstein & Bernstein, 1980, p. 87). Ambivalent or conflicting feelings may be expressed "not as a movement away from completely negative ones but as a basic problem as in a hard choice or dilemma" (Bernstein & Bernstein, 1980, p. 88). For example, a patient who has a choice of two different treatments may be both drawn to and repelled by each

choice, depending on the particular advantages and side effects of each possibility.

Generally speaking, positive, negative, and conflicting feelings fall into one of five major categories—anger (negative), fear (negative), uncertainty (negative), sadness (negative), and happiness (positive). Table 6-2 describes examples of affect words that make up these three categories. Becoming acquainted with these words will help you recognize them in patient messages; they will also serve as a vocabulary to use for rephrasing affect. After identifying the patient's emotion, determine which word best describes the feelings expressed in that message. The affect word you select should also be acceptable to the patient. As Hein (1980) notes, "many times we find that a word, such as *angry,* may be unacceptable for some patients, because to *them* it evokes feelings of violence, loss of control, or powerlessness. To be angry, therefore, is not a part of *their* behavior as *they* see it. These people may have acceptable substitutes for that feeling—words such as *annoyed, irritated, ticked off,* or *out of sorts*" (p. 60).

A second way to identify feelings is not just to listen for affect words but also to watch the patient's nonverbal behavior while he or she delivers the message. As we mentioned in the previous chapter, nonverbal behavior is often a more reliable clue to patient emotions than words because the nonverbal behaviors are less easy to control and are thus usually more accurate. Head, facial, and body movements, gestures, and voice quality give important data about a patient's underlying feelings. Some research has found that *head* cues communicate information about the *nature* of the emotion while both *head* and *body* cues provide data about the *intensity* of an emotion (Ekman & Friesen, 1967). These clues are not always easy to detect, and the meaning of nonverbal behaviors varies across cultures. Observing the patient's pattern or sudden changes in nonverbal behavior, however, can aid in developing accurate hunches about feelings. Nonverbal cues are especially important when the affect is only implied, not expressed directly by the patient. Once the affect reflected by the patient's words and nonverbal behavior has been identified, the next step involves rephrasing this affect using different or fresh words. Be careful not to use the same affect words as the patient; otherwise, "parroting" may result. The affect word(s) chosen should say no more or no less than what the patient expressed and should be at about the same level of emotional intensity. For example, if a patient says "I'm nervous," an interchangeable affect word that picks up this feeling at about the same level would be "You're feeling apprehensive (worried, concerned, tense)." However, affect words such as "afraid" or "fearful" very likely go beyond the intensity of the patient's expression and add something to the communication that was not present in the patient's expressed affect.

The third step in reflecting involves taking the selected affect word and adding it to a sentence stem that begins with the personal pronoun "you" (and also perhaps the patient's name) and words following that like "feel" or "seem." For example, the interviewer could say "Mary, you feel nervous," or "You seem nervous," or "You sound nervous." It's important to vary your sentence stem occasionally. Always saying "you feel" can detract from the effectiveness of the reflection response.

The fourth step in reflecting feelings is to tie in the situation or event to which the feelings pertain. The situation or event will be expressed in the cognitive component of the patient's message. For example, one health care provider might say:

> You feel *worried* [affect word] about being pregnant at your age [cognitive component: situation].

Or

> You seem *confused* [affect word] about all of these negative thoughts [cognitive component: situation].

Or

> You sound as if you're *down* [affect word] on yourself every time you overeat [cognitive component: situation].

A reflection can combine two or more situations as in the following example:

Table 6-2
List of Commonly Used Affect Words

Happiness	Sadness	Fear	Uncertainty	Anger
happy	discouraged	scared	puzzled	upset
pleased	disappointed	anxious	confused	frustrated
satisfied	hurt	frightened	unsure	bothered
glad	despairing	defensive	uncertain	annoyed
optimistic	depressed	threatened	skeptical	irritated
good	disillusioned	afraid	doubtful	resentful
relaxed	dismayed	tense	undecided	mad
content	pessimistic	nervous	bewildered	outraged
cheerful	miserable	uptight	mistrustful	hassled
thrilled	unhappy	uneasy	insecure	offended
delighted	hopeless	worried	bothered	angry
excited	lonely	panicked	disoriented	furious

You feel *concerned* about being pregnant at your age, having all these negative thoughts, and overeating.

What situation you reflect will depend on what part of the message you wish to emphasize in responding. In the preceding example, which mentions three concerns, the patient will probably respond to the situation she is most concerned about. In contrast, reflections that rephrase only one situation direct the patient to discuss her concern about that particular situation.

Here are some other examples of ways to phrase and respond with a reflection of feeling.

Patient, a 40-year-old man: I know both myself and my wife really want to have a child. But trying so long like this without having it happen is so discouraging. I've tried everything I know to do—have sex a lot, wear loose underwear, etc. Lately I've been thinking maybe I'm just too old.

Reflection: You sound *disappointed* about trying so long with no results.

Or

You seem to feel *pessimistic* about being able to have a child at this point.

Patient, a six-year-old girl: I can't help crying. I don't want to go to the hospital and have my tonsils out. Hospitals are for sick people and I'm not sick. Besides that, it might hurt really bad and I'm scared.

Reflection: You're *afraid* of going to the hospital.

Patient, a 40-year-old man: This clinic has got to be one of the most inefficient places I've visited. You have to sit around forever before anyone sees you. I just sit here all morning wasting my time when I could be at work.

Reflection of implied affect: You're feeling *irritated* about sitting here all morning and wasting your time. [Since there is no affect

word in the patient's message, the interviewer must rely on nonverbal cues.]

Or

You *resent* having to use valuable work time to wait for a checkup.

Patient, a 29-year-old woman: I wish I didn't get so many colds and sore throats. I've always thought I was in pretty good health overall. Most of the time I feel good—and pleased about the way my life is going. I try to take care of myself—take vitamins, eat the right foods, sleep regularly, take Geritol, etc. Still I seem to have four or five of these colds or sore throats each year—it's frustrating.

Reflection of conflicting affect: You feel *satisfied* about your overall health and lifestyle yet *bothered* by these frequent colds and sore throats. [Patient has expressed two different feelings in her message so reflection will rephrase both of these.]

The learning activity on page 118 will give you an opportunity to try out reflecting feelings.

Common Errors in Reflecting Feelings

Beginning interviewers often make the same errors in reflecting feelings. We describe a few of these problems below.

Misidentification or Mislabeling of Thoughts or Feelings

Most people have a natural tendency to respond to content, not feelings (Tyson & Kramer, 1981). Some beginning interviewers believe they are reflecting feelings when they actually have only rephrased the objective or cognitive component. This typically sounds like "You feel that." For example, the interviewer might say "You feel that you should be seen more quickly here." The way

○

┌──────────────── *LEARNING ACTIVITIES* ────────────────┐

Reflecting Feelings

In the previous learning activity you responded with paraphrase to the *content* portions of three patient messages. Your task here is to respond to the *affect* (explicit or implied) with a reflection of feeling response (Chapter Objective 3). Remember the four steps of building a good reflection. First, look for the affect word and imagine how the patient sounds and looks to identify the feelings expressed by the message. Second, rephrase the feeling using fresh words. Third, attach a sentence stem to the affect word—don't always use the same one. Finally, add the situation or events producing the feelings. Try out at least two reflections for each message. The first one is completed as an example. Feedback follows.

1. *A teenage girl:* You know it's hard to have much of an appetite when you're feeling the way I feel right now.

   Reflection of feeling: You're feeling kind of bad now. **Or** Right now you're not feeling very good.

2. *A middle-aged man:* It's hard for me to understand why I'm having so many problems with my teeth—it's pretty confusing. For years I've been taking care of them so well—brushing them, using floss—you know, the whole bit.

   Your reflections: _____

   _____

   _____

3. *An elderly man:* I don't know why I have to have this therapy. I think it is a waste of time.

   Your reflections: _____

   _____

   _____

4. *A young woman:* "I just feel so down. I keep thinking what's the use. And then I can't stop crying."

   Your reflections: _____

   _____

   _____

Feedback

Patient 2
You feel puzzled about all of these frequent problems with your teeth. **Or** You're uncertain about why all of these teeth problems have developed recently.

Patient 3
You feel annoyed about having to spend time doing this therapy. **Or** You're skeptical of this therapy.

Patient 4
You feel so depressed that it's hard to stop the tears. **Or** You're feeling very discouraged, like what really matters anyway.

---

the sentence begins is no guarantee of whether feelings are reflected. The above interviewer omitted any mention of affect in the response and rephrased only the content part of the message.

Misuse of Language and Vocabulary

The language used in reflections should be adapted to the patient and the situation. Avoid jargon, and develop a good affect word vocabulary. Many beginning interviewers tend to overuse a few of the more common affect words like *happy, anxious, frustrated,* or *angry* to describe feelings. "This limitation misses the broad range of emotions and its many nuances" (Bernstein & Bernstein, 1980, p. 89).

Longwindedness

Reflections have most impact when they are worded concisely. The longer the reflective response, the less powerful it may be in the interview. Try to say exactly what you mean and no more.

Inaccuracy or Feigning Understanding

Some beginning interviewers, for lack of practice in identifying feelings, either label the affect inaccurately or display false understanding. Reflecting a patient's feelings—but mislabeling the feeling—often has an acceptable result as long as the patient perceives the interviewer as trying to understand. Often the patient will then elaborate and describe the feelings more fully or accurately. If the health professional is very uncertain about the patient's emotional tone, it is generally better to use a clarification to "check it out" instead of a wrong reflection. "Such a response indicates an effort to be understanding, and not a failure to understand" (Bernstein & Bernstein, 1980, p. 88). These authors go on to assert that faking or feigning understanding can be detrimental. They state "one should never pretend understanding on the basis of ambiguous or minimal information. The patient may become skeptical or suspicious of 'mind reading' under the circumstances" (Bernstein & Bernstein, 1980, p. 89).

Inappropriate Timing

A major decision confronting interviewers is when to reflect feelings and when to deal with the non-affective parts of the message. At one end of the spectrum are interviewers who avoid reflecting feelings when reflection would be very appropriate. Typically out of insecurity they propose a solution or probe for more information and ignore the patient's feelings. At the other end of the spectrum are interviewers who focus too much on feelings and reflect feelings at inappropriate times. Jessop has suggested four guidelines to use in the timing of reflection (from Jessop, 1979, pp. 68–69):

1. *Phase of the patient/interviewer relationship.* Because discussion of feelings is generally considered to be more personal than content,

reflecting feelings very early in the relationship can make a patient feel uncomfortable and guarded.

2. *Patient level of readiness.* Readiness of patients can be determined by their willingness or reluctance to talk about and consider pertinent issues. Prematurely pushing a person to discuss an issue or reveal a feeling may make him or her unnecessarily defensive. "If you attempt to discuss feelings or content and are met with resistance it is generally best to refocus and try again at a later time" (Jessop, 1979, p. 68).

3. *Frequency of the skill.* Reflection should not be used to the exclusion of other interviewing responses. Overuse of it can be detrimental and can impede the progress of the interview.

4. *Goals of the interview.* Depending on the focus and nature of the interview, reflection may be functional or dysfunctional. In an interview emphasizing specific concrete tasks, the focus would be primarily on the objective or cognitive message. However, in an interview aimed at discussing a patient's reactions and adjustment to illness, a major focus on feelings would be quite appropriate.

Summarization

A summarization is a collection of several paraphrases and reflections that condenses patient messages or a series of sessions (Cormier & Cormier, 1979). Like the paraphrase and the reflection response, "summarization also rephrases what has been said or implied but does so from a much broader perspective" (Ivey & Simek-Downing, 1980, p. 75).

The summarization response can be used at various times. An interviewer can summarize several preceding minutes of an interview, an entire session, a previous interview, or even a series of interviews. Consider the following examples.

Example 1: Summarization of preceding few minutes of the interview:

I'd like to make sure I understand what you've been telling me the last few minutes. In spite of the fact that you've been eating less and exercising more, you're still gaining weight for no apparent reason, and this is very frustrating to you.

Note that this summarization combines two paraphrases *(you've been eating less and exercising more; you're still gaining weight)* and one reflection *(you're frustrated).*

Example 2: Summarization of the entire interview:

It seems that we've talked primarily today about your weight. We've discussed the possible effects your weight can have on your health, the difficulties you've had in controlling your weight, and the frustration you feel when your eating patterns control you instead of you controlling them.

Observe that this summarization has three paraphrases *(talked about weight, effects of weight on health, difficulties in controlling weight)* and one reflection *(frustration over eating patterns controlling you).*

Example 3: Summarization of a previous interview:

As you may recall, the last time we talked you felt very concerned about your weight and also somewhat out of control with respect to managing it. We discussed some options or plans for you to try out this week.

This summarization describes two reflections *(felt concerned about weight, felt out of control)* and one paraphrase *(options to try out).*

Example 4: Summarization of several preceding interviews:

I've noticed that the last four times I've talked to you, you always mention the weight issue. It seems to be something you feel concerned about, and you seem unsure as to how to manage it more effectively.

This summarization contains one paraphrase *(talked about weight issue)* and two reflections *(something you feel concerned about, feel unsure how to manage it).*

As you can see from these examples, summarization has various uses (see also Table 6-1). One purpose of summarizing is to tie together multiple elements of messages (Examples 1, 2, and 3). A second purpose is to identify a common theme or pattern that becomes apparent after a few minutes or several sessions. Topics that the patient recurrently brings up may follow certain themes. Such themes can be identified by listening to what the person repeats "over and over and with the most intensity" (Carkhuff, Pierce, & Cannon, 1977). Example 4 above depicted the use of a summary to identify a common patient theme from four previous interviews.

Another important way summarization can be used is to interrupt a patient who consistently rambles or engages in frequently "storytelling." Summarization is helpful at these points because it interrupts the rambling and provides focus to the interview. A fourth purpose of summarization is to regulate the pace of the interview, particularly to moderate the tendency to move along too quickly. As Foley and Sharf (1981) indicate, "intermittent summaries and transitions permit the patient to correct inaccuracies and add informa-

tion, and also provide some psychological breathing spaces during the course of the interview" (p. 27). A fifth purpose of a summary is to review progress that has been made during the interview(s) and to suggest areas that need to be discussed during future contacts (Hein, 1980, p. 61).

Summarization can be difficult to implement because it involves recall of messages and events over time and integration of material that is rephrased to a patient in a meaningful way. The following three-step sequence may help in mastery of this skill:

1. Recall the patient's messages over a course of one or more interviews.

2. Identify the major messages or themes during this time period.

3. Rephrase the themes or messages in similar yet different words in the form of a summary.

Try out this process in the following learning activity.

LEARNING ACTIVITIES

Summarization

In this learning activity we present four patient messages. Read each message carefully and try to recall the entire message. Identify the major parts or themes of the message, and rephrase these in the form of a summary (Chapter Objective 4). The first one is completed as an example. Feedback follows.

1. *A teenage girl:* You know it's hard to have much of an appetite when you're feeling the way I feel right now. I haven't felt this terrible before in my life.

   Summarization: Feeling lousy like you do now is something you're not accustomed to. It's certainly interfering with your appetite and maybe some other things, too.

2. *A middle-aged man:* It's hard for me to understand why I'm having so many problems with my teeth—it's pretty confusing. For years I've been taking care of them so well—brushing them, using floss—you know, the whole bit.

Your summarization: _____

_____

3. *An elderly man:* I don't know why I have to have this therapy. I think it's a waste of time.

Your summarization: _____

_____

4. *A young woman:* I just feel so down. I keep thinking what's the use. And then I can't stop crying.

Your summarization: _____

_____

Feedback

Check your summaries with the ones presented below:

Patient 2
   You're uncertain about why you're having all these problems with your teeth now, especially since you've always made an effort to take good care of them. [A summarization with one reflection—*You're uncertain*—and two paraphrases—*why you're having problems with your teeth; you've made an effort to take care of them.*]

Patient 3
   You're uncertain about what this therapy will do for you, and you resent having to spend time doing it. [A summarization with two reflections—*You're uncertain about what this therapy will do for you; you resent having to spend time doing it.*]

Patient 4
   You feel depressed and discouraged, like nothing seems to matter anymore. These thoughts and feelings make it difficult to stop crying. [A summarization with one reflection—*You feel depressed, discouraged; nothing matters*—and one paraphrase—*difficult to stop crying.*]

Chapter Summary

The four responses presented in this chapter form the foundation for understanding patient communication. *Clarification* is a tool to "clear up" any ambiguous patient messages in order to avoid misunderstanding or misinterpretation. *Para-*

phrase is used to focus on the nonaffective parts (cognitive) or patient messages. In contrast, *reflection of feeling* is used to highlight the affective or emotional tone of the message. The decision to focus on content or on affect depends on several factors, including the timing and sequence of the interview, the patient's attitudes, and perhaps most important, the goals of the interview. Chronic negative emotions, such as fear, anger, and dependency, should be clarified and discussed because of their potential role in the onset and maintenance of health and illness. *Summarization* is a collection of paraphrases or reflections and is used to link multiple messages together, to describe a theme or a pattern, to provide focus in an interview, to regulate the pace of an interaction, and to review progress. Because of the role these responses have in communicating understanding to patients, they are especially important in initial interactions with patients. The next chapter describes some responses that are particularly useful in subsequent patient interviews.

Suggested Readings _____

Bernstein, L., & Bernstein, R. *Interviewing: A guide for health professionals.* New York: Appleton-Century-Crofts, 1980. Chapter 7, "The Understanding Response," provides a useful discussion of the process of understanding patients, with particular emphasis on the reflection of feeling response.

Cormier, W. H., & Cormier, L. S. *Interviewing strategies for helpers: A guide to assessment, treatment, and evaluation.* Monterey, Calif.: Brooks/Cole, 1979. Chapter 5, "Listening Responses," describes selected listening skills such as clarification, paraphrase, reflection of feeling, and summarization.

Foley, R., & Sharf, B. The five interviewing techniques most frequently overlooked by primary care physicians. *Behavioral medicine,* 1981, 26–31. In this concise, information-packed article, these authors describe a number of useful but often overlooked interviewing techniques, such as the role of summarization to maintain control of the interview. An additional feature of the article is a "self-assessment checklist," which enables professionals to evaluate their interviewing techniques.

Hein, E.C. *Communication in nursing practice.* Boston: Little, Brown, 1980. Chapter 6, "Communication Skills in the Nursing Interview," discusses ways in which clarification, reflection, and summarization can be used effectively with patients.

Jessop, A. L. *Nurse-patient communication: A skills approach.* North Amherst, Mass.: Microtraining Associates, 1979. Section III, "Focusing the Interview," describes the skills of paraphrasing, reflecting feelings, and summarizing. The author's description of these skills is highlighted by numerous examples.

Long, L., & Prophit, Sister Penny. *Understanding/ responding: A communication manual for nurses.* Monterey, Calif.: Wadsworth, 1981. Chapter 5, "Reflective Listening," uses a series of dialogues and exercises with feedback to help the professional develop the skill of reflective listening.

Action-Oriented Responses: Questions and Confrontation

Objectives

After completing this chapter you will be able to do the following:

1. Write at least two examples of appropriate open-ended questions in response to four patient messages.

2. Write at least two examples of focused questions in response to four patient messages.

3. Given a written interviewer/patient dialogue, discriminate if the interviewer's questions are examples of open-ended, closed, focused, or laundry-list questions.

4. Write an example of a confrontation response for four patient messages.

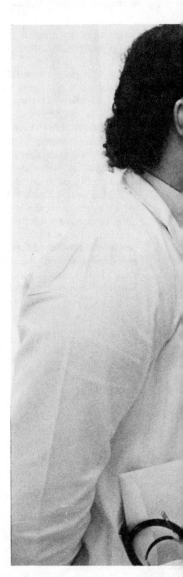

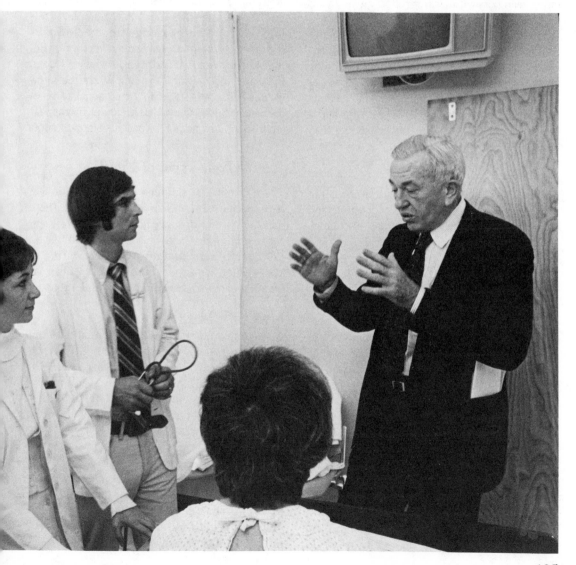

In the preceding chapters we have emphasized the importance of listening to and understanding patient communication. Listening and understanding are both important components of health care interviewing, but for the interview to have direction and for the interviewer to be able to make a diagnosis, additional interviewing techniques must be used.

This chapter describes two such techniques, known as action-oriented responses. These two responses, *questions* and *confrontation,* are active rather than passive, and they reflect a style that is more interviewer-directed than patient-directed. A primary consideration in using these action-oriented responses is *timing*—the point in the interaction when the interviewer decides to question and/or confront the patient. These two responses can be used effectively during patient interactions as long as the interviewer has first established a rapport through listening and understanding. If an interviewer probes for information or confronts a patient too quickly, the patient may become withdrawn, defensive, or otherwise noncompliant. However, once the patient has established confidence in the interviewer, the use of questions and confrontation may invite rather than discourage active patient responses.

Questions

Questions are an indispensable part of a health care interview. Interspersed effectively throughout an interview, appropriate questions encourage patient elaboration and elicit vital patient information. Lahiff (1973) regards the question as the "motor" of the interview. However, he and others are quick to point out that it is inaccurate to regard an interview as only a series of questions and answers (Lahiff, 1973; Smith & Bass, 1979). Questions are most effective when there is a specific reason for asking them and when they center on patient concerns rather than interviewer concerns. For example, suppose a new patient comes into an infertility clinic and reports that she has been trying to become pregnant for three years with no results. Appropriate questions would

include those that center directly around the expressed concerns of the patient such as "Have you ever been pregnant before?" "What is the pattern of your menstrual periods?" "How often do you typically have sexual relations?" and "What things have you tried so far in attempting to become pregnant?" Such questions reveal an immediate interest in the patient's problem and imply genuine concern on the part of the interviewer. Irrelevant questions, asked to satisfy the health professional's curiosity, to reduce the interviewer's anxiety, or to "buy time" to organize thoughts, may have a negative effect. For example, if this interviewer begins by asking "Are you divorced?" with the intention of establishing whether or not the patient is married and, if so, in a first or second marriage, the question may imply that the interviewer has some "stake" in the personal affairs of the patient. Such a question is irrelevant, may appear judgmental, and may inhibit patient communication.

Four Types of Question

There are several different types of question that have specific uses in health care interviewing. These include *open-ended questions, closed questions, focused questions,* and what Froelich and Bishop (1977) refer to as *"laundry-list" questions* (p. 24). This section describes the differences and purposes of each of these four types of questions.

Open-Ended Questions

Open-ended questions ask for information about an area of patient concern but do not direct the patient to reveal or discuss a particular issue (Hillman, et al., 1981). According to Ivey and Simek-Downing (1980), "an open-ended question must be answered with an explanation, requires discourse, and cannot easily be answered with a 'yes' or 'no' " (p. 15).

Table 7-1 summarizes the purposes of open-ended questions in a health care interview. First, open-ended questions are used to invite the patient to talk and to encourage them to explain, to elaborate, or "to tell a spontaneous story" (Hillman et al., 1981, p. 15). As such, they are very effective at the beginning of an interview ("What sorts of problems have you been having?" or "What problems bring you in here today?") and during the early stages of an interview ("What does the pain feel like?" "How have you been feeling lately?").

As Hein (1980) observes, the patient's expanded response to an open-ended question is used by the health professional to assess the importance of the event for the patient, the chronological order of events, and the patient's frame of reference for

Table 7-1
Definition and Purposes of Four Types of Question

Type of Response	Definition	Purposes in Interview
Open-ended question	A question beginning with "what," "how," "when," "where," or "who" that asks for information without specifying the content and requires more elaboration than a one-word response	1. To invite patient to talk at beginning of an interview 2. To encourage patient elaboration during early stages of an interview 3. To obtain specific examples of a patient problem 4. To inform patients of their illness and to determine the kind and amount of information they need 5. To assess type and level of vocabulary used by the patient
Closed question	A question beginning with words like "are," "do," "did," "is," or "can," which asks for a specific fact or piece of information and can be answered with one word or a short phrase	1. To obtain a specific fact or piece of information; or when a one-word answer is desired, as in "Review of Systems" in a health history 2. To narrow rather than broaden an area of discussion, as in introducing a specific area of history-taking, such as social or family history 3. To stop a patient who is rambling from overtalking
Focused question	A question often beginning with "have you," "can you," "do you," which narrows or defines the topic by asking for a specific response	1. To define a topic and request for a response in a more definitive manner than the open-ended question 2. To characterize a symptom or obtain descriptive information about a clinical sign or event
"Laundry-list" question	A question that provides the patient with a list of adjectives or descriptive phrases from which to choose	1. To obtain specific information about a symptom or illness by providing a series of choices 2. To obtain patient identification of a piece of information that has not been obtained from open-ended or focused questions

his or her observation or participation in the event (p. 43). Depending on the patient's response, the interviewer also can detect discrepancies or gaps in information provided (Hein, 1980, p. 43).

Open-ended questions may be used to obtain specific examples that shed light on a particular patient situation. For example, suppose a patient comes in and complains of "racing and pounding heart" (tachycardia). Open-ended questions such as "When was the most recent time this happened?" "Where does this typically occur?" or "What are you doing when this happens?" will encourage the patient to supply specific examples that may be useful in deciding on an eventual diagnosis and treatment regimen.

Another purpose of open-ended questions is to concentrate the patient's attention on a particular component of the message. Questions can focus on the cognitive or affective parts of a message. For example, an interviewer could use an open-ended question to seek the patient's opinion by focusing on the cognitive part of the message and asking "What do you think about these test results?" Or attention may be drawn to the patient's feelings by focusing on the affective part of the message with a question such as "How do you feel about this diagnosis?"

A fifth use of open-ended questions has been proposed by Froelich and Bishop (1977). These authors suggest the use of open-ended questions to inform patients of their illness (p. 37). Such questions as "What is your understanding of what is wrong with you?" "Our lab reports say . . . ; what do you know about this" or "What questions do you have about your illness?" can be used not only to relay a diagnosis to the patient but also to determine what information patients know and what information they need about their illness.

Another purpose of open-ended questions is to observe how the patient responds verbally and nonverbally during the information exchange. As Hein (1980) notes, "these opportunities assist us in assessing the type and level of vocabulary used by the patient as he discusses a situation, event, or idea" (p. 43).

Perhaps you have noticed from our examples that open-ended questions typically begin with the words "what," "how," "who," "when," or "where." "Why" questions are not recommended as they seem to discourage rather than to encourage patient elaboration. We will expand on this point later in the chapter when we discuss accusatory questions. The word that begins the question is important because certain words and phrases tend to elicit predictable responses. "What" questions often solicit facts and the gathering of information, whereas "how" questions are typically associated with the sequence and process of emotions (Ivey & Simek-Downing, 1980, p. 75). Similarly, "when" and "where" questions solicit information regarding time and place, and "who" questions are associated with information about people. Ivey and Simek-Downing (1980) stress the importance of using a variety of introductory words in the asking of open-ended questions. They note that interviewers frequently develop a routine of asking only one kind of open question, to the exclusion of others. Variety in wording is important because different responses illuminate different dimensions of patient problems. The final decision as to how to word questions depends on the goals and focus of the interview.

In spite of the importance of open-ended questions for obtaining patient information, it would not be realistic or feasible to use only open-ended questions during a patient interview. As Foley and Sharf (1981) point out, in addition to open-ended questions, "specific queries are needed to probe for more explicit meanings or to clarify data" (p. 27). More specific queries include closed, focused, and laundry-list questions. We discuss these in the next three sections; but first do the learning activity for open-ended questions.

Closed Questions

In contrast to open-ended questions, closed questions ask for a specific fact or particular piece of information that the interviewer needs. Closed questions typically begin with words like "are," "do," "did," "can," or "is" and can be answered

◯

┌─────────────────────── *LEARNING ACTIVITIES* ───────────────────────┐

Open-Ended Questions

Four patient messages are given below. Chapter Objective 1 asks you to write at least two open-ended questions you could use with each message. The first one is given as an example. Feedback follows.

1. *A middle-aged woman recovering from surgery:* "I've been having a lot of pain lately."

Examples: "What does the pain feel like?" "How long has this been going on?" "When do you notice the pain most?"

2. *An older man:* "I haven't been feeling very well recently so I thought I had better come in to see you."

Your open-ended questions: _____

_____

_____

3. *A young man:* "I'm worried about some sharp pains I've been having on the left side of my forehead."

Your open-ended questions: _____

_____

_____

4. *A 30-year-old mother:* "I'm very concerned about my daughter. She bruises and bleeds so easily and seems so tired much of the time. She doesn't seem to have the energy that her playmates do."

Your open-ended questions: _____

_____

_____

Feedback

The following questions are possible examples for open-ended questions to use in response to these patient messages. Your examples may be very similar or somewhat different.

Patient 2

What exactly has been bothering you?

How long have you been feeling under the weather?

What do you think might be wrong?

Patient 3

What exactly does this pain feel like?

When does the pain seem to be the worst?

How long does the pain last?

Patient 4

When did your daughter seem to develop these symptoms?

How long has this been going on?

What else have you noticed that makes you concerned about her?

---

easily with one-word responses such as "yes" or "no" or a short phrase such as "That's right," "I don't know," or some other phrase supplying the requested information. Froelich and Bishop (1977) note that closed questions usually do not add much information to what an interviewer already has, but at times "they may provide that crucial bit of information that is diagnostic" (p. 26).

There are several purposes for using a closed question deliberately in a health care interview. These are summarized in Table 7-1. Closed questions are most appropriate when either a specific bit of information or a short answer is desired. In such instances, closed questions are less time consuming. For example, as noted in Chapter 8, during the review of systems (ROS), the interviewer typically presents a rather long list to the patient and asks "Have you ever had or noticed _____?" All the interviewer really needs at this point is a one-word response—yes or no. The closed question is the most efficient way to obtain this information.

A second use of a closed question is to narrow the area of discussion (Ivey & Simek-Downing,

1980, p. 74). Open-ended questions broaden the range of discussion. In contrast, closed questions are most effective for narrowing or reducing the discussion to a particular area or topic. For example, in taking a patient's history, the interviewer may wish to focus on a specific section of the history such as social or family history. The interviewer can subtly signal or cue the shift to a new topic by using a closed question related to this particular topic—for example, by asking "Do you live alone now?" or "Are you working?" The interviewer may then decide to shift back to open-ended questions once the new area for discussion has been narrowed and defined.

A third use of a closed question is to unobtrusively stop or interrupt a patient who tends to ramble in a pointless and disorganized fashion (Ivey & Simek-Downing, 1980). For example, imagine that a patient has taken control of the interview and discussed five or six different topics for ten minutes. An open-ended question would only encourage greater patient elaboration. A closed question would prompt a short rather than a long-winded response. For example, consider the following interchange between a health professional and Mrs. Downs, a patient:

Health Professional: Mrs. Downs, you've talked now for about 15 minutes, and you've mentioned about six problem areas. I'm confused! Is your problem with your son what is bothering you the most?

Mrs. Downs: Yes, he's so disrespectful. I don't know how to handle him.

Hein (1980) recommends the use of a particular type of closed question with patients who are children, who have a limited vocabulary, or who are reticent to speak. This type of closed question is one that limits the patient's response by providing two choices such as:

Would you like to talk to me now or in 30 minutes?

Would you like to get out of bed now or in an hour?

As she observes, the implication is that the patient is expected to comply but is permitted some part in the decision. Such an approach is highly useful at bedside for patients who may not approach the required tasks for recovery with much enthusiasm (Hein, 1980).

It is important to use closed questions sparingly in an interview and only with a specific rationale in mind. Frequent use of closed questions may inhibit discussion, may allow the patient to avoid a sensitive topic, and may encourage the patient to respond too often with silence or minimal information (Ivey & Simek-Downing, 1980). With some patients there is also another danger in using too many closed questions, as Froelich and Bishop (1972) note. According to these authors, it is important to:

Remember that the interview is a professional, interpersonal interaction, and that the patient may answer the question in a way dependent more upon the immediate milieu than on the facts. When a question is asked that is answered with a "yes," you cannot be sure

what the "yes" means. Is it given to please you, to give you what the patient thinks you want to hear, to avoid discussing an area that he wants to avoid, or is it a factual response? (p. 33).

Of course, the same confusion exists with a "no" answer.

Focused Questions

Focused questions narrow or define the topic by asking for a specific response (Hillman et al., 1981). Focused questions are used when the patient is having difficulty responding to an open-ended question. They are also helpful "when trying to characterize a symptom or elicit descriptive data concerning a clinical sign or event" (Hillman et al., 1981, p. 15). Some examples of focused questions are:

Have you noticed anything that seems to make these complaints worse?

Can you describe that sensation of dizziness to me?

Can you tell me about the health history of your father's side of your family?

Do you know of any particular illnesses that tend to run in your family?

Focused questions can solicit the necessary information in an efficient manner. In contrast to open questions, focused questions define a topic and set limits on the patient's answer (Hillman et al., 1981). There is a fine line, however, between a focused and a closed question, thereby prompting a "yes" or a "no" response. For example, asking the patient questions like "Are you feeling dizzy?" or "Is your father in good health?" or "Is your family healthy?" probably will not elicit the kind of information you would be seeking with a focused question. The learning activity on page 132 gives you an opportunity to practice the use of focused questions.

Laundry-List Questions

Sometimes a patient may have difficulty responding to both open-ended and focused questions because of a lack of knowledge, vocabulary, or

LEARNING ACTIVITIES

Focused Questions

Listed below are four patient messages. For each message, write examples of at least two focused questions you could use with each patient (Chapter Objective 2). The first one is completed as an example. Feedback follows.

1. *A 16-year-old girl:* "I feel dizzy a lot of times. It seems worse after I move around suddenly."

Examples: "Can you describe the sensation of dizziness to me?" "Can you tell me what the dizziness feels like?" "Have you noticed anything else other than sudden movement that seems to make it worse?"

2. *A middle-aged secretary:* "I'm afraid I may be developing high blood pressure. I've had it up to here lately at work. I feel flushed and lightheaded a lot of the time."

Your focused questions: _____

_____

_____

3. *A 40-year-old woman:* "To tell you the truth, I'm sort of worried about getting breast cancer myself. After my mother and grandmother had it, it almost makes me feel like I'm next in line."

Your focused questions: _____

_____

_____

4. *A 45-year-old man:* "My left arm has felt numb now for some time. It's getting harder and harder to really do anything with it."

Your focused questions: _____

_____

_____

Feedback

The following examples represent possible focused questions to use in response to these patient messages. See if yours are similar.

Patient 2

Does high blood pressure or any other illness run in your family?

Can you describe your recent work situation to me?

Can you tell me more about how you feel when you are flushed and lightheaded?

Have you noticed anything else that makes you think you have high blood pressure?

Patient 3

Are you aware of any symptoms that you have which are similar to those your mother had?

Can you tell me more about the health history of your mother's side of the family?

Do you know of any illnesses other than breast cancer that tend to run in your family?

Patient 4

Can you tell me more about this numbness?

Can you describe more about the things you can't do now with your left arm?

Is there anything that seems to make the numbness better? Worse?

---

awareness to describe certain symptoms or sensations. In such cases, the interviewer can facilitate the patient's response with what Froelich and Bishop (1977) refer to as a "laundry list" question. They define a laundry-list question as one "that gives the patient a number of alternative adjectives or descriptive phrases to use" (p. 24). For example, in Chapter 8 (p. 154) the interviewer uses a laundry-list question to ask Mr. Green to describe his pain after he already had used a focused question to ask Mr. Green "to describe what the pain feels like." Because Mr. Green had difficulty responding to the focused question, the interviewer asks the following laundry-list question: "Would you say the pain is cutting, shooting, sharp,

boring, stinging, aching, burning—or none of those terms?" Mr. Green replied that the pain was both stinging and burning, information that was vital to the health professional's eventual diagnosis.

With laundry-list questions, it is important not to provide any verbal or nonverbal clue about what answer is expected. Froelich and Bishop (1977) point out that one way to avoid suggesting the answer is "to scramble the logical sequence of items" (p. 25). Another way that the interviewer in the above example did not bias Mr. Green's response was to give the patient an "out." If the interviewer's words did not describe the pain accurately, the patient could say "None of those terms" or "It is more like _____." Laundry-list questions are not used as frequently in health care interviewing as open, focused, or closed questions. However, occasionally an opportunity arises when the laundry-list question is the most efficient and effective way to obtain the desired information from a patient who otherwise may have difficulty identifying the precise data needed.

Regardless of the type of question used, it is important to allow sufficient time for the patient to respond. Patients should not feel coerced or pressured into answering questions before they are ready to do so. As Hein (1980) notes, the feeling of having to supply an answer can be threatening to patients and either inhibit their responses or force them to make up answers that please the interviewer (p. 43).

Guidelines for Wording Questions

Regardless of the type of question asked, the interviewer should phrase each question carefully. Wording of questions can be very important. Inaccurate or incomplete patient information may result from poor wording. There are several basic guidelines to follow regarding appropriate wording of questions, as summarized in Table 7-2. First, avoid jargon and medical terminology. Adapt the language to each patient so that the patient has no problem understanding the question. Second, keep each question brief and concise. Long questions

Table 7-2
Guidelines for Wording Questions

1. Phrase questions simply—avoid medical jargon.
2. Phrase questions concisely—avoid long-windedness.
3. Ask only one question at a time—avoid "stacking" questions.
4. Phrase questions in a nonaccusatory way, using "what" or "how." Avoid "why" questions.
5. Phrase questions so they do not suggest or influence patient answers. Avoid parenthetical phrases or sequences of words that suggest a particular symptom, illness, or diagnosis.

are confusing, and patients may be uncertain about what information the interviewer is actually requesting.

Another important guideline is to ask only one question at a time. Although this may sound simple, in actual practice it is difficult to do. It is especially troublesome for beginning interviewers who, in their desire to obtain all the proper information, may overload the patient with two or more questions simultaneously. Asking more than one question at a time has been referred to as using multiple or compound questions (Hillman et al., 1981) or double-barreled questions (Bernstein & Bernstein, 1980). We use the term *stacking questions* here. The interviewer presents two or three questions at a time without allowing the patient time to respond. Stacked questions can be very frustrating or annoying, because often patients are not sure which questions they should answer. As an example of stacking questions, the interviewer might say "How are you feeling today?" "I mean, are you feeling better?" or "Are you still in pain?" It would have been much more productive just to ask the open-ended question "How are you feeling today?" and then pause and let the patient reply.

A fourth guideline to follow is to avoid the use of "why" questions. Questions that begin with the word "why" such as "Why aren't you taking your medicine?" or "Why aren't you eating?" sound accusatory or antagonistic. Such questions may imply to patients that they are being asked to justify or account for their behavior. Some patients may not know "why." Others may know but prefer not to discuss the reasons, causes, or motives. The primary disadvantage of "why" questions is the tendency to make patients defensive. In most instances the same information can be obtained with a "what" or a "how" question, and overtones of antagonism or accusation can be avoided.

The fifth guideline is to be alert for any wording of questions that may bias or influence the patient's response. Questions that seem to suggest or influence the patient's response are called "suggestive questions" (Hillman et al., 1981, p. 15), "leading questions" (Hein, 1980, p. 47), or "loaded questions" (Bernstein & Bernstein, 1980, p. 77). Such questions suggest or imply an expected response or make it more likely for a patient to give one answer instead of another. Try to phrase questions so that they do not prejudice the patient's answer. In addition, interviewers should avoid suggesting an expected response by their demeanor, tone of voice, or other nonverbal behavior (Enelow & Swisher, 1979, p. 64).

There are two common wording errors associated with suggestive or loaded questions. The first involves the use of a parenthetical phrase at the end of the question. Notice the unwritten or implied message in the following dialogue between a woman at her first prenatal visit and her obstetrician as the social history is being obtained.

Obstetrician: You don't smoke, do you?

Patient: No, I don't!

It is apparent that the obstetrician has a predetermined "right" answer for the question. Many patients could easily be intimidated by the question into giving such a response and, in doing so, be less than truthful (Bernstein & Bernstein, 1980).

A second error involving suggestive or loaded questions is the question that, because of its wording, seems to suggest a pattern, diagnosis, or illness to a patient. For example, suppose a health professional says to a patient "As I recall, your mother died of cancer of the ovary. Didn't she have an abdominal pain very similar to the one that you describe?" This question may suggest two things to the patient—first, that the interviewer expects her to confirm that the pain she is having is similar to her mother's, and second, that there is a link between her pain and ovarian cancer. Immediately the patient may jump to conclusions about a diagnosis or treatment regimen that may or may not eventually be accurate or necessary. A more effectively worded question would be a straightforward open-ended one—"How would you describe this sensation of pain?"—or a focused one—"Tell me about illnesses or surgery on your mother's side of the family."

Bernstein and Bernstein (1980) observe that the effects of suggestive questions can be especially serious in a health care setting. They note that if a patient gives an unexpected but inaccurate response, this "can then lead to a misunderstanding of the complaints and consequent diagnostic errors" (Bernstein & Bernstein, 1980, p. 78). They point out that this process can interfere with the development of an effective patient/interviewer relationship. As they suggest, "the patient may feel that he has been inadvertently 'trapped' into giving incorrect answers and, aware of the serious results of misinformation, feel guilty, concerned, and angry" (p. 78).

Sequence of Questions in a Health Care Interview

Every health care interview has at least two purposes. One is to allow the patient to present and explain concerns; the other is to provide focus, direction, or structure to the process. Encouraging patients to talk is especially critical in initial interactions or in the first phase of the health history interview. Later in the history interview or in subsequent interactions the interviewer is concerned more with discovering specific details. This process is best accomplished by a sequence of questions that begins initially with general, broad open-ended questions, followed by more specific and detailed questions such as closed or focused questions. Bernstein and Bernstein (1980) refer to this sequence in questioning as "narrowing" (p. 77).

Initial questions can be general, designed to encourage patients to identify their immediate health concerns and to encourage them to speak as freely as possible (Enelow & Adler, 1979; Engel & Morgan, 1973). The purpose of general questions is to open rather than limit the topics of discussion. Then, by building on the material the patient provides, the interviewer can follow up general questions with more specific and detailed questions until the topic is clear and the necessary information obtained. At this stage, it is still important to utilize questions that follow or are on the same track as the patient's messages. As Engel and

◯

================= *LEARNING ACTIVITIES* =================

Types of Question

In this learning activity, a brief health professional/patient dialogue is presented. According to Chapter Objective 3, you are to decide whether each of the interviewer's responses is an example of an open-ended question, a closed question, a focused question, a laundry-list question, or some other response. Indicate your answer by placing a check in one of the five blanks provided. The first one is completed as an example. Answers follow the learning activity.

1. *Health Professional:* What brings you here today, Mrs. Strong?

   __✓__ Open _____ Closed _____ Focused _____ Laundry List
   _____ Other
   Patient: Well, I thought maybe I needed a general check-up.

2. *Health Professional:* OK, I see. Well, how have you been feeling recently?

   _____ Open _____ Closed _____ Focused _____ Laundry list
   _____ Other
   Patient: Not too bad, I guess. Sometimes kind of run down, though.

3. *Health Professional:* What do you mean by 'run down'?

   _____ Open _____ Closed _____ Focused _____ Laundry list
   _____ Other
   Patient: Well, like I just sort of go along and all of a sudden, I don't have any energy and I feel like I need to sit or lie down for a while.

4. *Health Professional:* So once in a while your energy seems to run out on you?

   _____ Open _____ Closed _____ Focused _____ Laundry list
   _____ Other
   Patient: Umm-hmm, that's right.

5. *Health Professional:* How long has this been going on?

   _____ Open _____ Closed _____ Focused _____ Laundry list
   _____ Other
   Patient: Well, for about the last six or seven months, I think.

6. *Health Professional:* Have you noticed anything else that concerns you about your health other than this fatigue and lack of energy?

   _____ Open _____ Closed _____ Focused _____ Laundry list
   _____ Other
   Patient: Not really. Well, sometimes I have trouble sleeping, and I guess that doesn't help the fatigue.

7. *Health Professional:* Anything else you can think of you'd like to bring up or discuss?

    _____ Open   _____ Closed   _____ Focused   _____ Laundry list
    _____ Other

    Patient: No, not right now. It's mainly the fatigue and not always sleeping well.

8. *Health Professional:* OK, let me ask you a few things about your sleeping patterns. How often do you have trouble sleeping—on the average— say, in a given week?

    _____ Open   _____ Closed   _____ Focused   _____ Laundry list
    _____ Other

    Patient: Oh, probably about three nights a week.

9. *Health Professional:* What sorts of sleeping difficulties do you have on these nights?

    _____ Open   _____ Closed   _____ Focused   _____ Laundry list
    _____ Other

    Patient: Well, it's mainly that I just can't get to sleep—it seems like it takes forever.

10. *Health Professional:* Do you have more trouble sleeping on certain nights?

    _____ Open   _____ Closed   _____ Focused   _____ Laundry list
    _____ Other

    Patient: No, not really.

11. *Health Professional:* Do you always sleep in the same place?

    _____ Open   _____ Closed   _____ Focused   _____ Laundry list
    _____ Other

    Patient: Yes.

12. *Health Professional:* And do you have a certain routine you follow before bed?

    _____ Open   _____ Closed   _____ Focused   _____ Laundry list
    _____ Other

    Patient: Yes, I do.

13. *Health Professional:* Could you describe that routine to me?

    _____ Open   _____ Closed   _____ Focused   _____ Laundry list
    _____ Other

Feedback

2. Open-ended	6. Focused	10. Closed
3. Open-ended	7. Focused	11. Closed
4. Other (paraphrase)	8. Open-ended	12. Closed
5. Open-ended	9. Open-ended	13. Focused

Morgan (1973) note, the interviewer who follows the lead of the patient "avoids the disruption of the patient's train of thought and important associations emerge naturally under such conditions" (p. 39). Questions that follow the patient's thinking are another indication of the interviewer's overall attentiveness. The process of narrowing is illustrated in the dialogue in the learning activity on pages 136–137.

Confrontation

A confrontation is a verbal response in which the interviewer describes a discrepancy or contradiction in patients' words and behavior or directs patients' attention to something they may not be aware of (Cormier & Cormier, 1979; Enelow & Adler, 1979). As Ivey and Gluckstern (1976) note, "in a confrontation individuals are faced directly with the fact that they may be saying other than that which they mean, or doing other than that which they say" (p. 46). It is easy to misconstrue the actual purpose of a confrontation because of the typical meanings associated with the word "confront." In a helping interaction, confrontation does not mean a punitive act or an attack on someone for his or her own good. It does not mean telling patients they are wrong or are bad people (Ivey & Simek-Downing, 1980, p. 102). Rather, it is a description of present behavior or communication as perceived by the interviewer. Confrontations are based on what the interviewer has observed about the patient rather than on inferences about the patient's motives or emotional state (Enelow & Adler, 1979, p. 49).

The primary purpose of confrontation is to identify discrepant or distorted messages or areas of communication. In an interview, a patient expresses a variety of verbal and nonverbal messages. There are four common types of mixed messages that patients express (Cormier & Cormier, 1979): (1) discrepancies between words (verbal statements) and actions; (2) discrepancies between two verbal messages (stated inconsistencies); (3) discrepancies between words (verbal statements) and nonverbal behaviors; and (4) dis-

crepancies between two nonverbal messages (apparent inconsistencies). For example, frequently patients are unaware that they are talking about the importance of maintaining their health yet are actually inviting illness because of constant unhealthful behaviors. A woman who states emphatically "Good health is extremely important to me," yet shows evidence of being overweight, chain smoking, and leading a sedentary life may not realize the apparent discrepancy between her words and actions or she may be unsure of the relationship among obesity, smoking, lack of exercise, and particular kinds of health problems. A confrontation might sound something like: "You've said that you place a lot of value on your health although you've also indicated you smoke heavily, don't exercise, and need to lose weight. Do you see any problem or contradiction in this situation?"

A confrontation helps the patient see the discrepancy, and through the interviewer's careful choice of words and supporting nonverbal cues, it is conveyed to the patient in a noncritical manner. One way to hear the inconsistency expressed in two verbal messages (stated or expressed inconsistencies) is to listen to the conjunction the patient uses to connect two or more ideas. Consistent or congruent messages typically are connected with the word "and," whereas mixed or incongruent messages often are connected with words like "but," "however," or "although." Noting the consistency (or inconsistency) of patient messages can be important because mixed messages often reveal conflicting feelings or inaccurate or distorted information.

There are two types of mixed message associated with nonverbal behavior: (1) verbal and nonverbal behavior; and (2) two nonverbal messages with apparent distortions or inconsistencies. For example, a patient may say "I want to have my tubes tied," but while she is saying this, she is staring at the floor, squirming in her seat, and speaking in a barely audible voice tone. These nonverbal behaviors are inconsistent with her verbal message. In these instances, the nonverbal message is usually the more representative one "... because it is less likely to be masked or controlled" (Long & Prophit, 1981, p. 33). Another patient may state that his forthcoming operation does not worry him; as he says this he smiles (nonverbal message one) and his hands tremble (nonverbal message two) at the same time. These two nonverbal behaviors are inconsistent with each other.

In a confrontation for mixed messages it is often helpful to describe both parts of the discrepancy. For example, a patient may say "I feel very comfortable talking to you" yet be very silent, withdrawn, and fidgety. The confrontation would be worded like this: "You say you feel comfortable [one part of discrepancy] yet it also seems hard for you to talk about this" [second part of the discrepancy]. After hearing both parts of the contradiction, patients can note the discrepancy and examine their rationale for the contradictory behavior. Patients who are totally ignorant of their incongruent behavior will gain new knowledge by simple follow-up on the segments of the confrontation.

A second use of confrontation is with patients who present distorted or inaccurate perceptions or information. For instance, perhaps a pregnant woman has revealed having inaccurate information about the effects of smoking on the fetus. According to Egan (1975), "people who cannot face things as they are tend to distort them" (p. 160). This patient may naively assume that smoking during pregnancy has little or no effect on the developing child. In this instance, a confrontation could be used to describe the apparent distortion or misinformation. One interviewer might say something like:

> From your comments I have the impression you believe that smoking is a safe thing to do during pregnancy. I feel uncomfortable hearing this because I have seen some of the effects the mother's frequent smoking has had on infants. Did you know that smoking is associated with babies of low birth weight?

An interviewer can confront a patient's distorted messages by (1) describing them and by (2) indicating alternative ways to view or handle the situation (Cormier & Cormier, 1979, p. 82). For example, suppose a patient states:

> Sure, I'd like to have 10 or 15 more good years. But what is the point in even thinking about a possible cure—or even a remission? I might as well just think I'm going to die very soon.

The interviewer might respond with a confrontation in the following way:

> It seems important to you to be able to live as long as possible, yet you seem to already have given up on yourself and the treatment [description of patient's present view of situation]. Perhaps believing in the treatment and your body's ability to heal itself would be one way to extend your life a little longer [alternative way to view the situation].

Guidelines for Confronting

Confrontation is hardly ever a neutral response; it typically evokes some reaction from a patient. It is important therefore to use confrontation with some specific guidelines in mind. The guidelines presented here are adapted from Egan (1975), Johnson (1981), and Cormier and Cormier (1979) and are summarized in Table 7-3. The decision to use confrontation must consider the patient's present ability to handle the confrontation. Confrontations are probably inappropriate when a patient is confused or highly anxious. The use of confrontation also depends on the degree of rapport that exists between the health care provider and the patient. If little rapport exists, confrontation is not advisable. Once the interviewer has decided that the timing is appropriate, the confrontation should be made with care, with empathy, and with the proper motivation (Egan, 1975, p. 165).

The interviewer's primary aim in using confrontation should be to help the patient, not to flaunt authority, to punish, to get even, or to put the patient in his or her place. Only on very rare occasions should confrontation be used to express the interviewer's own frustration about or toward a patient. In these situations the interviewer's irritation with the patient's behavior may be the cue that suggests the need for confrontation (Enelow & Adler, 1979, p. 51). Or the presence of persistent negative feelings on the part of the interviewer toward the patient may prompt such a confrontation. The following example of one health professional's confrontation may clarify this principle.

> Mr. Franklin, I'm having trouble in controlling feelings of irritation while discussing your problems with you. You have telephoned me now three nights in a row after midnight, you have asked my opinion on what you should do to reconcile your differences with your wife, and now you are upset because I cannot extend our interview today to discuss these problems further. Furthermore, you have indicated you have made no effort to reduce your salt intake and have not been taking your medicines for blood pressure! I'm confused. You continue to seek my advice about your health, yet you don't follow my suggestions. It seems to me that you would prefer a nurse or physician whose suggestions you are willing to follow. Right now we're wasting your money and my time. I wonder if you would not be more satisfied by finding another physician or nurse?

Mr. Franklin has apparently been overbearing, inconsiderate, and noncompliant. In circumstances where good rapport has been established, such a confrontation may be very therapeutic for a manipulative patient. Health professionals can "put all their cards on the table," tell patients that their manipulations are counterproductive to the professional/patient relationship, and indicate that unless changes occur, it is useless to continue. Once this strategy is in effect, patients either tend to agree that their actions are not therapeutic and will strive to change or transfer blame for the failure to the professional and seek care elsewhere. Either outcome, if sought judiciously, may have a therapeutic effect—either by encouraging change in the patient's approach to his or her own health or by finding another health professional who may serve the patient more effectively.

A confrontation should be descriptive rather than evaluative and concrete rather than vague. Specific discrepancies or distortions should be mentioned and vague or ambiguous inferences avoided (Cormier & Cormier, 1979). The confrontation also should focus on behaviors the patient can do something to change. In the following dia-

Table 7-3
Confrontation: Guidelines for Use and Patient Reactions

Definition	Guidelines	Patient Reactions
Confrontation—a verbal response used to describe and identify a discrepancy or distortion apparent in a patient's communication	1. Offer with care and with empathy and to help, not to punish, the patient. 2. Be descriptive rather than evaluative and concrete rather than vague. 3. Direct the confrontation toward situations and behaviors that the patient can change. 4. Deliver confrontation in "small doses;" avoid two successive confrontations. 5. Word the confrontation tentatively. Request but do not demand change. 6. Confront only when there is sufficient time to hear and understand the other person's reactions to the situation.	1. Denial and anger 2. Confusion 3. False acceptance 4. Real acceptance

logue, a dietitian is speaking with the unemployed mother of eight children.

Dietitian: Today makes the third time that we have discussed the use of all the food groups in a healthy diet. But when I look at the diet diaries you have kept, I notice that you continue to feed the children three or four meals a week consisting of starches—beans, cornbread, and spaghetti. I'm hoping we can find a way for you to include more meats, fruits, and vegetables in their diets.

Patient: I am sorry that I don't give the kids more variety in their meals. But since I only have an income of $285.00 a month, there's not much money left for other kinds of foods.

In this situation, the problem lies not in the unwillingness of the patient to change her dietary habits but rather in her inability to change because of her income. A successful outcome under these circumstances is beyond the patient's control. It is pointless and demeaning to confront behaviors or situations that the patient cannot change.

Confrontation should be delivered in "small doses." According to Enelow and Adler (1979), two successive confrontations in one interview about the same or related observations may be too overwhelming and should be avoided. Confrontation threatens the basic professional/patient relationship; since it is based on the interviewer's perception of the patient, the patient may construe it as judgmental. The professional is attempting to induce patients to see or hear their incongruent words or actions. Confronters strive to enable confrontees to see themselves as others see them, and too much introspection may overwhelm the patient. Consequently, when confrontation has been used, time should be allowed to recement the rapport that may have been strained so that the professional relationship will not be jeopardized.

Confrontations should be presented tentatively by the use of word or voice cues that suggest questions, provide the patient with the opportu-

nity to disagree, and convey general support and genuine understanding. In using confrontation, an interviewer may *request* but should never *demand* changes from the other person (Johnson, 1981). A common management technique for dealing with situations requiring a confrontation is to point out positive aspects of a relationship or treatment program and reserve the confrontation until last. This tactic enables the patient to see the positive aspects of the interaction and to retain these during the ensuing confrontation. Further, it is well established that subjects first covered in an interview or teaching session are best remembered, followed by subjects that are discussed later. Such a format provides the confrontee with a positive self-image that carries over through the confrontation so that rapport is not lost.

Finally, confront only when there is sufficient time available to discuss the conflict and situation jointly. It is unfair for the patient to be confronted by a "hit and run" interviewer who gives her or his views about the situation and then disappears or leaves before the patient can respond (Johnson, 1981, p. 231). Schedule sufficient time for the patient to share his or her reactions to the confrontation.

Patient Reactions to Confrontation

Although the interviewer may make a very effective confrontation, patients' reactions may vary greatly. Interviewers can be better prepared to handle the effects of confrontation by anticipating possible patient reactions. Typically, a patient may respond to a confrontation in one of four ways: denial, confusion, false acceptance, or real acceptance (Cormier & Cormier, 1979). A patient who does not want to acknowledge or agree to the interviewer's perceptions may deny the confrontation. Egan (1975) describes four ways a person may deny a confrontation.

1. Discredit the interviewer ("How do you know—have you ever had this illness yourself?").

2. Persuade the interviewer that he or she misinterpreted the patient ("I didn't really say that; you didn't hear exactly what I said.").

3. Diminish the importance of the topic or the situation ("This isn't worth discussing now; let's go on to something more important.").

4. Seek support from other sources ("No one in my family has ever noticed it.").

Patients who deny the substance of a confrontation may also respond with anger toward the interviewer. The anger tends to impugn or malign the interviewer and rarely has any connection with the problem under consideration, as in the following dialogue.

Health Professional: John, over the past two years we have discussed your weight problem on numerous occasions. You've indicated that it is important to you to lose weight. Nevertheless, you still are not exercising at all, and you continue to consume large amounts of alcoholic beverages. All of these things continue to aggravate your weight problem.

John: Well, who the heck do you think you are? If I want to stay at this weight, that's my business. Also, if *I* want to drink a few beers, what's that to you? You health nuts are all the same! Just because you run five miles a day, you think everybody should. Well, I think that's for the birds. And besides, you don't really care what happens to me, you just want to collect my money every time I come in here!

Health Professional: Well, I guess I can understand some of the frustration you must feel at trying to lose weight. It is very difficult because you are really trying to change a habit pattern that you have followed for many years. Nevertheless, if you will recall, you did come to see me the first time asking me to help you lose weight. So, I have been working on the assumption that you still want to take off some pounds. Am I mistaken?

John: No, you're right. I'm sorry. I just get so upset with all this weight. But I can't seem to walk past the refrigerator without getting something to eat, and I can't stop having a few drinks with the guys every night after work.

Certainly the interviewer is tempted to respond to John's unreasonable accusations in similar fashion. A good rule to remember under such circumstances is the old maxim "Count to ten." Then proceed, perhaps after a short silence, by ignoring the derogatory personal references and concentrating on the problem that prompted the outburst. Once again, if good rapport exists between patient and professional, the angry intrusion should pass quickly and the interview can proceed.

Some patients may appear to be genuinely puzzled or confused by the content of a confrontation. If the patient is genuinely uncertain about the meaning of confrontation, the wording may have been vague, unclear, or couched in jargon, or the patient may be honestly ignorant of the material being presented. Consider the following dialogue.

Health Professional: Ever since I saw your baby when he was six months old I have been encouraging you to have a sweat chloride test done on your baby to see if he has cystic fibrosis. Now he is sick again, and I find out from his chart that the test has never been done. You've said it is very important to you to have a healthy baby, yet you haven't made arrangements for this rather simple test.

Patient: Zachary has been sickly ever since he was about two weeks old. I just can't stand to put him through any more painful tests. Besides, a test on sweat glands sounds like quackery to me. I just don't see any reason for it.

The resolution of this confrontation should be immediately apparent. The health professional must spend time educating the patient. Informed and educated patients are more likely to comply with instructions and to utilize a confrontation effectively.

On occasion it may be difficult to ascertain whether or not a patient is genuinely ignorant or is feigning ignorance and confusion to avoid responding to a confrontation. Under such circumstances further inquiry will usually reveal the degree of ignorance, and the interview can proceed.

Some patients may respond to confrontation with what seems to be acceptance. The interviewer must decide whether the acceptance is genuine or feigned. If the patient acknowledges the confrontation and seems ready to deal with it, he or she may genuinely accept the intent of the confrontation. However, if the patient seems to agree only to distract the interviewer with another topic, this is probably false acceptance. Once again, further questioning will expose the ruse.

There is no one "right" way of dealing with patient reactions to confrontation. However, some of the understanding responses presented in Chapter 6 may be very helpful. Paraphrase and reflection of feeling are effective ways of dealing with a patient's denial, anger, or confusion following a confrontation. For example, the interaction may go like this:

Interviewer: You're saying that it's very important to you to lose weight, but you've also indicated you have not been exercising or following the diet plan we agreed to. Do you see any problem or contradiction? [confrontation]

Patient: What do you mean? I'm not sure what you're saying. [denial, confusion]

Interviewer: You're feeling uncertain about what I said—and perhaps upset also. [reflection of feeling]

Whatever the response, it is important to allow the patient to express his or her reactions and to take time to understand the patient's feelings about the situation (Johnson, 1981).

Confrontation with Families and Colleagues

Because confrontations are a form of feedback, they are particularly useful in certain interactions with families of patients and with colleagues. For example, suppose the family of a patient recovering from abdominal surgery continually tries to defy the patient's prescribed diet by bringing in hamburgers and french fries for the patient. The health professional could effectively confront this behavior in a tactful and descriptive manner by saying something like the following:

> I know from talking with you how eager you are to have your father recover speedily from surgery. I'm also aware you've been bringing him things to eat that really aren't in his best interest at this time. Perhaps you aren't aware of how much these kinds of foods could interfere with his recovery.

In another situation, a health professional may have a colleague or a subordinate who talks a great deal about good patient care yet fails to demonstrate any real commitment to patients. Perhaps the colleague is repeatedly late to work, refuses to carry his or her share of the workload, hesitates to respond to patient calls, or fills out records and charts improperly. If such actions continue without apparent notice, patient care is affected and other members of the health care team are likely to feel increasingly annoyed. As Johnson (1981) observes, if an interpersonal conflict is to be resolved, a confrontation will be necessary. A supervisor could confront this team member by saying something like this:

> Jack, I know you're always talking about how important it is for you to work directly with patients and how much you believe in giving good patient care. Yet I've noticed that you continue to get behind in filling out your charts and when you do catch up and complete them, sometimes rather important items like medication dosage are omitted. Perhaps you haven't realized how much this also can be a critical part of overall patient care.

In confrontation with families or colleagues, it is also important to be descriptive and supportive rather than punitive. If it seems important to express your feelings of anger as part of the con-

LEARNING ACTIVITIES

Confrontation

In this learning activity, we present four examples of patient communication. Your task is to write an example of a confrontation response for each patient message (Chapter Objective 4). The first one is completed as an example. Feedback follows.

1. *A hospitalized 45-year-old woman:* Who said anything about being upset with this hospital? [in a loud, shrill voice]

Confrontation: Mrs. Johns, perhaps it is difficult to talk about your feelings concerning the hospital. I know you said you hadn't mentioned feeling upset, yet I realize you were speaking in an upset tone of voice.

2. *A young child:* I feel very, very upset about this [while smiling broadly]

Your confrontation: _____

_____

3. *A 60-year-old man:* This high blood pressure is really annoying to me—can't you fix it up quickly? [while reporting he occasionally forgets to take the prescribed medication]

Your confrontation: _____

_____

4. *A young woman:* Of course I want to lose weight. I would feel and look so much better. But when you've been fat since you were a little child like I've been, it's a hopeless battle.

Your confrontation: _____

_____

Feedback

Patient 2

You've just said you feel so upset about this, and I noticed as you spoke that there was a big smile on your face.

Patient 3

[confrontation for a discrepant message] On one hand you're indicating you want to get your blood pressure under control as soon as possible, yet you've already said that you occasionally forget to take the medicine that will help you do that.

Or

[confrontation for distorted message] You seem to want us to be responsible for managing your high blood pressure, yet we can't always be around to remind you what to do, like taking your pills. Perhaps if you put yourself more in charge of this problem you would find it getting under control more quickly.

Patient 4

You've said that you want to lose weight but also that it seems hopeless—like you've already given up. Is that right?

---

frontation, remember to "focus your anger on issues and conditions that can be changed with reasonable amounts of effort and time, not on the other person" (Johnson, 1981, p. 232). In addition to expressing anger, also remember to express your commitment to the relationship and to resolution of the conflict. Remember that an effective confrontation is intended to help another person examine the consequences of his or her behavior, not to make that person defensive. Also, be alert and receptive to the reactions of the other party, which probably will be very similar to the patient reactions we discussed previously.

Chapter Summary

This chapter has discussed the role of two action-oriented responses in health care interviewing. *Questions* are a critical part of interviews. They encourage patient explanations, and they help obtain important patient information. Health care interviewers use four types of question: *open-ended, closed, focused,* and *"laundry-list" questions.* The sequence of questions in a typical health care interview begins with open-ended, general questions, and proceeds to more specific questions such as the closed, focused, and laundry-list. This process of moving from general to specific questions is called *narrowing.* In order to be most effective, questions should use simple, understandable language, should be concise, and should not be accusatory or suggestive.

A *confrontation* is important for describing a discrepancy or distortion in the patient's communication. An effective confrontation is descriptive, specific, tentative, and offered gradually or in "small doses." Patient reactions to confrontations can vary from denial, anger, and confusion to feigned or genuine acceptance of the impact of the confrontation. A general rule of thumb for responding to patient reactions is to use the understanding responses, such as paraphrasing and reflecting.

These action-oriented responses are an indispensable part of health care interviewing because they elicit information from and encourage actions by the patient. The effectiveness of these skills varies with the degree of concern and the good judgment of the interviewer. These responses should be made with care and empathy and should be grounded in good rapport.

Suggested Readings _____

Bernstein, L., & Bernstein, R. *Interviewing: A guide for health professionals*. New York: Appleton-Century-Crofts, 1980. Chapter 6, "The Probing Response," discusses the use of a variety of questions in a medical interview.

Cormier, W. H., & Cormier, L. S. *Interviewing strategies for helpers: A guide to assessment, treatment, and evaluation*. Monterey, Calif.: Brooks/Cole, 1979. Chapter 6, "Action Responses," discusses the purposes and guidelines for using open-ended questions and confrontation in an interview setting.

Egan, G. *The skilled helper: A model for systematic helping and interpersonal relating*. Monterey, Calif.: Brooks/Cole, 1975. Chapter 5, "Integrative Understanding/Dynamic Self-Understanding," has an excellent discussion of the ways in which confrontation can be used effectively in a helping interaction.

Enelow, A. J., & Swisher, S. N. (Eds.). *Interviewing and patient care*. New York: Oxford University Press, 1979. Chapter 3, "Basic Interviewing" (contributed by Enelow & Adler), and Chapter 4, "Obtaining Additional Specific Information," discuss the role of questions in medical interviewing.

Froelich, R., Bishop, F., & Dworkin, S. *Communication in the dental office*. St. Louis: Mosby, 1976. Chapter 6, "Obtaining Specific Information," describes the role of probing, closed, and laundry-list questions in an interview setting.

Johnson, D. W. *Reaching out: Interpersonal effectiveness and self-actualization*. Englewood Cliffs, N.J.: Prentice-Hall, 1981. Chapter 11, "Confrontation and Negotiation," presents an excellent discussion of the role of confrontation in negotiating and resolving interpersonal conflicts.

Obtaining a Health History_____

Objectives

After completing this chapter, you will be able to do the following:

1. Using the mnemonic PAST MED and a telegraphic style of writing, write the patient's past medical history based on a patient/interviewer dialogue.

2. Given a patient interview dialogue, record the patient's family history in telegraphic style and with a genetic diagram.

3. Using the mnemonic MOLEST and telegraphic style, write the patient's social history based on a patient/interviewer dialogue.

4. Given a patient/interviewer dialogue, record a portion of the patient's review of systems using telegraphic style.

5. Using the mnemonic P^2QRST and a narrative style of writing, be able to write the patient's history of present illness based on a patient/interviewer dialogue.

6. Given a hypothetical patient description, conduct a 30-minute role-play health history interview with a classmate and then record and assess the results using the format given in the Guide for the Health History (p. 180.)

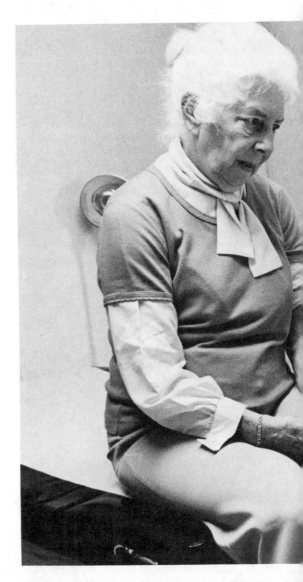

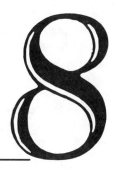

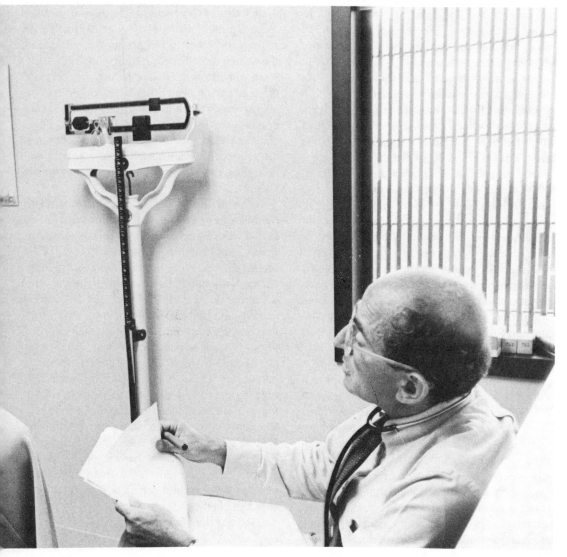

Regardless of the area of specialization or the type and degree of training of the health professional, the obtaining of a health history requires extraordinary communication with the patient. Rarely does the patient present to the health professional without some degree of illness, discomfort, or personal anxiety that tends to obfuscate the finest efforts at communication. Add to such feelings a tendency to deny personal illness, a lack of objectivity about one's personal shortcomings, anger with health professionals because their services are required, and fear of the unknown compounded by medical terminology and jargon, and it is not difficult to understand why encounters between patients and health professionals are frequently unsatisfactory for both parties.

"The most frequent and serious errors [in eliciting a medical history] arise from a lack of a system rather than from failure to detect, or interpret correctly some [historical or physical] finding, which has been sought" (Sleeth, 1975, p. 1). It is essential for health professionals to develop a systematic approach to assessment that they plan to follow throughout their professional career. The quality of care rendered to patients and the continued professional growth of the practitioner will vary directly with the use of a systematic approach.

There are several reasons for following a systematic line of inquiry during the assessment and history interviews. First, the systematic interviewing pattern contributes to the gathering of reliable information, with less chance for oversight and omission than a random interviewing technique. This style has proven both economical and effective at insuring completeness.

A second reason for the systematic approach is that the content is recorded in writing in great detail. Whereas interviewers such as vocational counselors or family therapists rely largely on notes outlining general trends or concepts, the health care record contains specific, detailed information to be shared with other health professionals who may participate in the care of the patient. The standardized record organization becomes very important as it provides a ready index to specific information. For example, the obstetrician who

wants to know the previous obstetric history of a new patient will know immediately that the information is recorded in the section Past Medical History and that the Past Medical History immediately follows the History of Present Illness.

Notice that a new parameter for the evaluation of a good health history has entered the picture—namely, that the eliciting of the desired data and the recording of that data have assumed equal importance. If health professionals are unable to write or dictate the results of their interviews succinctly, they have failed in a substantial portion of their purpose. They will not be able to communicate their findings to others who may participate in the patient's care. The proper composition of the written record is outside the scope of this text. It is assumed that the reader, having once obtained the appropriate health data base, will be competent to record that information in a clear and concise fashion. Therefore, for the remainder of this chapter, we do not distinguish between obtaining the appropriate information from a patient and recording that information appropriately in the patient's chart.

A third reason for the use of the standard interview format is that much writing can be eliminated. Convention dictates where specific information should appear. Consequently, users of the record will recognize essential elements of information without additional detailed written interpretation. A great deal of data can be quickly recorded in short phrases, telegraphic style, omitting unnecessary words (except for the History of Present Illness, as described on pages 152–157).

Finally, there is one overriding reason to adhere very closely to the established pattern of eliciting and recording a health history. By following such a rigid outline from the start, health professionals quickly gain familiarity with the content. Consequently there is a substantial decrease in interview time and anxiety, they will rapidly develop confidence in their capabilities, interview records will be complete and accurate, and supervisors will applaud their efforts.

Despite the importance of uniformity and convention, it should never be construed that the interviewer's "hands are tied" during the course of taking a history. Either the patient or the health professional may digress from the specific sequence. Since important and relevant information may be aired at any time, the wise interviewer pursues such information with subsequent related questions even though the sequence of the interview is disrupted. However, once the topic has been exhausted, the interviewer returns to the original line of questioning.

We should re-emphasize here that any information elicited from patients is to be held in strict confidence, and patients must be reasonably assured that all such information will be regarded as privileged and confidential. This understanding creates a special "bond" between patients and health professionals and greatly aids health professionals in arriving at accurate diagnoses.

Components of the Health History

The health history-taking process, although similar to general interviewing techniques in many ways, has evolved through tradition and convention into a relatively fixed pattern of inquiry. Although the specific content and sequence may vary from examiner to examiner, the basic interview always consists of seven components, with the content of the parts elicited in a specified sequence. The seven parts are (1) patient identification, (2) chief complaint, (3) history of present illness, (4) past medical history, (5) family history, (6) social history, and (7) review of systems.

The patient identification provides a very brief overview of the physical, the psychological, and the environmental aspects of the patient's problem (see Chapter 4 and the three focus areas of the interview). Depending on the nature of the chief complaint, the history of present illness and past medical history may concentrate on any of the three focus areas of a health history. For example, in a patient complaining of signs and symptoms compatible with heart disease, the focus will largely be physical. Alternatively, interviews regarding problems associated with depression or child abuse would be more likely to concentrate on the environmental or psychologic focus areas. Obviously, there are great areas of overlap in these three spheres, regardless of the nature of the presenting complaint.

Part I: Patient Identification

Patient identification frequently is abbreviated in the written chart as ID (identification) and is usually a single sentence that provides the reader with a general description of the patient. It typically makes reference to the name, age, sex, race, occupation, and general health status of the patient— for example, "Mr. Green is a 49-year-old Caucasian, male, coal miner, ambulatory, and in general good health." Notice that the recorded information informs the reader of the physical, psychological, and environmental status of the patient. One can continue reading the record or begin the interview with a reasonable point of reference for many aspects of the patient's problems.

Part II: Chief Complaint

Chief Complaint is usually abbreviated in the written record as CC. The chief complaint usually consists of a concise description of the nature of the problem or reasons that prompted the patient to present for health care. It is preferably transcribed in the chart as a verbatim quote from the patient. This practice tends to remove any bias in the health professional's interpretation of what the patient has said. It also allows a reader of the record to understand the problem more from the patient's point of view. Notice how the following example, in dialogue, is eventually recorded in the chart.

Health Professional: Good morning, Mr. Green! What prompts you to come in this morning?

Mr. Green: Well, for the past nine or ten days, I've had to urinate about every five minutes. And when I do, it hurts and I can't seem to get my bladder empty.

The chief complaint might be recorded in the following fashion:

> For the past nine or ten days, I've had to urinate about every five minutes . . . it hurts . . . and I can't seem to get my bladder empty . . .

Notice that the complaints are recorded in the patient's own words and that symptoms appearing to be linked to the same bodily system are recorded together. Complaints referable to other systems would be recorded in a similar fashion as additional chief complaints. Also, observe that, although the chief complaints are quoted verbatim, the writer has assessed the problems and has already ranked them to some degree. Finally, notice that the writer has abbreviated the record of the patient's complaints while still retaining enough of the patient's own words to transmit the exact meaning.

Part III: History of Present Illness

The History of Present Illness is usually abbreviated in the written remarks as HPI. Unlike the other six parts of the history, HPI is recorded in a narrative, prose style rather than a telegraphic style of writing. The history of present illness connotes the most recent episode of illness or an accumulation of symptoms (regardless of the time span) that have finally prompted the patient to seek health care services. For clarity, the history of present illness characteristically describes each complaint in a chronological fashion and defines and describes symptoms in objective terms.

For each symptom admitted by the patient, the interviewer obtains information in at least each of the six following categories: provocative-palliative factors, quality, region, severity, and temporal characteristics. The information may be obtained in any sequence. The mnemonic P^2QRST was devised by DeGowin and DeGowin (1976, p. 31) to describe the diagnostic attributes of pain. (The letters in the mnemonic describe the six categories listed here and described below.) Although the areas reflected by the mnemonic work most

precisely with pain, the categories also can be easily adapted to fit most symptoms if the questions "who, what, when, where, and how" are answered.

Provocative Factors (P)

DeGowin and DeGowin (1976) write that provocative factors are factors associated with, or which aggravate, a symptom. Body position, exercise, or body functions such as breathing, urination or defecation, alcohol ingestion, emotional upset, or intercurrent illness may serve as provocative factors (p. 31).

Palliative Factors (P)

These are conditions that tend to alleviate symptoms or to reduce pain. Examples are the effects of medication, therapeutic procedures, foods, relaxation, rest, body position, or body functions.

The following dialogue shows how an inquiry into provocative and palliative factors might progress with Mr. Green.

Health Professional: Mr. Green, you said that for the past few days you have been bothered by frequent urination. When you say "frequent" urination, how often do you mean that you must urinate?

Mr. Green: Well, I feel as if I have to go all the time. But, when I do get to the toilet, I can only make a few drops. I'll bet I try, though, about every half hour. Then the pain hurts so much that I have to sit down to rest.

Health Professional: You said you have pain when you urinate. Have you noticed anything that seems to make that problem worse?

Mr. Green: Well, I have noticed that if I don't drink many fluids, the burning gets worse and I don't seem to make as much water, and my urine smells bad.

Health Professional: Have you noticed anything besides drinking more fluids that relieves the symptoms?

Mr. Green: Well, one time I had a urinary tract infection and my family doctor told me to drink cranberry juice and to take some little red pills three times a day. I still had a few of the pills left, so I took them and they helped quite a lot. But I only had a few of them and now they're gone.

Health Professional: Do you know what those pills were called?

Mr. Green: No, but they made my urine look orange-colored.

Health Professional: OK, that's helpful. Have you found anything else that seems to relieve your symptoms?

Mr. Green: No. I've tried all the other home remedies I know and nothing seems to help—including the cranberry juice!

Health Professional: Can you explain why you feel that your bladder does not empty completely?

Mr. Green: Well, like I said before, even though I make urine I still feel as if there is more and I can't get it out.

Quality (Q)

Once the provocative and palliative factors have been described adequately, the health professional makes a transition and begins to inquire about the quality of the pain. Three general types of pain are usually described (DeGowin & DeGowin, 1976, pp. 31–32):

1. Cutting, knifelike, lightning, shooting, or sharp pain;

2. Burning, hot, or stinging pain; and

3. Aching, boring, gnawing, throbbing, pressure, or pounding pain.

Pain is further described as being superficial or deep. Superficial pain usually includes the types of pain described in 1 and 2 above and occurs in the tissues near the surface of the body. The site can be accurately delineated, by pointing a finger, and frequently the tissues causing the pain can be "picked up" and held between the patient's or examiner's fingers. Associated complaints may include abnormal sensations such as itching or "pins and needles."

Deep pain, the type indicated in item 3 above, is more difficult to localize and is more persistent. Associated descriptive terms may include throbbing, cramping, and so on. Note that, although the types of pain are generally well established in medical and health literature, there may be no association between the type of pain that is anticipated from a given set of circumstances and the type of pain that the patient actually perceives. For example, although the examiner might anticipate that a stab victim would experience "sharp, cutting, or knifelike pains," the victim may claim the wound was "painless" or of a "burning, throbbing" quality. Individual perceptions may differ markedly. It is best to avoid "putting words in the patient's mouth" regarding the nature of pain or any other symptoms.

The following dialogue might occur between the health professional and Mr. Green regarding the quality of his pain.

Health Professional: Mr. Green, you said earlier that "it hurt" when you passed your urine. Can you describe the type of pain you felt a little more specifically?

Mr. Green: Oh, I don't know! It's kind of hard to put in words. I guess it was a stinging or a burning sensation. It was the same kind of pain I had when I had the urinary tract infection before.

On occasion, patients will not be able to describe their sensations of pain. In such cases, the health professional can make some suggestions to the patient. However, to avoid biasing the patient's reply, it should be done by providing the patient with several terms from which to choose.

The terms should include adjectives that apply to both superficial and deep pain. For example:

Health Professional: Mr. Green, you said that "it hurts" when you pass your urine. I'm going to suggest several terms to you which may describe your pain. Please tell me which ones fit most accurately. Would you say that the pain is cutting, shooting, boring, stinging, aching, or burning—or none of those terms?

Mr. Green: Oh, there's no question! It burns and stings.

Region (R)

The next attribute of a symptom that must be inquired about is region (R) (DeGowin & DeGowin, 1976). Region is the term applied to the portion of the body where the symptom is localized. It usually is best defined by having the patient point to the area concerned—for example, the patient outlines the area under the right breast. The health professional would then record the location of the pain in anatomic terms, such as "the right fourth and fifth intercostal spaces," or in terms of objective measurements from fixed anatomic landmarks—that is, "a region measuring 3 cm × 3 cm and located 2 cm to the right of the tip of the breastbone."

In addition to describing the region in which a pain is located, it must be remembered that pain may be sensed either "locally" or "referred." "Local pains are pains felt over or in the vicinity of the pathologic process. Referred pains are pains which are not felt at the area of the disease process, but are referred and felt at some distant point on the body or extremities" (Major & Delp, 1963, p. 25). For example, the pain of angina pectoris (chest pain caused by heart disease) is usually sensed over the region of the sternum and the inner aspect of the left arm. Consequently, when asked about the regions affected by pain, patients should be asked if the pain travels along a specified course, follows a particular pattern, or is sensed at any other locations. Note this line of inquiry in the following dialogue.

Health Professional: Mr. Green, where do you notice the burning pain that you mentioned a moment ago?

Mr. Green: Well, it feels as if it starts right up inside me [Mr. Green points to the region of his pubis] and runs all the way down through my penis.

Health Professional: Does pain appear in any other areas of your body—for example, in the legs or the back—or does it seem to travel anywhere else?

Mr. Green: No, it is just where I mentioned before.

Health Professional: Are there any other symptoms associated with this pain?

Mr. Green: None that I know of!

Health Professional: Have you noticed any discharge associated with the pain?

Mr. Green: What do you mean by discharge?

Health Professional: Well, does any pus or any bloody material come out of the penis?

Mr. Green: No, I don't think I've seen anything like that.

Health Professional: Have you noticed any discoloration or blood in your urine?

Mr. Green: No.

Severity (S)

Severity estimates the quantity or degree of pain or disability produced by a given symptom. On occasion, a comparison may be useful, such as "like a toothache," or "the worst headache I've ever had." Other indications such as "My chest hurt so badly that I had to stop pushing the lawn mower" or "I was so dizzy that I had to lie down in the mall before I fell down" also may serve as bits of quantifying information indicating relative severity. Notice this line of inquiry in the continuation of the example dialogue:

Health Professional: Mr. Green, can you tell me how painful it is when you pass your water?

Mr. Green: Well, it's so painful that I have to hold onto the towel rack for something to squeeze—like biting a bullet—whenever I make water. It feels as if I'm passing red hot iron!

Temporal (T)

Temporal characteristics also are necessary in the definition of a symptom. Did the symptom begin suddenly or gradually? How long has the symptom persisted? Is the symptom present all the time or intermittently? If intermittent, is it related to the season of the year (for example, allergies), time of day (for example, early morning headache may be associated with brain tumors), sleep and/or wakefulness (such as bedwetting), or certain daily activities or bodily functions (for instance, gastric ulcer pain may be most pronounced about one hour before mealtime). Observe the assessment of temporal characteristics in the dialogue with Mr. Green.

Health Professional: Mr. Green, when did you first notice this pain?

Mr. Green: As I said, it was about two weeks ago.

Health Professional: How did this pain begin?

Mr. Green: Well, I was doing just fine, but one night the pain started very suddenly, and it has done nothing but get worse.

After inquiring about the specific characteristics of the chief complaint, the skilled interviewer requests answers to additional questions that relate to the body system under consideration in the chief complaint. Since the male genitourinary tract is the system involved in Mr. Green's complaint, additional pertinent questions for the genitourinary tract will be posed. A guide for appropriate questions can be found in the section on the Review of Systems, page 174.

Health Professional: Mr. Green, we've spoken in some detail already about your immediate problem. I'd like to ask you some more questions relating to that body system.

Mr. Green: OK.

Health Professional: You said that you do have some burning and a need to urinate more urgently and frequently than usual. Do you also have some difficulty in starting your urine stream or totally emptying your bladder? [retention]

Mr. Green: Yes, recently, because it burns so much!

Health Professional: Do you have a problem with dribbling urine after you have finished voiding?

Mr. Green: Well, I don't seem to dribble much more than usual. But now it seems that no matter how hard I try, I just can't ever seem to get my bladder completely empty and there always seems to be a few more drops.

Health Professional: Have you ever had problems with holding your urine during the day or night? [enuresis]

Mr. Green: No, that's never been a problem. In fact, recently I can't wait long enough between trips to the bathroom to allow any real amount of urine to accumulate.

Health Professional: Have you had any problem with severe back pains [colic], fever, or chills?

Mr. Green: No.

Health Professional: Have you ever had a kidney stone?

Mr. Green: No.

Health Professional: You already told me that you have not noticed any discolored [smoky] or bloody [hematuria] urine. Is my memory correct?

Mr. Green: Yes, you are right.

Health Professional: Have you ever been told that you had albumin, protein, or sugar in your urine?

Mr. Green: No.

Health Professional: How is your sexual life? Do you have the urge to have sexual contacts? [libido]

Mr. Green: Well, yes, I don't think that my sexual life is much different than usual. I certainly am interested if that is what you mean.

Health Professional: Yes, that's what I was getting at. In that same context, are you able to achieve and maintain an erection? [impotence]

Mr. Green: Yes, that's not a problem either.

Health Professional: Have you ever had a sexually transmitted disease or a venereal disease—VD—of any type?

Mr. Green: Heck no! What kind of person do you think I am? I haven't even thought about VD since I saw those movies when I was in the Army.

The interviewer sensed that Mr. Green responded in a nervous, embarrassed, reactionary, and uncomfortable fashion to the last question. The health professional now has the option of retreating temporarily from the sensitive material or pursuing the matter at once. Since this is an initial interview and because not enough time has elapsed to establish sufficient rapport, the interviewer elects to overlook the response and return to the matter at some later point in the interview.

Health Professional: I'm sorry to have embarrassed you with my last question. However, venereal disease is one of the ailments that could explain most of the symptoms that are bothering you now.

Therefore, I felt that I had to at least inquire to see if you had any concerns about VD. Let's just go on. I have a number of other questions to ask you. OK?

Mr. Green: I guess so. This really takes a long while, doesn't it!

In the preceding paragraphs, the process of obtaining a history of present illness was demonstrated for a simple problem. The process would now be repeated for any additional chief complaints relating to other body systems or problem areas. In other words, for each chief complaint or symptom identified by the patient, the interviewer would obtain information about P^2QRST factors and also would ask questions from the Review of Systems that were pertinent to that complaint.

Although the mnemonic P^2QRST does not apply directly to every problem as neatly as it applies to pain, the gist of the mnemonic can be applied—for example, P^2 = provocative and palliative factors related to crying: What causes the crying and what can be done to relieve it? Q = quality: Is it a constant sobbing or just a sad feeling? R = region: Does not apply specifically. S = severity: Is the patient forced to stay in bed, miss work, and so on because of crying spells? T = temporal: How long do the spells last? Are the spells related to other problems?

Another way to approach a problem that is less specific than pain, such as a psychosocial complaint, is to seek answers to the questions who? what? when? where? and how? For example, "Who causes you to be angry? What causes you to become angry? When do you get angry? Where are you most likely to become angry? How do you act when you become angry?"

In general, if the P^2QRST mnemonic or the "who, what, when, where, and how" questions and the appropriate review of systems are applied religiously to each chief complaint, it is unlikely that any substantial information relating to the complaint will be overlooked.

As we mentioned previously, the history of present illness should be recorded in a narrative, prose style in the medical record. The remainder of the written record, however, is recorded in telegraphic style. In other words, approved and generally accepted abbreviations are used extensively, punctuation is frequently substituted for conjunctions, and phrases rather than full sentences are the rule.

Part IV: Past Medical History

Past Medical History, often abbreviated as PMH, or simply PH (past history), is the next part of the health history or assessment process. The PMH focuses primarily on the physical sphere and attempts to determine significant events in the patient's health history that may have a bearing on the present illness. Once again, a mnemonic serves as a memory device to help recall the essential elements of information from the past medical history. Such a mnemonic is PAST MED:

P = Preventive medicine history; desirable immunizations history and dates of injections for usual childhood diseases, especially tetanus and diphtheria (DT) in adults.

A = Allergy history; inquire about allergic reactions to medications, especially penicillin and the "mycins." If a reaction has occurred, describe the type of reaction—for example, rash, shortness of breath, and so on.

S = Surgical history; list surgical procedures done in the past with dates, locations, and physicians' names, if possible.

T = Transfusion history; note transfusions received and any reactions to the blood products, as well as "why" the transfusions were required.

M = Medication history; include questions about all current medications either by prescription or over the counter (OTC). Ask specifically about aspirin, vitamins, iron, and birth control pills. These medications are used frequently but often are not considered as medications by patients.

E = Earlier illness history; include questions on serious illnesses, accidents, broken bones, and hospitalizations. Ask specifically about long-lasting childhood illnesses like rheumatic fever, scarlet fever, diphtheria, or illnesses that required long absences from school if diagnosis is unknown.

D = Delivery history; inquire about pregnancies, labors, deliveries, abortions, premature babies, and any problems associated with pregnancy and childbirth. Contraceptive history may be recorded here. Alternatively, all items in this section may appear as portions of the Family History, or Review of Systems, "Female Reproductive."

Notice that the information required in this section is relatively "cut and dried." Straightforward, simple questions are usually most effective for eliciting the necessary information.

The transition from History of Present Illness to Past Medical History (and to the other sections of the medical history) should be effected smoothly so that the flow of the interview is not disrupted. This can be accomplished best by some simple phrase that alerts the patient to the change in perspective of the interview and at the same time provides an explanation for pursuing the new line of questioning. The following dialogue might be one way to obtain a past medical history on Mr. Green:

Health Professional: Mr. Green, we've talked now quite a bit about your present health problems. I'd like to ask you a number of questions about your past health history to see if there is any connection with the new problems.

Mr. Green: Fine. Go ahead.

Health Professional: OK. Can you tell me when you had your last shots? Specifically, how about your last tetanus shot?

Mr. Green: Well, I don't remember exactly. I had a lot of shots when I was in the Army, but that was almost 30 years ago. I think I did have a tetanus shot when I got hurt in a mine accident about three years ago. Nothing serious, though.

Health Professional: Fine. Have you ever had the flu or pneumonia vaccine?

Mr. Green: Not that I recall.

Health Professional: OK. Do you know of any allergies that you have? Especially to any medicines?

Mr. Green: You remember I said that I had a urinary tract infection once before? Well, my doctor gave me an antibiotic, I think it was sulfur—or something like that....

Health Professional: Do you mean sulfa?

Mr. Green: Yes, sulfa, that's it! Anyway, I broke out with the worst case of hives you ever saw. I almost scratched my skin off! I've never used sulfas since that time.

Health Professional: It sounds as if you really got a bad case of the hives! It also sounds as if you may be quite allergic to sulfa drugs. Do you have any allergies to any other medicines? Especially penicillin?

Mr. Green: No. I seem to end up with a bad cold once in awhile. I have taken penicillin for that without any problems.

Health Professional: Have you ever had any surgery done on you?

Mr. Green: Just my tonsils and my appendix were taken out.

Health Professional: Can you tell me when and where this surgery was done?

Mr. Green: Well, both operations were done when I was six or seven years old. I think it was done at Brown Memorial Hospital, but I don't remember the doctors.

Health Professional: Have you ever had any other surgery done?

Mr. Green: Just a few stitches in my arm from a mine accident three years ago. I just had a cut on my right arm.

Health Professional: Did you require any blood transfusions with any of the surgery?

Mr. Green: I don't know of any.

Health Professional: Mr. Green, do you take any medicines now on a regular basis?

Mr. Green: No, just an occasional aspirin for headaches or aches and pains.

Health Professional: What about vitamins or iron pills?

Mr. Green: Neither.

Health Professional: It sounds as if you've been pretty healthy! Have you had any serious illnesses during your life?

Mr. Green: Well, when I was in grade school I missed about six weeks of school because I had rheumatic fever. For a couple of years after that they thought I had a heart murmur, but it went away by the time I entered the Army. I have been in pretty good health.

Health Professional: Well, that pretty much finishes this part of our interview. Now, if you're in agreement, I'd like to ask you a few questions about your family's health history to see if there are any indications that your illness may be related to some hereditary process.

The following is an excerpt from a dialogue with Mrs. Swift, a healthy, 42-year-old woman who is being seen on her initial visit by a gynecologic assistant prior to a routine annual examination.

Health Professional: Mrs. Swift, we have discussed your present state of health and have reviewed most of your past medical history. Now, I'd like to inquire about your previous pregnancies. (Go to page 160.)

LEARNING ACTIVITIES

Past Medical History

Using the preceding dialogue and the mnemonic PAST MED, construct a written example of a Past Medical History for Mr. Green, using a telegraphic style of writing. P (Preventive) is completed as an example. Feedback follows.

P = (preventive)—usual military shots—19___(date), tetanus shot—19___(date)

A = (allergy)

S = (surgery)

T = (transfusions)

M = (medications)

E = (earlier illnesses)

D = (deliveries)

Notice from the feedback that is shown below that the information from the dialogue has been (1) condensed extensively, (2) recorded in a chronologic and tabular form using the mnemonic as a guide, and (3) recorded using frequent abbreviations in a telegraphic writing style. Also, notice how successfully the relevant information in the dialogue was culled from the extraneous conversation and then written simply and concisely so that the significant events become immediately obvious. A working knowledge of the entire past medical history can be gained almost at a glance.

If the patient is female, inquiry into pregnancy, labor, and delivery histories can be made at this point or can be reserved until the Review of Systems (ROS). The total number of prior pregnancies (gravidity), the total number of children previously born (parity), and significant details of previous pregnancies, such as character and length of labor, type of delivery, complications, infant status, and birth weight comprise a minimal obstetrical history.

Feedback

P = (preventive)—usual military shots—19___(date), tetanus shot—19___(date).

A = sulfas—hives; no penicillin allergy

S = Brown Memorial Hospital; tonsillectomy—age 6 or 7; appendectomy—age 6 or 7; laceration of right arm—age 46

T = none

M = aspirin; 2 tabs occasionally for headache or minor pain

E = rheumatic fever as child, no residual problems

D = since the patient is male, there is no past medical history for delivery. Therefore, the item would be omitted in the write-up.

Mrs. Swift: Go right ahead.

Health Professional: Can you tell me how many times you've been pregnant?

Mrs. Swift: Four times, as far as I know.

Health Professional: Did all of those four pregnancies result in term deliveries?

Mrs. Swift: Well, the first time I was pregnant I started bleeding after about six weeks and lost the baby. Then I had to have surgery—a D and C. About a year later, I got pregnant again and delivered my first son without a hitch. Two years after that, I had my daughter. My "baby" son, who is now 16 years old, arrived about five weeks early. He did just fine, though, and I was able to take him home after about two weeks, when he gained some more weight.

Health Professional: You've implied that two of the pregnancies were entirely normal and that labor and delivery were totally uncomplicated. Is that correct?

Mrs. Swift: That's right.

Health Professional: Do you have any idea or do you recall if your doctor had any opinions as to why you lost your first baby?

Mrs. Swift: No, we don't know. I guess nature just intended it that way!

Health Professional: What reasons were you given for the early delivery of your son?

Mrs. Swift: Well, I was in an auto accident that brought on early labor. So I suppose that was the problem. Neither one of us was hurt, though.

Health Professional: Do you recall how much each of your children weighed at birth?

Mrs. Swift: I've got it written in the baby book, but I don't recall exactly, except for Tom, who arrived early. He was four pounds and ten ounces, and they made him stay in the hospital until he was almost five

pounds. The other two were over six pounds.

Health Professional: That's fine. You have a good memory. I would assume, on the basis of your age, that you still have regular menstrual periods. Is that correct?

Mrs. Swift: Yes, it is.

Health Professional: I'd like to inquire about your menstrual history in more detail later. However, if you still have regular periods, you could still become pregnant. Are you using any method of contraception?

Mrs. Swift: Oh yes! I don't know what I'd do with another baby now. I'm too old! I've been using a diaphragm and jelly for most of my married life.

Health Professional: Very well. It sounds as if you're quite satisfied with that method of contraception.

Mrs. Swift: Well, I'm afraid to take "the pill," and I don't like the thought of having a piece of plastic inside me, so IUDs are out. I'm quite satisfied with the diaphragm.

Health Professional: OK, Mrs. Swift. That finishes this part of the interview. Do you want to add anything about your babies or birth control that I have not covered?

Mrs. Swift: No, that's all there is to it, as far as I know.

The obstetrical history is usually expressed in the chart as a four-digit number representing the number of term deliveries, premature deliveries, abortions (both therapeutic and spontaneous) and number of living children. For example, in Mrs. Swift's chart, the history would be recorded as:

2:1:1:3 (2 term deliveries, 1 premature delivery, 1 spontaneous abortion, 3 living children)

Another common system for recording obstetric history uses the concepts of *gravidity* (total number of times pregnant), *parity* (number of living offspring), and *abortuses* (number of aborted pregnancies). For Mrs. Swift, the chart entry would read simply:

G4; P3; A1

Details of the premature birth and the miscarriage would be noted as above.

Other aspects of D (delivery) might be recorded for Mrs. Swift as follows:

- = uncomplicated labor and delivery × 2; birth weights 6+ pounds

- = premature infant probably as result of auto accident; five weeks early; wt. 4# 10 oz.; discharged from hospital after gaining weight to approx. 5#

- = miscarriage (spontaneous abortion) at 6 weeks; cause unknown

- = contraception: diaphragm and jelly

(Now do the learning activity on page 159.)

Part V: Family History

After the past medical history has been obtained, the examiner concentrates on the family history, often abbreviated in the records as FamHx. Usually, this process is accomplished by inquiring about each family member in turn, from the grandparents through the children of the patient in question. If suggestion of hereditary disease is present, then the questioning is extended to include even more distant family members. In addition to the age and sex of family members, information usually is obtained about the general state of health and chronic or present illnesses (if the person is living) or the cause of death if the individual is dead.

Two basic patterns of recording such data are common. The first is by using the telegraphic format. A second method is the use of a genetic diagram. Much more information can be grasped in a short time using the standard format of a genetic diagram. In such a diagram, the various family generations are depicted on horizontal lines and the type of relationship is indicated by vertical lines. The standard symbols used on most genetic diagrams are shown below.

□ = male   ○ = female   ╱ = dead

↗ = patient being interviewed (propositus)

◇ = unknown sex or unknown status

□——○ lines connecting individuals signify marriage (husband and wife)

⌐□   ○⌐ lines bracketing individuals signify siblings (brother and sister)

The basic symbols can be annotated to provide additional information about the individual concerned. Note the following examples.

43 □ diabetes = 43-year-old male with diabetes

49 Ø breast cancer = dead 49-year-old female with breast cancer

53 ○ ↗ = 53-year-old female (patient interviewed)

◇₂ = two unknown individuals

The following dialogue shows one method by which a family history could be obtained by interviewing Mr. Green:

Health Professional: Mr. Green, I'd like to ask you a few questions about the health of the other members of your family.

Mr. Green: OK, go right ahead.

Health Professional: In order to help me organize things a bit better, tell me about your father's side of the family first. Is your father's father—your grandfather—still living?

Mr. Green: Oh no! He was killed in a mining accident when he was about 39. I hardly ever knew him.

Health Professional: How about your father's mother? She'd be your grandmother on your father's side.

Mr. Green: She's dead too. Hmm, I guess she was in her 70s when she died. She had cancer that spread all over her—started from her breast.

Health Professional: Did your father have any brothers or sisters?

Mr. Green: There were, let's see, seven of them altogether, but I only knew Uncle Ralph and Uncle Hal. They're both alive. Ralph is about 73 and he has some kind of arthritis that makes his hands knot up like an old tree trunk. Hal's about 59 or 60 and I think he's OK. There were three or four other brothers and sisters, but I don't know anything about them.

Health Professional: Is your father still living?

Mr. Green: No, he died about seven years ago. He had cancer of the prostate that went to his bones. He was 64 when he died.

Health Professional: You have a good memory. Now, about the other side of the family. Are your mother's parents, your maternal grandparents, alive?

Mr. Green: Well, I haven't seen her for many years, but I think mother's mother is still living.

Health Professional: All right, tell me about your grandmother. How old is she and what is her state of health?

Mr. Green: Well, as I said, I haven't seen her for a long time. She's living in a nursing home. I think she's in her 90s now—but she's as healthy as a horse, as far as I know. She just won't quit!

Health Professional: Good. How about her husband? That would be your maternal grandfather, right?

Mr. Green: Yeah, he was a no-good! Couldn't hold a job and used to beat his wife and family. I never heard of a guy with so many girlfriends! His drinking finally got to him when he was 56 or so, and he swelled up like a toad and died! They said he had cirrhosis.

Health Professional: Is your mother still living?

Mr. Green: Yes. She's 68 though, and she has a lot of chest pain—angina, or something like that. She has hardening of the arteries and diabetes too! She's pretty miserable most of the time.

Health Professional: Does your mother have any brothers or sisters?

Mr. Green: She had one sister, but she's dead now.

Health Professional: Do you know what caused her death? What was her age at the time of her death?

Mr. Green: I didn't know Aunt Bertha very well because she and Mom didn't get along. I guess she was about 60 when she died. She was a chain smoker and her lungs finally gave out.

Health Professional: OK, now that brings us to your family. You're 49, right?

Mr. Green: Yes, 49 and holding! Ha, ha!

Health Professional: Do you have any brothers or sisters?

Mr. Green: I had one brother, but he drowned when I was about eight years old. He was only five then.

Health Professional: Is there a Mrs. Green, and how old is she?

Mr. Green: We've been split for nine years. She's 46.

Health Professional: Is your ex-wife in good health?

Mr. Green: I guess. I haven't seen her for a couple of years.

Health Professional: Did your ex-wife have any brothers or sisters?

Mr. Green: No! Her parents quit after they got her!

Health Professional: OK, did you and your wife have any children?

Mr. Green: Yes, we had two. Ellen is 24. She has a two-year-old and another baby on the way. John is 28 and works for the government. Both kids are healthy.

Health Professional: OK, Mr. Green. That should hold us for family history. Other than the two cases of cancer, your father and your paternal grandmother, do you know of any illnesses that tend to run in your family? For example, diabetes, high blood pressure, heart disease, kidney disease, alcohol or drug problems, or TB?

Mr. Green: Well, my mother has diabetes.

Health Professional: Yes, I forgot about her. And you also mentioned your grandfather who died of cirrhosis of the liver. Any others?

Mr. Green: No, I don't think there is much left to talk about. I feel as if I've told you everything I ever knew!

Health Professional: Well, I hope I haven't totally worn you out. We're getting to the end, but we're not through yet. If you're still willing, I'd like to talk to you about your social history and your lifestyle.

Mr. Green: Let's get on with it!

(Now complete the learning activities that start on the bottom of this page.)

Now that you have composed a family history using both the telegraphic style and the genetic diagram, examine the results of your efforts and compare them with the examples. Both types of recording convey similar information to a reader. However, "the picture is worth a thousand words" in defining the relationships that exist. Also, the diagram can be drawn and annotated very simply and conveniently as you are eliciting the family history. Consequently, many practitioners prefer the graphic representation, and most readers find it easier to use. If patients understand the purpose

_____ *LEARNING ACTIVITIES* _____

Family History (Telegraphic Style)

During the introductory paragraphs on family history, we stated that the family history could be recorded in two general ways. The first is to use the telegraphic phrase format. As a learning activity to reinforce this technique, refer back through the dialogue on Mr. Green's family history and record his family history in the telegraphic phrase format using the following outline. "Paternal grandfather" is completed as an example. Feedback follows.

Grandparents—Paternal grandfather: killed, age 39; mining accident

Paternal grandmother:

Maternal grandfather:

Maternal grandmother:

Parents—   Father:

            Father's siblings: (1)

                               (2)

            Mother:

            Mother's siblings: (1)

Patient—   Patient's siblings: (1)

            Patient's spouse:

            Patient's children: (1)

                                (2)

Now that you have written Mr. Green's family history in telegraphic style, compare your work with the feedback. You may have organized your record in a slightly different fashion. As long as the basic information is present, any organization that conveys a logical progression is acceptable.

Feedback

Grandparents: Paternal grandfather: killed; age 39; mining accident
              Paternal grandmother: dead; age 70s; breast cancer with
                                     multiple metastases
              Maternal grandfather: dead; age 56; alcoholism (cirrhosis)
              Maternal grandmother: living; age 90s; well in nursing home

Parents: Father: dead; age 64; cancer of the prostate, bone metastases
              Father's siblings: (1) male; age 73; arthritis
                                 (2) male; age 60; well
                                 four siblings unknown
              Mother: living; age 68; angina pectoris; diabetes mellitus;
                  arteriosclerosis
              Mother's siblings: (1) female; dead; age 60; lung disease

              Patient: male; age 49
              Patient's siblings: (1) male; dead; age 5; drowning
              Patient's spouse: divorced × 9 years; age 46; well
              Patient's children: (1) male; age 28; well
                                  (2) female; age 24; well

The second method of recording the family history is with the use of the genetic diagram. Re-examine the standard symbols on page 161 and complete the following learning activity.

Family History
(Genetic Diagram)

For practice in recording a family history using the genetic diagram technique, construct the family history for Mr. Green using such a diagram and the information from the dialogue on pages 161–163. The outline below may help you get started. "Grandparents" is completed as an example. Feedback follows.

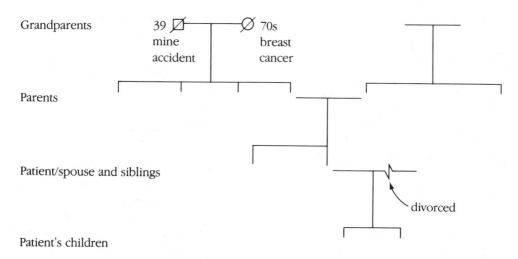

Grandparents

Parents

Patient/spouse and siblings

Patient's children

Feedback

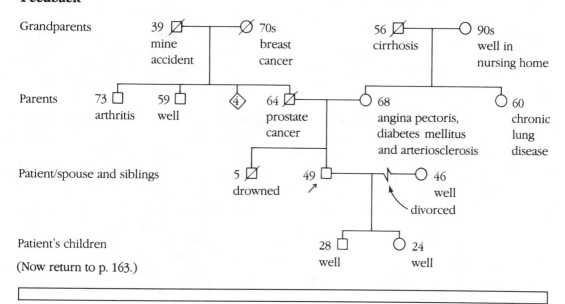

Grandparents

Parents

Patient/spouse and siblings

Patient's children

(Now return to p. 163.)

of the diagram, few will object to the examiner drawing and recording information as the interview progresses.

Part VI: Social History

The sixth portion of the health history is the Social History, abbreviated in the written record as Soc.

Hx. The social history focuses primarily on the environmental and psychological aspects of the patient's daily routine. Once again, a simple mnemonic is helpful in eliciting all the necessary information. The mnemonic is MOLEST, which stands for six categories: M = Marital status; O = Occupation; L = Lifestyle; E = Ethanol consumption; S = Smoking; and T = Travel history.

Marital Status (M)

Note if the patient is presently or was formerly married, duration of marriage, and the number of years passed since the loss of spouse through divorce, separation, or death. At the same time, attempt to make some assessment of the effects of the marriage or divorce on the patient's lifestyle. In initial interviews, broad, open-ended, nonjudgmental questions such as "How do you feel about your marriage?" or "To what degree is your marriage a happy marriage?" provide the interviewer with insight into the patient's degree of marital satisfaction.

In subsequent interviews, if the patient alludes to marital dissatisfaction or when the patient admits to a problem area, more penetrating questions can be posed, such as "You said that you are not very happy in your marriage. Can you tell me more specifically what is bothering you?"

Some suggestions for obtaining a marital history are demonstrated in the following dialogue with Mr. Green.

Health Professional: OK, we're making good progress, Mr. Green. We'll be done in a few more minutes. Next, I'd like to inquire about your social history and your lifestyle so that I can learn a bit more about you than just the medical side of your life.

Mr. Green: Do you really have to ask me more questions? I'm about talked out!

Health Professional: I realize you're probably feeling bushed. We need to consider a few more areas so that we won't overlook some aspect of your life that has an important bearing on this problem.

Mr. Green: OK, go ahead.

Health Professional: You indicated that you are not married. Is that correct?

Mr. Green: Yes, my wife left me about nine years ago—after we'd been married almost 23 years.

Health Professional: How have you gotten along since she has been gone?

Mr. Green: Well, we hadn't gotten along for a number of years. I guess when she left I wasn't really too surprised. I'm doing just fine.

Health Professional: Have you since been divorced?

Mr. Green: Oh yes! The divorce was final about six months after she left. Since we didn't own much property and she didn't want our house, I just bought out her half of the house, and she took her things out, and that was it!

Health Professional: So, are you saying that the divorce wasn't too traumatic?

Mr. Green: Well, it was sort of hard to tell the kids, but I guess they knew it was coming too. Worst thing was that the house was awfully lonely when I got home from work.

Health Professional: Lots of divorced people mention that problem. I guess it would make you feel pretty alone.

Mr. Green: Well, it really bothered me for a while, and I just wouldn't go home. I'd stop down at Ralph's Place and spend the whole evening drowning my troubles in beer and shooting pool. Eventually several of us guys who were there every night talked Ralph—he's the owner of the bar—into sponsoring a softball team. We did pretty good—got into the semi-finals. Best part was that I made a few new friends and we started going out together, and I would invite them over to watch TV or something. So, I finally got out of the rut. Took me about two years though.

Health Professional: So, now you feel you are reasonably happy with things as they are?

Mr. Green: Yeah, they're not too bad.

Health Professional: Are you doing any dating?

Mr. Green: Well, I went out with a number of women, especially right after the divorce. I spend most of my time now, though, with Angie. She's divorced and has two kids.

Health Professional: How often do you see Angie?

Mr. Green: Almost every day. I practically live at her place. I suppose I'd move in if it weren't for the kids. I'm not sure I can handle them. They're teenagers and uncontrollable. She doesn't discipline them very well.

This portion of the social history may also provide an opportunity for obtaining a sexual and contraceptive history. Current sexual trends have expanded the range of sexual "normality" enormously. In a general sense, any sexual expression between consenting adults that is enjoyed by all parties (when there is no physical or psychological pain inflicted on anyone involved) must be considered normal by an interviewer. It is frequently difficult to remain objective where sexuality is concerned because it is so entwined with cultural, religious, and moral beliefs. Since so many different sexual practices can be considered normal, it can be difficult for interviewers to conceal their personal biases from the start. Heterosexuality, homosexuality, various forms of sexual gratification by mechanical means, extremes of sexual frequency, and numerous other practices unfamiliar or even repulsive to the interviewer may be encountered. In order to maintain a therapeutic relationship, the interviewer must not allow his or her biases to interfere with the interview process.

Additionally, interviewers must frequently reflect on their own reasons for pursuing certain lines of questioning. Are the questions relevant, and is the information necessary for the molding of a therapeutic relationship? Or is the interviewer pursuing a certain line of questioning for personal satisfaction, personal curiosity, or even voyeurism?

Smith and Leversee (1980) assert that a sexual history is easier to obtain if the health professional "has a conviction that sexuality is an important area in the patient's total health" (p. 120). According to these authors, inquiry into sexual matters is important in any complete history or physical examination, when the patient presents an overt sexual problem, when an organic disease demands attention to the area of sexual functioning, or when a sexual problem is suspected to be involved with the patient's presenting concern (p. 120). The content of the sexual history will vary with the nature of the chief complaint. At the very least, however, the interviewer will inquire about sexual preference, gender preference, extent of sexual activity, degree of sexual satisfaction, and particular sexual problems or dysfunction. Notice this line of inquiry in the dialogue with Mr. Green:

Health Professional: I'd like to ask you a few questions about your sexual practices and preferences. I gather from what you've told me already about Angie that you have established a sexual relationship with her. Is that correct or not?

Mr. Green: Yes, as I said, we practically live together—especially on weekends. We have a pretty good sex life.

Health Professional: So, you seem to feel pretty satisfied then with your sexual relationship.

Mr. Green: Yes, you could say so!

Health Professional: Are there any problems or concerns about your sexuality that you would like to mention?

Mr. Green: No, things are going smoothly, I think, for both of us.

Health Professional: OK. Do you have sexual contact with anyone other than Angie?

Mr. Green: Heck no! (defensively) I don't cheat on her and she doesn't cheat on me. We have an understanding about that.

Health Professional: Fine. One more question and that will wrap up this part of the interview. In the past, have all or most of your sexual contacts been with women?

Mr. Green: Absolutely! I guess I don't care what other people do, but that gay stuff sure isn't for me!

Notice that the interviewer proceeded to gather all the necessary sexual history data in an on-going, matter-of-fact style. Questions in this portion of the interview were asked routinely in exactly the same fashion as all the preceding questions, and they were nonjudgmental and free of personal opinions.

Occupation (O)

Goldman and Peters (1981, p. 2833) suggest three essential points to be incorporated into a routine occupational history: (1) a listing of current and past jobs; (2) a key screening question such as "Do you now (or some time in the past) have exposure to fumes, chemicals, dust, loud noises, or radiation?" and (3) determination of whether a relationship exists between the chief complaint and activities at work or in the home, jobs and possible toxic exposures, and other contributing factors such as smoking, medication, and so on. In addition, some estimate of job satisfaction can be elicited by asking "How much do you enjoy the kind of work you do?"

Notice how the interviewer pursues these questions in continuing the social history with Mr. Green.

Health Professional: OK. A few more questions and we'll be finished with this interview. Can you tell me about your work history?

Mr. Green: Well, I've been a coal miner for 26 years now.

Health Professional: What kind of job do you have at the mines?

Mr. Green: I've done everything. I can run the motor, or a continuous mining machine,

or a roof bolter—you name it! I'm the section chief now and have 12 men working for me.

Health Professional: Have you worked anywhere else beside the coal mines?

Mr. Green: No, I've worked for the same company ever since I started.

Health Professional: I would assume that you come into contact with a lot of dust and fumes in the mines. Is that correct?

Mr. Green: Well, there is some dust, but you get used to it.

Health Professional: Do you use a respirator on the job?

Mr. Green: Occasionally when the dust is really bad. Usually though, none of us wear them. They're a nuisance. You can't breathe right, and it's about impossible to run the section because you can't tell the men what to do 'cause you can't talk right.

Health Professional: Do you use ear plugs to protect yourself from all the noise in the mines?

Mr. Green: No, you get used to that noise, too!

Health Professional: Have you ever mined any radioactive substances?

Mr. Green: Nope. Only coal.

Health Professional: How do you like your work?

Mr. Green: I love it! Otherwise I wouldn't have stayed this long. The mines sort of grow on you. When I retire I'll have over 40 years with the company.

Lifestyle (L)

Obtain information about the patient's "CDEF" (Castle, Diet, Exercise, Fun). Regarding the Castle, determine the type of home in which the patient lives, the number of occupants, status of ownership, plumbing and heating facilities, and general location. Some answers may suggest further questions regarding possible environmental causes of illness. For example, tenements may be associated with infectious diseases such as tuberculosis, or decrepit plumbing facilities may be associated with outbreaks of viral hepatitis.

Next, the patient's Diet and its adequacy need to be explored. Does the patient get enough to eat? Does he or she choose foods from each of the major food groups and in sufficient variety? Does the patient follow any unusual or "fad" diet, eating only certain types of foods (for example, vegetarian) or poor quality foods (junk foods)? Similarly, inquire about the intake of coffee, tea, cola, and other caffeine-containing beverages.

To evaluate Exercise, determine if the patient is primarily sedentary (little or no physical activity), moderately active (occasional participation in vigorous exercise), or active in both work and leisure activities (sustained physical exertion such as walking briskly, running, lifting, or carrying at least three times weekly).

Fun includes an assessment of the patient's leisure time activities, pastimes, sports, hobbies, and so on. Be particularly alert to the presence of physically risky pastimes (auto racing, motocross, scuba diving, rock climbing) or possible toxic exposure (fiberglass, epoxy resins, fumes, lead, pigments). Also notice if the patient has no leisure time pursuits at all. An illustration of the process of obtaining this portion of the social history follows.

Health Professional: How about your home? You mentioned that you lived in your own house since your wife left you. Do you own that home now?

Mr. Green: Almost. I still owe a small mortgage. I bought out her half and then fixed it up all by myself. It's really pretty nice now.

Health Professional: Do you live in town?

Mr. Green: Just outside of town, but I get city water, gas, electric, and sewer.

Health Professional: Tell me about your eating habits.

Mr. Green: Well, cooking is not one of my favorite pastimes. I seem to be able to burn water when I boil it! I eat most of my meals at Angie's, and she's a good cook. A couple of times a week I just run out and get a bite to eat. Pizza and beer at Ralph's Place are my real weaknesses.

Health Professional: Do you feel that you eat a pretty well-balanced diet?

Mr. Green: Oh, yes! I make sure that I get some vegetables, potatoes, and meat at least several times each week. I'm a basic steak and potatoes man.

Health Professional: Can you tell me about how many cups of coffee and tea you drink each day?

Mr. Green: Well, I'm not a tea drinker at all. I suppose I have seven or eight cups of coffee, though, each day. I take a thermos in my lunch pail and that holds a quart. Then I usually have a couple of cups of black coffee to help pry my eyes open before I leave for work and a couple of cups of coffee with supper.

Health Professional: About how many Cokes or soft drinks do you drink each day?

Mr. Green: I'm not much of a soda pop drinker. I might have two or three bottles of Coke a week at the most—when I'm down at Ralph's.

Health Professional: What do you do for exercise?

Mr. Green: Well, as a section chief in the mines I do a heck of a lot of walking every day. Then, I mentioned the softball team. Also, I'm a pretty good bowler, and I play in a league. In the spring I spend a lot of time fishing, and I usually manage to get a deer and a few rabbits during the hunting season.

Health Professional: Well, it sounds as if you keep yourself pretty busy. Do you consider yourself to be sedentary, moderately active, or very active?

Mr. Green: Oh, probably moderate. I don't do as much vigorous exercise as I used to. But, then, I'm not as young as I used to be!

Health Professional: Do you do anything else for fun? I mean, do you have any hobbies or other pastimes?

Mr. Green: No, I don't have any hobbies except that I am a loyal professional baseball and football fan. I don't miss many games on TV.

Ethanol Consumption (E)

Try to estimate the amount of alcohol (beer, wine, or hard drinks) the patient consumes daily, and determine the duration of this drinking pattern. This information may have significant bearing on the diagnosis and may frequently surprise the interviewer. (It has been said that to quantitate alcohol consumption one should double what the patient admits and halve what other family members claim!)

One way to approach such questions is to suggest an unlikely high level of consumption—for example, "How much alcohol do you consume—a fifth of whiskey a day, or a case of beer daily?" Virtually everyone who consumes less than the suggested amount will laugh and say "Oh, no, not that much!" and then try to estimate actual consumption.

Sometimes, however, the patient will admit "Yes, at least a fifth of whiskey a day." Other patients with alcohol problems may be reluctant to admit to actual levels of consumption and occasionally deceive the interviewer and admit only partial consumption. Therefore, the interviewer should ask about each general class of alcoholic beverage specifically. For example, with the patient above, the conversation may continue "OK, you claim that you consume about a fifth of whiskey a day. Do you also use any beer, rum, vodka, or other alcoholic beverages?" Unfortunately, under the best of circumstances and with the most skillful inter-

viewers, patients with alcohol problems still frequently succeed at hiding the truth.

The following dialogue illustrates this line of questioning.

Health Professional: Do you frequently drink alcohol?

Mr. Green: Well, I don't usually drink very much—except right after my wife left. Then I really drank heavily.

Health Professional: Can you tell me about how much you consume? Would you usually drink a fifth of whiskey or a case of beer daily?

Mr. Green: No way! I wouldn't be able to go to work! I did drink about that much a few years ago, after the divorce, but I've really tapered off since. I was gaining too much weight.

Health Professional: You say you've "tapered off" in your beer consumption. How much beer do you usually drink each day?

Mr. Green: Well, I occasionally have a beer when I get home from work, but that's about it. I don't like to drink alone. But when I go to play ball or bowl or something with the boys, I'll have two or three beers. I guess I drink about two six-packs a week.

Health Professional: Do you use any rum, wine, or other alcoholic beverages?

Mr. Green: No hard liquor at all. Occasionally I may have a little wine with dinner for a special occasion, but that's all.

Health Professional: So, except for about two years following your divorce, when you drank very heavily, you now consume mostly beer and limit your intake to about 12 bottles weekly. Is that pretty accurate?

Mr. Green: Yes, that's about right.

Smoking History (S)

Determine the number of "pack years" that the patient has smoked, especially cigarettes. (Number of pack years = number of packs per day × the number of years smoked.) Smoking, particularly of cigarettes and to a lesser extent cigars and pipes, is associated with many medical conditions and diseases. Consequently, information about smoking habits may be very useful. It is also convenient and may be appropriate to inquire at the same time about the smoking of substances other than tobacco. If the patient admits to use of marijuana, then a reasonable follow-up question concerns the use of other nonprescription, prescription, or recreational drugs with abuse potential. In this confidential and nonjudgmental setting, an astute interviewer can elicit a great deal of information. The following dialogue illustrates this line of questioning.

Health Professional: Are you a cigarette smoker?

Mr. Green: Yeah, I smoke too many cigarettes.

Health Professional: How many cigarettes do you smoke?

Mr. Green: Oh, two-and-a-half packs a day.

Health Professional: How long have you smoked that much?

Mr. Green: Ever since I started working in the mines.

Health Professional: So, you've smoked two-and-a-half packs a day for the past 26 years?

Mr. Green: I'm afraid that's so.

Health Professional: That's a lot of cigarettes—that's 65 pack years! Have you ever considered giving up smoking?

Mr. Green: Not seriously. As long as I'm healthy I'll probably keep on smoking.

Health Professional: Do you ever use cigars or pipes?

Mr. Green: Just when my friends give 'em to me after they have babies!

Health Professional: You have pointed out that you are quite a heavy cigarette smoker. Do you smoke anything other than tobacco?

Mr. Green: You mean marijuana? No way!

Health Professional: Have you ever used any other drugs or chemicals for recreational purposes?

Mr. Green: No way! Dope's not for me!

Health Professional: OK, that wraps up my questioning on smoking. As an aside here, I would like to offer you one suggestion. There is an overwhelming amount of evidence that links cigarette smoking to all kinds of lung problems. Consequently, anything that you can do to reduce the number of cigarettes you use would certainly be in your best health interest. Maybe we can talk further about this matter a little later when we have completed this history.

Note that the health professional has digressed from the pattern of the questioning to interpose some patient education. Such a digression interrupts the monotony of the interview process and performs an educational function at the same time. The health professional's suggestion is not offensive, even for patients who are not interested in following it. For those seriously interested, the health professional has left the door open for further discussion at a later time in the interview.

Travel History (T)

Find out where the patient has traveled, particularly to foreign countries that may have associated health hazards, such as malaria, dysentery, or penicillin-resistant gonorrhea. Also, inquire about local travel or pastimes that may expose the patient to specific disease processes (for example, backpackers may drink contaminated water). Additional immunization history also may be acquired in this context. The interviewer might pursue Mr. Green's travel history as follows:

Health Professional: Mr. Green, have you recently done any traveling outside the United States where you might have come into contact with any unusual causes for illness?

Mr. Green: No, except for going to the beach in the summer, I pretty much stay close to

LEARNING ACTIVITIES

Social History

Using the preceding dialogues between the health professional and Mr. Green and keeping in mind the mnemonic MOLEST, devise and record an appropriate social history using the telegraphic style of writing. M (marriage) is completed as an example. Feedback follows the learning activity.

Marriage = married 20 years; now divorced × 9 years; resettled into own lifestyle; dating steadily

Occupation =

Lifestyle: Castle =

Diet =

Exercise =

Fun =

Ethanol consumption =

Smoking =

Travel =

Feedback

M = married 20 years; now divorced × 9 years; resettled into own lifestyle; dating steadily

O = miner × 26 years; runs motor, continuous miner, or roof bolter; presently section chief with 12 men in section

L: C = owns home; just out of town; city gas, water, electric, and sewer

D = good quality and variety of foods; no tea; drinks 7–8 cups coffee daily; several bottles cola weekly

E = walks, plays softball, bowls regularly; hunts and fishes; "moderate exercise"

F = no hobbies; professional sports fan

E = drank heavily × 2 years after divorce; drinks two six-packs of beer weekly; no other alcohol except wine with special dinners only

S = 65 pack years cigarette smoking; no cigars or pipes; no marijuana or other drugs

T = Far East with military post-war

home. Oh, I was in the Far East with the military after the war, but that was a long time ago.

Part VII: Review of Systems

The last part of the complete health history is the Review of Systems, usually abbreviated ROS. The review of systems is a series of questions concerning symptoms and signs that might be produced by or associated with abnormalities in each of the body systems. The examiner usually memorizes these questions and then recites them in rote fashion to patients. Patients are instructed beforehand to stop the examiner at any time when a question brings up a problem they have experienced. In this way, the examiner can "screen" very quickly for the major symptoms and signs that may indicate disease in a particular body system. In contrast to the other parts of the health assessment interview, the review of systems is based on a number of "closed" questions so that a large amount of material can be considered in a relatively short period of time.

The review of systems is recorded in the chart in an abbreviated, telegraphic style. To indicate that the questions have been asked, each system is named and pertinent responses are listed. If the response suggests an incidental finding, such as the presence of false teeth, the fact is simply noted in the ROS. On the other hand, if the response suggests some significant new information, with major implications for the patient's care, or reveals the existence of a previously unrecognized problem, the new information is considered as an additional chief complaint and the process previously described for the History of Present Illness (HPI) should be applied for the new problem. (This involves the techniques of P^2QRST or who, what, when, where, and how.) In such cases, the new information is recorded in the HPI either as an elaboration on problems already established or as an entirely new problem.

Each major system is tabulated in the review of systems. If detailed information regarding that system has been previously obtained and recorded,

the review of systems entry indicates simply "(see HPI)" or "(see PMH)" to direct the reader to that information. In general, the review of systems that is pertinent to the system in the HPI is included as a portion of the HPI. Further, a complete review of systems must include not only a notation indicating the presence of signs and symptoms but also a notation indicating the absence of any anticipated findings.

The content of a review of systems varies from examiner to examiner and may reveal the areas of the interviewer's greatest interest. The ROS for the cardiovascular system, when compiled by a nurse in the coronary care unit, may be very extensive. At the same time, that nurse may pay little attention to the ROS for the GU (genitourinary) system. On the contrary, the urologist would likely elicit a detailed ROS on the GU system but a less detailed one of the cardiovascular system. In addition, the need to obtain specific information may vary among interviewers depending on the reason for the interview. The dentist considering the prospect of extracting impacted wisdom teeth will be much more concerned about a history of prolonged bleeding and easy bruising than will a physical therapist who is involved in maintaining joint range of motion.

A good review of systems, then, contains a comprehensive list of questions designed to detect significant abnormalities in the system under consideration, but it should accomplish this end without going into excessive detail. The review of systems list on page 174 is one example (Sleeth, 1975). Although the example uses medical terminology, remember that patients may not be familiar with the terms. Therefore, instead of asking patients "Have you ever had diplopia, strabismus, or excessive lacrimation?" the question should be phrased "Have you ever had double vision, a lazy eye, or increased tearing?" The descriptive terms should be used with the patients, and the appropriate medical terminology should be recorded in the written record.

For ease of memorization and recollection, the ROS progresses "from head to toe," except for questions relating to the emotional or mental sta-

A Review of Systems*

Skin
Acne, furuncles, exanthem, ulcers, dryness of skin or hair, pruritis, bruising, dermatitis, bleeding, tumors

Head and Neck
Eyes—Vision, diplopia, pain, strabismus, cataract, injury, lacrimation, dryness, scotomata
Ears—Hearing, pain, otorrhea, tinnitus, vertigo
Nose—Olfaction, rhinorrhea, obstruction, epistaxis, injury, sinus trouble, allergic rhinitis
Mouth—Gustation, teeth, dentures, gingivae, tongue, ulcer, growth
Throat—Voice, tonsils, pharynx, larynx, hoarseness, masses
Neck—Pain, stiffness, tenderness, masses, goiter

Allergies
Eczema, urticaria, hay fever, asthma, congestion, sneezing, known drug or food sensitivities

Respiratory
Chest pain, pleurisy, cough, sputum (appearance and amount), pneumonia, hemoptysis, wheezing, dyspnea, cyanosis, fever, chills, night sweats; dates and results of any chest X-rays

Cardiovascular
Dyspnea, edema, cyanosis, orthopnea, paroxysmal nocturnal dyspnea, palpitation, heart murmurs, pain, previous electrocardiograms (dates and details); claudication, varicosities, stasis dermatitis or ulcer, etc.

Gastrointestinal
Pain, dysphagia, regurgitation, nausea, vomiting, hematemesis, ulcer, previous X-rays, jaundice, dark urine, pruritus, cholelithiasis, belching, gas, constipation, diarrhea, laxatives abuse, tenesmus, painful defecation, hematochezia, melena, fatty or acholic stools, diet restrictions or idiosyncrasies, anorexia and change in appetite

Weight
Current, recent change (+ or −, amount, over what period), highest, lowest (with dates), weight at age 25

Endocrine-Metabolic
Polydipsia, polyphagia, polyuria, diabetes (insulin, oral agents, or neither), hair growth and distribution, age at puberty, goiter, exophthalmos, sweating, nervousness, heat or cold intolerance, change in appearance or voice

Genitourinary
Frequency (day/night), urgency, dysuria, retention, dribbling, enuresis, colic, stone, fever, chill, oliguria, smoky, cloudy, or bloody urine, venereal disease, stricture, history of albumin, glycosuria, nephritis, libido, impotence

Female Reproductive
Age at menarche, menstrual interval, regularity, duration, flow, last normal menstrual period (LNMP), pain, spotting, menopause and symptoms, post-menopausal bleeding, discharge, itching, libido, dyspareunia; list pregnancies in sequence by year, nature of outcome, complications; contraceptive methods

Breasts
Lumps or masses, swelling, pain, galactorrhea, details of any biopsy

Musculoskeletal
Trauma and sequelae, arthritis, gout, spasm, pain, backache, weakness, deformities

Neurological
Head or spine injury, paralysis, weakness, parasthesias, anesthesia, vertigo, faintness, syncope, seizures, coma, memory defect, stroke, aphasia, tremor, ataxia, headache

Emotional
Personal profile and self-evaluation; insomnia, depression, crying, anxiety, phobias, amnesia, delusions, hallucinations, history of "nervous breakdown" or of psychiatric treatment

*Underlined terms are defined in the ROS Glossary at the back of the book.

tus, which are purposely reserved until the end. This ordering of the questions allows patients to become comfortable with and fully understand the process of the ROS so that they are not offended by and reluctant to answer questions pertaining to their psychological state.

A portion of the ROS for the skin, head, and neck areas for Mr. Green appears in the following dialogue. Notice how the health professional effects the transition into the ROS and provides Mr. Green with specific instructions regarding his possible answers.

Health Professional: Mr. Green, we have finally gotten to the last part of this interview. In this final section I want to make sure that I have not missed some important fact. So, just hang in there for a few minutes, OK?

Mr. Green: I guess so—but I'm getting hungry!

Health Professional: Mr. Green, I'm going to ask you a series of questions about yourself and any other symptoms you may have had that we have not previously discussed. I am interested in only those problems that may occur or recur on a repeated basis. I will recite a long list of possible complaints. Please interrupt me if I mention a problem that you have experienced. Do you understand what I mean?

Mr. Green: You mean that I should stop you only if I have had the problem myself or if the problem has occurred a number of times?

Health Professional: That's right. Here we go! Have you ever had problems with acne, boils, shingles, rashes, ulcers, dry skin or hair, itching, bruising, bleeding, or other problems with your skin?

Mr. Green: I had seven boils during my last year of high school, but that's all.

Health Professional: OK, how about your head and neck? Have you ever had problems with your eyes, including difficulty in

seeing, double vision, eye pain, a "lazy eye," cataracts, injuries, tearing, dryness, or blind spots?

Mr. Green: Well, I've seen double a few times when I've left Ralph's Place, after a few too many, but that's all!

Health Professional: Yes, I understand that can be a problem—but not too worrisome if it goes away by the next morning, right?

Mr. Green: I guess so.

Health Professional: How about your ears? Have you had any problems with hearing, pain, discharge, ringing in your ears, or a sensation that you were spinning?

Mr. Green: Nothing.

Health Professional: Have you had trouble with your nose giving you smell problems, a discharge, blockage, nose bleeds, sinus trouble, or hay fever?

Mr. Green: I have hay fever in the spring and fall. I think I'm allergic to grass and goldenrod.

The ROS continues methodically probing into each of the body systems. If positive items are revealed, the examiner may stop and discuss the items in detail using the P^2QRST factors once again. Imagine that the ROS on Mr. Green has now progressed to the items pertaining to the genitourinary tract. No significant new information has been obtained so far from the ROS.

Health Professional: Mr. Green, we spoke earlier in some detail about your kidneys and urinary tract, which seem to be the system most affected by your present illness. Also, you admitted that you have some burning and a need to urinate more urgently and frequently than usual. But, then, you seemed a bit upset when I asked you about venereal disease. Does the possibility of having a venereal disease concern you?

Mr. Green: Who, me? Oh no, nothing like that. I told you I haven't even thought about VD since they showed us all those movies in the Army.

Again, the health professional senses that Mr. Green is uncomfortable in talking about VD. In view of Mr. Green's complaints, it appears increasingly likely that a venereal infection may be related to the symptoms. Rather than badgering the patient, the interviewer proceeds with a different tack on the problem.

Health Professional: As I recall from our earlier conversation, you mentioned that you have dated a number of times since you have been divorced. Does my memory serve me correctly?

Mr. Green: Yes, that's true.

Health Professional: Did you have sexual contact with any of your dates?

Mr. Green: Yes, several of them.

Health Professional: How long ago was your last sexual contact?

Mr. Green: Why are you pushing me so hard on this business about my sex life? I don't see why you need to know these things.

Health Professional: Well, I'm sorry if it makes you uncomfortable. I asked you earlier whether or not you had ever had VD, and you appeared a bit embarrassed about it. Also, very early in this interview I asked you if you had noticed any kind of a discharge from the penis, and you said you had not seen a discharge. It appears that you are reluctant to talk about the possibility of VD. However, from the story that you have told me about the burning and frequency of urination and the fact that you have had sexual contact with a number of women, I am concerned that VD could be a possibility. Are you scared that you may have VD and can't bring yourself to talk about it?

Mr. Green: Well, I guess I have thought about it. But don't you always have a lot of discharge with VD?

Health Professional: With some types of VD you may have a lot of discharge. Not all types, however. And not every person has the same symptoms.

Mr. Green: Well, that does bother me some.

Health Professional: Let me ask you a few more questions about your sexual contacts. When was your last sexual contact?

Mr. Green: Well, I went bar-hopping with one of my buddies one weekend about a month ago. Angie had to work. We met two girls, got loaded, and spent the night at their apartment.

Health Professional: Did you have sexual contact with either of the girls?

Mr. Green: Yes, I slept with one, and my friend slept with the other one. That was the first time I ever cheated on Angie and. . . .

Health Professional: What happened since that time?

Mr. Green: Well, about three days afterwards I started getting this burning every time I tried to urinate. I was going out of my mind. I couldn't find the nerve to go see my regular doctor. I was too embarrassed. So, I kept putting off getting an appointment, and the burning got worse and worse. About the same time I also developed a thick, yellow discharge from my penis. The discharge disappeared after three or four days, except for little traces of it on my underwear. Well, I thought I had gonorrhea, and I didn't want to give it to Angie. I couldn't tell her what had happened, and she can't understand what she did to me because all of a sudden I won't stay overnight at her place. Well, I finally got up my nerve and picked a number out of the phone book, and you were it. Do you think I could have VD?

That's why I haven't slept with Angie, 'cause I thought I might give it to her!

Health Professional: Well, your story made me wonder about the possibility of gonorrhea—or one of the other types of VD. Now the combination of your symptoms and the discharge seem to make a more plausible story. It won't be difficult to try to confirm the diagnosis. Then we will know more about how to proceed. First, though, I'll need to examine you when we are done here to see what

physical findings we may be able to discover.

Note from the preceding dialogue how adroitly the interviewer was able to switch from the ROS concerning the genitourinary tract back to social history. This contributed substantially to resolving the perplexing history of the present illness. The logical, deliberate progression of the questioning and the nonjudgmental posture of the interviewer reassured Mr. Green that there was no need for embarrassment while discussing sensitive and personal material. Further detail such as the exact

LEARNING ACTIVITIES

Review of Systems

Using the foregoing dialogue between Mr. Green and the health professional and a telegraphic style of writing, record an appropriate ROS for the skin, head, and neck using the following outline. "Skin" is completed as an example. Feedback follows the learning activity.

      Skin: 7 boils while in high school

      Head and Neck: Eyes—

             Ears—

             Nose—

Feedback

      Skin: 7 boils while in high school
      Head and Neck: Eyes—normal
             Ears—normal
             Nose—"hay fever" in spring and fall with possible
                     allergy to grass and goldenrod
(Skip through the review of systems to genitourinary.)
Genitourinary: (see HPI)
Note: Since the entire ROS for the urogenital tract is germane to Mr.
          Green's HPI, the information is recorded only in the HPI and the
          ROS contains only an index reference.

Now you have read the chapter and assimilated the dialogue with Mr. Green. You should be able to complete the following learning activity for History of Present Illness and conduct a health history practice interview.

History of Present Illness

The preceding pages have elucidated a method for taking the medical history. Using the technique described in the chapter and the Guide for the Health History presented on page 180 of this chapter, write the history of present illness for Mr. Green as revealed in the dialogue throughout the chapter. Write in your best narrative prose style and organize the write-up chronologically using the following blank space or a separate sheet of paper. Feedback follows.

Feedback

Approximately one month ago, Mr. Green had sexual intercourse with a female other than his regular sexual partner. Three days later he noted the onset of pain and frequency of urination. About the same time a thick, yellow penile discharge appeared. The symptoms have continued to the present time, but the discharge has largely disappeared.

The pain is described as a "stinging or burning" sensation present most of the time in the pubic area and through the penis. It is aggravated by the passage of urine but is localized to the region described and does not radiate to other areas of the body, including the legs or back. It causes such excruciating pain that he feels as if he's "passing red hot iron." He has had trouble in initiating the urine stream due to the pain. The urge to urinate occurs approximately every 30 minutes. When urine does flow, the amounts are extremely small, only a few drops at a time. When the few drops have passed, he has a continued urge to urinate and feels as if his bladder has ₙot totally emptied. In addition, the pain is so severe that he finds he must lie down and rest after an attempt to urinate.

He claims that the only factors tending to aggravate the pain are the act of urination and a reduced fluid intake. When his fluid intake is reduced he also notices that his urine output is lowered and the urine has a foul odor. Some relief is obtained by ingesting a small "red pill" (unknown) previously prescribed for treatment of a urinary tract infection, which he took three times a day. The pill tends to render the urine "orange colored."

Associated with the pain, urgency, and frequency was a thick, yellow penile discharge. The amount of discharge was sufficient enough to stain his underwear for 3 or 4 days. Then it disappeared except for traces of discharge that occasionally stained his underwear. He denies any problems with dribbling (other than with the present illness) and has noted no hematuria.

Notice in the HPI how the information from all seven parts of the medical interview is woven together to create a chronological, narrative story. Also notice how each of the items from the ROS was placed in the HPI either as a "positive" or "negative" finding.

Health History Practice Interviews

In order to practice the process of obtaining a health history, conduct a role-play interview using a friend or classmate as the patient. Using the mnemonics given in this chapter and the Guide for the Health History (p. 180), conduct your interview to include (1) ID, (2) CC, (3) HPI, (4) PMH, (5) Family History, (6) Social History, and (7) ROS. Complete the role play in 30 minutes or less.

To assess the adequacy of your technique, write down the results of your interview, and then compare your record with a tape-recorded playback or have your classmate critique your write-up, using the Guide for the Health History as the device for assessment.

Suggested role-play patient problems are:

1. Any acute or chronic personal medical problem of the patient.

2. A 20-year-old black female college student who works 28 hours a week as a waitress has a three-week history of dull, throbbing headaches located in the back of the neck and into the scalp. The headaches are absent in the morning and become increasingly severe as the day wears on. They are particularly incapacitating when she must wait tables for the evening meal and are also aggravated by the menses, stress, and lack of sleep. Recently, her usual boyfriend has become interested in another coed. Rest, weekends, and three aspirin tablets are the only factors that have provided relief.

3. A 19-year-old white male prisoner in the county jail complains of inability to eat the jail food, as it causes him nausea, vomiting, and diarrhea. The symptoms also are associated with cramping and mid-abdominal pain. He has had no relief from several antacids. He denies any blood in the stool and indicates that his diarrhea recurs several times daily with "watery stools." Several other prisoners have similar complaints.

Guide for the Health History

I.D.   Name [ ]   Sex [ ]   General health status [ ]
        Age [ ]   Race [ ]   Occupation [ ]

C.C.   State in patient's own words.

H.P.I. For pain: provocative [ ]   palliative [ ]   quality [ ]
                  region [ ]   severity [ ]   temporal characteristics [ ]
        For psychosocial problem: who [ ]   what [ ]   when [ ]
                                     where [ ]   how [ ]

P.M.H. P = Preventive medical Hx = immunizations [ ]   last diphtheria immun. [ ]
                                                          last tetanus immun. [ ]

        A = Allergy history =   penicillin [ ]   mycins [ ]
        S = Surgery history =   procedure [ ]   when [ ]   by whom [ ]
        T = Transfusions =   with what procedure [ ]   blood reaction [ ]
        M = Medications =   name [ ]   strength [ ]   dose schedule [ ]
        E = Earlier history =   name [ ]   time lost from work/school [ ]
        D = Delivery history =   gravida [ ]   preemies [ ]   abortions [ ]   parity [ ]

Fam. Hx (genetic diagram)
              marriage   siblings
        [ ]———————O   45 ⊠ dead 45-year-old   ◇7 7 siblings unknown
       male   female   male, stroke

Soc. Hx   M = Marriage = # years married [ ]   divorced [ ]   separated [ ]
                          # years since death of spouse [ ]
                Heterosexual [ ]   Alternate sexual lifestyle [ ]
                Sexually active [ ]   Not sexually active [ ]
          O = Occupation = list of current and past employment [ ]
                Exposure to fumes [ ]   chemicals [ ]   dust [ ]   noise [ ]   radiation [ ]
          L = Lifestyle: Castle: own/rent [ ]   utilities [ ]   urban/rural [ ]
                         Diet: amount [ ]   variety [ ]   food fads [ ]
                         # cups coffee [ ]   tea [ ]   cola [ ]   /day
                         Exercise: sedentary [ ]   moderate activity [ ]   marked activity [ ]
                         Fun: none [ ]   high risk [ ]   toxic exposure [ ]
          E = Ethanol consumption = type [ ]   amount [ ]   frequency [ ]   duration [ ]
          S = Smoking = cigarettes [ ]   cigars [ ]   pipes [ ]
                        pack/day [ ]   × years [ ]   = pack years [ ]
          T = Travel =   USA [ ]   outside USA [ ]   camping, etc. [ ]

ROS: Check against list on page 174.

dates and names of contacts probably would be easily elicited by following this line of questioning, after the importance of tracing the contact had been explained. In a similar fashion, additional questions could be posed regarding unconventional sexual practices if these were germane to the problem under discussion.

Chapter Summary

This chapter listed and discussed the seven major parts of a health history interview. In sequential fashion these are (1) Patient Identification, (2) Chief Complaint, (3) History of Present Illness, (4) Past Medical History, (5) Family History, (6) Social History, and (7) Review of Systems. In addition, mnemonics for the History of Present Illness (P^2QRST or Who, What, When, Where, and How), Past Medical History (PASTMED), and Social History (MOLEST) were defined. We presented guides for writing the Patient ID, Chief Complaint, Family History, and Review of Systems, and, in addition, we provided a Guide for the Health History for evaluation of practice interviews.

Differences in the sequence of obtaining and recording the health history were pointed out, and the example demonstrated the synthesis of all the historical information into the recorded HPI. In addition, we discussed the variations that may occur in an interview because of examiner bias, interview purpose, and so on. The need for a narrative record of the identification (ID), chief complaint (CC), and history of present illness (HPI) was compared and contrasted with the telegraphic style of recording utilized for the past medical history (PMH), family history (Fam. Hx), social history (Soc. Hx), and ROS. In addition, we emphasized the need for accurate, succinct, and concise records without duplication of information.

The systematic use of the seven traditional components of a health history allows interviewers to progress through an interview in a deliberate fashion that augments rapport with patients and reduces patient anxiety. At the same time interviewers gain a large amount of reliable, detailed health history data in a short time. Finally, the standardized format allows interviewers to record the results of their efforts in a way that is readily accessible to and understandable by other members of the health team so that improvement in patient care may result. (Now do learning activity on p. 177).

Suggested Readings _____

DeGowin, E. L., & DeGowin, R. L. *Bedside diagnostic examination*. New York: Macmillan, 1976. Chapter 2, "A Practical Discussion of the Medical Record, the History Taking Process and the Diagnostic Attitudes of Pain (P^2QRST)," describes in further detail some of the concepts presented in this chapter.

Goldman, R., & Peters, J. The occupational and environmental health history. *Journal of the American Medical Association*, 1981, *246*, 2831–2836. The authors suggest a practical and succinct method for obtaining an occupational history.

Hillman, R. S., Goodell, B. W., Grundy, S. M., McArthur, J. R., & Moller, J. H. *Clinical skills: Interviewing, history taking, and physical diagnosis*. New York: McGraw-Hill, 1981. Chapter 2, "Adult History and Medical Record," and Chapter 3, "Pediatric History and Medical Record," provide concise descriptions of the features of the health history in interviewing adults and children.

Lipkin, M. *The care of patients: Concepts and tactics*. New York: Oxford University Press, 1974. Chapter 3,

"Diagnostic Problems: Methods and Pitfalls of Collecting Information," emphasizes, in easy, readable fashion, the importance of history taking, of establishing rapport, of defining terms, of avoiding the tendency to equate symptoms with complaints, of avoiding medical jargon, and so on.

Morgan, W. L., & Engel, G. L. *The clinical approach to the patient*. Philadelphia: Saunders, 1969. A good standard reference regarding the interviewing of patients.

Reiser, D., & Schroder, A. *Patient interviewing: The human dimension*. Baltimore: Williams and Wilkins, 1980. Chapter 8, "Components of the Medical History," gives an excellent discussion of the various parts of a thorough health history interview.

Walker, H. K., Hall, W. D., & Hurst, J. W. *Clinical methods*. Boston: Butterworth, 1976. Chapters 1, 4, 5, and 6 give a very concise discussion with suggested formats for conducting a health interview.

Instructions, Information Giving, and Patient Compliance

Objectives

After completing this chapter you will be able to do the following:

1. Using a written example, evaluate in writing the interviewer's delivery of instructions based on nine criteria.

2. Using a written case, evaluate in writing the interviewer's delivery of information based on five criteria of effective information giving.

3. In a simulated activity, present information to a role-play patient demonstrating at least four out of five criteria for effective delivery of information.

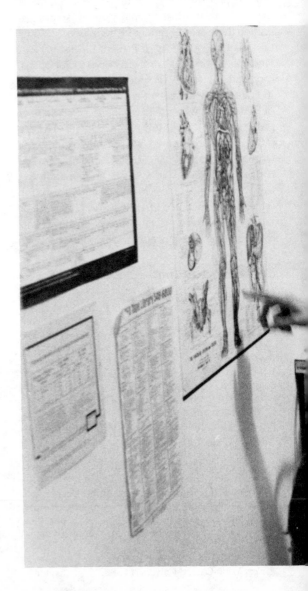

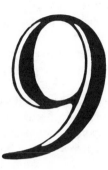

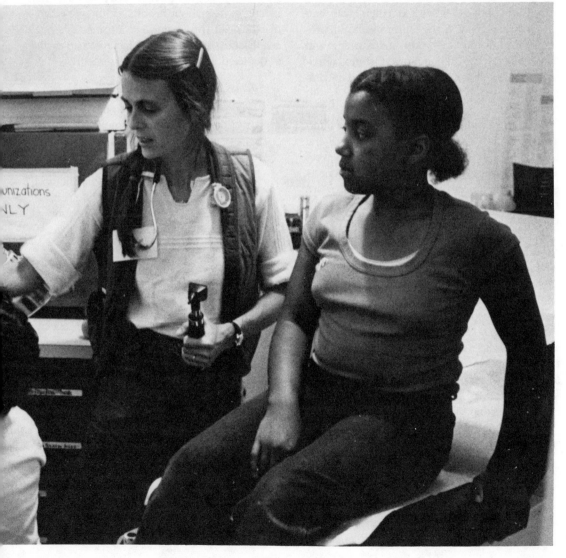

One of the major tasks confronting health professionals is how to give appropriate and useful instructions and information to patients. A great deal of any health professional's time is spent giving instructions to patients about treatment regimens, laboratory tests, medications, life management, and so on. Health care providers are also constantly faced with the challenge of providing important information to patients concerning their diagnoses, clinical findings, nature of the illness, management of the illness, alternative treatments, and prognoses. Patients both need to know and are legally entitled to know about their health and illness management. At the same time, health professionals rely on their skill at informing and instructing patients to encourage them to participate actively in their own health care and to comply with the advice and suggestions of the health professional.

This aspect of the professional/patient interaction involves some of the most frequent and frustrating problems for patients and interviewers alike. Patients are annoyed because their requests for information seem to fall on deaf ears or are met with an inadequate response. From a patient's perspective, too little or incomplete information is worse than no information or too much information. At the same time, health professionals, who have many demands on their time, find it difficult to gauge how much information to give to patients and how to give it effectively and efficiently. This chapter will describe two interviewing skills, *providing instructions* and *information giving,* and will discuss the use of these skills in promoting patient compliance. Patient compliance is manifested by: (1) entering into or continuing treatment; (2) keeping follow-up or referral appointments; (3) taking medication as prescribed; and (4) restricting or changing behaviors such as smoking, diet, and exercise (Kasl, 1975, p. 6).

Instructions

Instructions or directions are verbal statements in which the interviewer instructs or directs the patient to do something. Instructions have both *influenc-*

ing and *informative* effects. According to Cormier and Cormier (1979), "instructions should help to encourage and influence a person to respond in a certain way and should also provide information that helps a patient perform a certain task" (p. 101).

Unfortunately, in health care management instructions do not always serve their intended purpose. Many patients do not follow the directions given to them by their health care provider. Some of the reasons for this are out of the interviewer's control. For example, the patient may hold certain beliefs about his or her illness or habits that the health professional cannot modify directly and that the patient shows no inclination to change, as depicted in the following example:

Health Professional: Chuck, will you consider reducing the amount you smoke or totally stopping your cigarette smoking?

Patient: Well, I spent twelve years in the submarine service and then nine years working in a penitentiary. Taking all those risks didn't kill me, so I guess the risks associated with cigarettes won't get me either.

Guidelines for Giving Instructions

However, patients may also disregard instructions because of the way in which the instructions are presented to them. Although use of effective instructions represents only one way to promote compliance, recognition of and adherence to the following guidelines will increase the likelihood of patient compliance. These guidelines are summarized in Table 9-1.

First, specific instructions are more effective than general ones (Doster, 1972; McGuire, Thelen, and Amolsch, 1975; Stone & Gotlib, 1975). Consider the differences in the following two sets of instructions given to a patient by a nurse practitioner:

It's very important that you take care of yourself, especially in the first few weeks of breast feeding while your milk supply is being established. Or—

It's very important in these first few weeks of breast feeding that you take care of yourself in certain ways to help establish your milk supply. Try to drink a lot of fluid—any kind except alcohol—and get adequate rest. Lie down for 15 or 20 minutes twice a day. Even if you don't sleep, the rest will help.

In the first example the instructions "take care of yourself" are too vague. The patient's interpretation might be very different from what the nurse

practitioner had in mind. In the second example, the nurse specifies how the patient should take care of herself—by drinking a lot of fluids and getting adequate rest, including two rest periods during the day.

Brief and concise instructions are easier to follow than lengthy directions (Doster, 1972; McGuire, Thelen, & Amolsch, 1975; Stone & Gotlib, 1975). It is better, for example, to provide instructions to hospitalized patients in "small doses" than to give one lengthy set of directions just prior to discharge.

Table 9-1
Instructions: Purposes and Guidelines for Use

Definition	Purpose	Guidelines for Use

One or more verbal statements in which the interviewer instructs a patient to do something	1. To influence a patient to respond in a particular way
	2. To inform a patient how to perform a certain task or regimen
		1. Be as specific as possible.
		2. Keep instructions brief and concise.
		3. Deliver instructions as suggestions, not commands, in a friendly, not dogmatic, manner.
		4. Confirm whether the patient understands the instructions.
		5. Supplement oral instructions with written or typed "take home" instructions.
		6. Some oral instructions may need to be supplemented with modeling or demonstrations.
		7. Motivate the patient to use the instructions—for example, invite patient participation in the process of giving and following instructions, as in the use of contracts, self-monitoring, or daily logs.
		8. Link compliance of instructions to positive or rewarding consequences:
		  a. Simplify the treatment regimen as much as possible.
		  b. If possible, arrange the regimen so that compliance to it will provide some rapid relief of symptoms or complaints.
		  c. Arrange for positively reinforcing events—or for social support—to follow patient's compliance with the treatment.
		9. Follow up your instructions by a telephone call or note or in person at your next contact or visit. Followup may be provided by you or by a colleague or aide.

Instructions also are more likely to be followed if they are worded and delivered in a friendly rather than a dogmatic manner. As Long and Prophit (1981) note, instructions should "take the form of suggestions, not commands" (p. 178). Many patients dislike being told what to do or not to do concerning their health (Matthews & Hingson, 1977). They will automatically resist and resent instructions delivered by a "drill sergeant." If you word your instructions carefully and the patient still rejects them, the instructions were probably offered before the patient was ready to accept them.

The interviewer should remember that, although good instructions have been given, there is no guarantee that patients will understand them. After giving the directions, verify whether or not patients really understand what you are asking them to do. Simply ask the patient to repeat the instructions back to you, with emphasis on how to follow the prescribed regimen (Cormier & Cormier, 1979; Matthews & Hingson, 1977; Shulman, 1974).

To aid the patient's understanding and recall of instructions, supplement your oral instructions with written or typed summaries that patients can take home with them (Bernstein & Bernstein, 1980; Matthews & Hingson, 1977). Suggest to patients that they put the instructions in a highly visible place, such as on a mirror or the refrigerator door. Written contracts that spell out the professional's instructions as well as the patient's agreement to follow them have been found effective with hypertensive patients (Stekel & Swain, 1977). Melamed and Siegel (1980) note that "a key point of this procedure was to encourage the patients to write the contract and to assist them in analyzing the process into manageable steps" (p. 119).

Some oral and written instructions may still be unclear to patients unless supplemented by modeling and demonstration. For example, a new mother may not understand a nurse's oral instructions on how to induce the sucking reflex in her newborn infant. However, if the nurse models this process either by demonstrating with the infant or by showing the mother pictures or slides, then the mother may understand exactly what to do. Similarly, a father who will be giving insulin injections to a diabetic child will need to observe the procedure and practice his skills before actually administering the injections.

Patient Compliance with Instructions

Health care professionals must motivate the patient to follow the instructions once they are understood. Increased patient participation in the process of developing, giving, and following instructions may be one way to increase patient motivation. In the study mentioned above with hypertensive patients, all patients complied with the terms of the contracts that they had helped prepare (Stekel & Swain, 1977). In another study with hypertensive patients (Haynes, Sackett, Gibson, Taylor, Hackett, Roberts, & Johnson, 1976), half of the patients (comprising the experimental group) were taught a method for monitoring and charting their own blood pressure and scheduling their medication. In addition, they were seen by a paraprofessional health worker every two weeks to review their charts and to encourage their progress. The control group received no such instruction or follow-up. Six months later, an evaluation of the control group revealed a 1.5 percent *reduction* in compliance, whereas the experimental group demonstrated a 21.3 percent *increase* in compliance. According to Bernstein and Bernstein (1980), "apparently the opportunity to observe the benefits of medication on their self-recorded blood pressures provided the necessary motivation" (p. 34).

Another effort to motivate patients to follow instructions by increasing their decision making and participation was suggested by Zifferblatt (1975), who recommended the use of a written log or diary to record adherence to a treatment regimen. Patients are more likely to keep a log if the entries to be made in it are brief. Epstein and Masek (1978) were successful in having patients write down the times when they took their medication. These authors found that such self-recording of medication times improved compliance.

Instructions are more likely to be followed if they are linked to positive or rewarding consequences (Melamed & Siegel, 1980; Shulman, 1974). Melamed and Siegel (1980) explain the role of positive consequences as follows:

> Consequences that immediately follow the desired behavior also affect the probable occurrence of that behavior. If the consequences are pleasant or reinforcing, the health-related behavior is more likely to occur, whereas compliance with the therapeutic regimen is less likely to occur if the compliance behavior results in either no reinforcing consequences or aversive events (p. 115).

Positive consequences may include improvement in health or function and the use of positive reinforcement for adherence to instructions.

There are several ways in which this principle can be implemented practically. First, simplify the instructions and regimen that the patient must follow as much as possible. Second, arrange the regimen so that compliance with it is likely to make the patient feel better in a fairly short time. As Bernstein and Bernstein (1980) note:

> If the prescribed regimen is likely to be a complex one, begin with one or two items that are likely to give relatively rapid relief. When the patient observes the benefits from this simple compliance, he will be more likely to accept and follow additional instructions that may make greater demands on him and take longer to effect results ... (p. 32).

Unfortunately, as Zifferblatt (1975) observes, not all medical regimens bring rapid relief. Some regimens have negative side effects, and others, such as those prescribed for preventive reasons, have neutral and very few, if any, noticeable positive consequences. The solution to this problem is to contrive positive consequences, either in the form of positive reinforcing activities or events or social reinforcement or support. For example, a patient might engage in an enjoyable activity, such as reading the newspaper, talking on the telephone, or watching television, only after taking the prescribed medication or after completing some other part of the prescribed treatment program. This principle has been effective in increasing compliance in young children as well as adults. Patients who receive strong doses of social reinforcement, such as support and encouragement from their spouse and a health professional, are more motivated to comply with medical instructions (Caplan, Robinson, French, Caldwell, & Shinn, 1976). Stuart and Davis (1972) refer to such persons as *social allies*—individuals with whom the patient has fairly frequent contact and who can remind patients about their treatment and positively reinforce them for complying with treatment regimens. The principle of the social ally is the keystone of organizations such as Alcoholics Anonymous and Weight Watchers International.

Follow-up: Repeating and Reviewing Instructions

Finally, once instructions have been given, follow-up is very important. Encouraging patient understanding of and compliance with instructions is a cumulative process that develops over time and with repeated patient contacts. Bernstein and Bernstein (1980) state that "instruction of patients is not a one-time event. Follow-up shortly after the instructions increases the likelihood of remembering" (p. 33). For example, a dental hygienist who has instructed a new patient on how to brush and floss her teeth can recheck the patient's technique at their next contact. Frequently, health professionals assume that long-term patients still remember initial instructions that may have been given months or years ago. It is not uncommon, for example, for health professionals to nearly overwhelm a mother-to-be with all sorts of instructions on self-care during pregnancy. Yet when the same patient returns four years later during a subsequent pregnancy, the health professional may assume that new instructions or a review of previous instructions are not necessary. All patients need repeated reminders about instructions in order to assure continued compliance. Such follow-up does not always have to be initiated by the attending professional. A supporting team member, a colleague, or an aide can take responsibility for follow-up.

These guidelines for the use of instructions in patient care are also applicable to interactions with families and colleagues. Often practitioners will need to instruct a patient or another family member in aspects of patient care when the patient is too young, too ill, or too confused to understand and follow the directions without assistance.

Effective delivery of instructions is critical in interactions with other members of the health care team as well. A subordinate's or colleague's failure to follow your instructions may be due not to carelessness or insubordination but rather to vague or overly complicated directions. Demonstrations of procedures are especially important for new team

LEARNING ACTIVITIES

Instructions

In the following dialogue a dental hygienist is giving instructions to an eight-year-old patient about care of the teeth. Your task is to evaluate the hygienist's instructions using the nine criteria listed in the learning activity on p. 189 (Chapter Objective 1). Check the accuracy of your evaluation with the feedback presented following the learning activity.

Dental Hygienist: John, I'd like you to take really good care of your teeth. Know what that means?

John: Yeah—making sure I brush them.

Dental Hygienist: Right. Brush them at least two times a day—it doesn't matter when as long as whenever you do it becomes a habit for you. When do you usually remember to brush your teeth?

John: Well, I always brush them after breakfast when I'm getting ready for school. Once in a while on weekends I forget. And I usually do it every night before I go to bed.

Dental Hygienist: Great. Those are two really great times. And the idea of a habit or schedule helps you remember. As you said, it is easier for you to remember on school days because it is part of your daily routine. Now let's make sure you know how to brush them—up and down like this, not across [shows John the strokes with a toothbrush]. It's important to have a routine to this, too. Start in the same place instead of skipping around. How does that sound?

John: OK, I think I've got it.

Dental Hygienist: OK, now you try it. [John practices while hygienist observes.] That's great, you're doing a good job. Now—one more thing. This piece of string—called floss—gets into the cracks between your teeth where the brush can't reach. It's very important that you use this floss in each crack at least one time each day. Let me show you how it works [demonstrates with floss]—see, it works, even in these back teeth. You try it now.

John: OK, but this flossing is harder for me to do.

Dental Hygienist: Give it a try. It takes some practice. That's good. OK, you just need a little piece. Sometimes a big piece gets in the way, but if it's too long, wrap the floss around your finger. Now before you leave can you tell or show me how you're going to take care of your teeth at home?

John: Well, I need to get in a routine of making sure I brush them twice a day and floss once a day. I need to remember to floss. Here's how I'm going to brush [shows hygienist]. The floss should go like this [shows hygienist].

Now assess the hygienist's instructions by answering the following questions (check the appropriate blank):

1. Were the instructions specific?

   _____ Yes   _____ No

2. Were the instructions concise?

   _____ Yes   _____ No

3. Were the suggestions given in a friendly manner and worded as suggestions?

   _____ Yes   _____ No

4. Did the hygienist confirm whether the patient understood the instructions?

   _____ Yes   _____ No

5. Did the hygienist give the patient written or typed "take home" instructions to supplement the oral ones?

   _____ Yes   _____ No

6. Did the hygienist supplement the oral instructions with modeling or demonstration?

   _____ Yes   _____ No

7. Did the hygienist suggest ways to help the patient participate in complying with instructions (contracts, logs, monitoring, and so on)?

   _____ Yes   _____ No

8. Did the hygienist attempt to link patient compliance with the instructions to positive consequences (relief of symptoms, social support, positively reinforcing event)?

   _____ Yes   _____ No

9. Did the hygienist arrange for a follow-up to determine the patient's understanding of and compliance with the instructions?

   _____ Yes   _____ No

Based on your evaluation of the hygienist's instructions, what suggestions would you make to this person to improve her or his giving instructions in the future?

Feedback

1. The instructions were specific—the hygienist told John precisely the ways in which he could take care of his teeth.
2. The instructions were concise—the hygienist said exactly what the patient needed to know and no more.
3. Although we could not see the hygienist's nonverbal behavior, the wording indicated that the instructions were delivered as suggestions and were given in a friendly manner.
4. The hygienist did confirm whether John understood the instructions by asking him questions and by asking him to repeat back the instructions at the end of the scenario.
5. The hygienist apparently did not give John take-home instructions.
6. The hygienist did use demonstration on two different occasions—showing John the correct way to brush and to floss his teeth.
7. The hygienist did not suggest ways to help John participate in complying with instructions.
8. The hygienist did not link John's compliance to any positive consequences.
9. The hygienist apparently did not arrange for a follow-up.

The hygienist met five of the nine criteria. Areas of improvement would include use of take-home instructions, suggestion of ways for the patient to participate in compliance, linking of compliance with positive consequences, and use of a follow-up. The following example depicts how the hygienist might incorporate these elements into another set of instructions about care of your teeth. The hygienist would say everything said in the previous example given on pp. 188–189 with the following addition:

> OK, that's great. John, one hard part is remembering to brush at least twice a day and to floss at least once a day. But if you do that each day your teeth will be less likely to decay and you can come in for just a check-up and not have to worry so much about getting all those cavities filled [linking compliance to a positive consequence—no or fewer cavities]. Here's something you can do to help you remember how often to brush and floss. You can take this sticker chart home and put it by your bathroom mirror. Each time you brush or floss your teeth, take one of these "smiley" stickers and put it over here—by the picture of the toothbrush for brushing or by the dental floss for flossing [suggesting a way for patient to participate in compliance via monitoring]. Also, I'm going to give you this picture to take home that shows the correct way to brush and floss—just like we practiced today. Keep it near the place where you usually brush your teeth [using take-home instructions]. And I'm going to reschedule you for another visit in six months—then we can see how you're doing.

Note that the sticker chart and pictorial instructions can be used even with patients who cannot read.

members who may be inexperienced or unaccustomed to the way in which a procedure is done in your service or setting. Supplementing oral instructions with written summaries and demonstrations helps to ensure accuracy and precision and to avoid costly errors in patient care. (Now do learning activity on p. 188).

Information Giving

In contrast to giving a patient instructions about a particular task or treatment regimen, information giving consists of verbal communication of data or facts to a patient. Effective information giving requires the health care provider to recognize when a patient needs information and what information he or she needs. Information giving is the cornerstone of patient education. A lack of information at a critical time may exacerbate patient problems in any or all three spheres described in Chapter 4—physical, environmental, and psychological. As Bernstein and Bernstein (1980) suggest, "a patient can feel genuinely reassured when given correct information at the time he needs it by someone he trusts" (p. 63).

Information giving serves a number of different purposes in patient interviewing. First, information tells a patient about his or her options in a given situation. For example, a patient who has been diagnosed as having a small cancer in her left breast with metastases should be informed about all of the available treatment options.

Second, information can help a patient envision outcomes from the available options and evaluate and select the best alternative. In the example above, information should be provided that will increase the patient's knowledge about the effects, risks, side effects, and benefits of treatments such as radical or conservative surgery, radiation, chemotherapy, and so on.

A third purpose of information giving is to correct misconceptions and to dispel myths. For example, if the patient above should assume or believe that a miracle cure for breast cancer had been discovered—for example, laetrile—the interviewer must make certain the patient's information about this drug is as reliable and accurate

as possible. Another patient might decide not to have surgery because of ignorance about the uses and advances in prosthetics following a mastectomy.

A fourth purpose of information giving is to increase the likelihood of patient compliance. As Matthews and Hingson (1977) note, if patients are not given feedback about their condition, they are less likely to comply with the health professional's requests.

The purposes of information giving are summarized in Table 9-2. An additional purpose, the use of preparatory information to reduce patient anxiety and apprehension, is discussed later in Chapter 13.

Note that information giving in this context differs from *advice giving*. In advice giving, someone recommends that another person follow a particular solution or course of action. In contrast, information giving consists of presenting a number of different alternatives and details about those alternatives. The final decision about which course of action to pursue rests with the patient. Consider this difference in the following example, in which a health professional is talking to a young adult who has had several sore throats in the past year.

Health Professional: I believe you'd better have your tonsils out as soon as we can arrange it because of all the sore throats you've been having. [advice giving]

Health Professional: You have now had three serious sore throats this year, all caused by the germ known as the streptococcus, or strep. Many authorities feel that such a series of serious infections may be sufficient reason to take out your tonsils. There is no single cut-and-dried right answer to this dilemma. But if you have more recurrent strep throats, you may want to consider having your tonsils removed. Right now, since you are well again, let's just wait and see what happens. OK? [information giving]

In the first example, advice giving, the health professional categorically recommends one and only one course of action and even fails to provide a rationale for the recommended procedure. In the second example, information giving, the professional cited alternative courses of action. And although the interviewer gave the patient some guidance, the patient could either concur with or object to the treatment that was presented.

There are several dangers associated with advice giving that make it a trap the wise health professional will avoid. First, the patient not only may reject the advice but may overreact and reject any further efforts or suggestions from the health professional. Second, if the patient accepts the advice and the advice leads to an unsatisfactory outcome, the patient is likely to blame the health professional. Finally, if the patient follows the advice and is satisfied with the outcome, he or she may become overly dependent on the health professional in subsequent interactions.

There are three general principles to consider in effective information giving. These can be referred to as the *when, what,* and *how* of giving

Table 9-2
Information Giving: Purposes and Guidelines for Use

Definition	Purposes	Guidelines for Use

Verbal communication of data or facts to a patient	1. To inform patient of possible options
	2. To help patient evaluate possible outcomes of all options and to select the best alternative
	3. To correct misconceptions
	4. To increase the likelihood of patient compliance
		1. When
		  a. Identify information presently available to the patient—is it sufficient?
		  b. Assess the accuracy and validity of the patient's present information; is there inaccurate information that needs correcting?
		  c. Look for signs of patient receptivity to additional or new information before presenting it—is the patient ready to hear the information?
		2. What
		  a. Determine the kind of information useful to each patient—including unpleasant information.
		  b. Identify the most reliable source to deliver the information to the patient.
		  c. Identify whether the information should be presented all at once or in a certain sequence.
		3. How
		  a. Limit the amount of information given at one time—two different pieces of information but no more.
		  b. Present the information as clearly as possible; avoid jargon.
		  c. Deliver the information in a sensitive and friendly manner.
		  d. Be realistic, but avoid scare tactics.
		  e. Ask for and discuss patient reactions to the information.

information. *When* refers to recognition of the patient's need for and readiness to hear information. *What* refers to the kind of information the patient needs, as well as the source and sequence of the information. *How* refers to the effective delivery of information to the patient. These principles are described in more detail in the following three sections and are summarized in Table 9-2.

When to Give Information

Knowing when to give information requires that health professionals recognize the patient's need for information. If a patient has incomplete or inaccurate information, then such a need exists (Cormier & Cormier, 1979, p. 106). There are three principles the interviewer can use to evaluate the patient's need for information. First, identify the information presently available to the patient and determine what, if any, vital information the patient lacks. Second, assess the information the patient currently has—is it accurate? Valid? Data based? Determine if the patient has inaccurate, invalid, or non-data-based information that needs to be corrected. But don't be in a hurry to give information or to correct inaccurate information prematurely. Look for some indication that the patient will be receptive to the information. If information is introduced too early in an interview, the patient may ignore it. Consider this process in the following example.

> The laboratory tests support a diagnosis of hyperthyroidism. The patient states she realizes this means she has an overactive thyroid gland and indicates she is aware of some of the symptoms, including increased heart rate, difficulty in sleeping, nervousness, and diarrhea. She indicates a desire to learn more about the illness, particularly its etiology, and also states that she has been told that hyperthyroidism is always a benign illness with no risks and one that usually requires only short-term medication in order to be "cured."

In this example, the patient seems to have sufficient and accurate information about the nature and symptoms of her illness. She also seems receptive to being given additional information because she has indicated she wants to learn more about the disease. However, her information about the prognosis, effects, and treatment for the illness seems somewhat inaccurate, as if it is information she has gained from talking with friends. For example, she seems unaware that hyperthyroidism may cause congestive heart failure or that untreated hyperthyroidism can, over a period of time, have other severe consequences. She also believes that a very short period of medication will cure the illness. Although this may be true for some patients, it should be pointed out that other patients may require a long-term medication regimen that manages rather than cures the illness. The patient also may be unaware of other possible treatments, such as surgery and radioactive iodine.

What Information to Give

Knowing what information to give requires that health professionals be able to identify the kind of information the patient needs and to determine a sequence in which to impart that information. There are several guidelines interviewers may follow to determine what information the patient needs. First, they may try to determine the kind of information that will be most useful for the patient. One patient may need information about the etiology of an illness, while another may need information about the alternative treatments available. It is important not to underestimate the ability of patients to understand and assimilate information about their health. When professionals do underestimate their patients, they tend to share less information, thereby depriving the patient of useful knowledge.

The interviewer also must be careful not to present only positive or pleasant information to patients. All of the relevant facts should be given, which at times will include unpleasant information. In most cases, health care providers do more harm than good by protecting patients from negative information. Most patients and their families prefer to know at the outset that a particular illness has been diagnosed, that the illness is chronic, that the prognosis may be poor, or that there are no good treatments presently available. Patients' faith in the professional may be shaken if they discover later that certain information was withheld, and they may feel the professional has been deceptive. Giving patients unpleasant information, however, always should be done in a sensitive and considerate manner, as described in the section of this chapter on the delivery of information.

A second guideline concerns the source or provider of the information. Where can the required information be obtained, and who should present it? Generally, a patient is more receptive to information given by someone in whom the patient already has confidence and faith (Bernstein & Bernstein, 1980; Matthews & Hingson, 1977). If interviewers do not have accurate or complete information available, they should not hesitate to say "I don't know." Then the patient may need to be referred to another source in order to obtain the needed information. For example, an obstetrician may prefer to have an older mother-to-be talk to a genetic counselor about the risks of a possible chromosomal abnormality. If the interviewer prefers to deliver the information and is uncertain of its accuracy or completeness, he or she should validate the information with expert sources before presenting it to the patient. In the example above, the obstetrician might consult with the genetic counselor first and then deliver the information personally. Accuracy of information can be an important factor in patient compliance. In a study conducted by Svarstad (1976), patients who were given accurate information complied far better (60%) than those who had misinformation (17%).

A third important guideline involves identifying whether the information the patient needs should be presented all at once or in some particular sequence. For example, a patient may need to have a certain information base before other facts will make sense. Consequently, the interviewer will have to sequence the information carefully in order for the patient to grasp it fully.

The previous example of the woman with the diagnosis of hyperthyroidism may help clarify this process. First, the patient has expressed a desire to know more about the causes and treatment of hyperthyroidism. The best source for such information is probably the health professional who is primarily responsible for the patient's care. The health professional should not hesitate to discuss the known causes, methods of treatment, or possible consequences of hyperthyroidism that is untreated. However, if the interviewer feels insecure about answering the patient's questions, he or she should arrange a consultation with another health professional who could provide the patient with the desired responses. Further, the interviewer must decide if the patient's questions can be answered all at one time or should be answered in "small doses" that the patient can more easily understand. One method may be to present the most important information first, since evidence suggests that initial information is what patients remember best (Bernstein & Bernstein, 1980). Therefore, in this example, the interviewer may choose to discuss the effects of the untreated illness first, followed by the information about the etiology of hyperthyroidism.

How to Give Information

Giving information effectively requires the interviewer to be aware of various psychological conditions and effects of information giving. There are five guidelines for the effective delivery of information (see also Table 9-2).

First, limit the amount of information given at one time. Do not overload or overwhelm the patient with a great many facts during a single interview. One study (Ley, 1976) found that the more information patients were told at one time, the less they remembered. This same study reported that patient recall of information was best when only one or two pieces of information were presented at one time; recall was poorer when three or four facts were presented at the same time. Thus a good rule of thumb is to limit the information presented on any occasion to only two items.

Second, present the information as clearly as possible in language that is understandable to the

LEARNING ACTIVITIES

Information Giving

Written activity

The following example dialogue depicts a health professional giving information to a patient about various treatment approaches for diabetes. Your task is to evaluate the interviewer's delivery of information based on the five criteria listed on p. 197 (Chapter Objective 2). Check your evaluation with that provided in the feedback following the learning activity.

Health Professional: Mrs. Green, I have received the results of your laboratory studies, and I think I know why you find it necessary to get up so often in the middle of the night to go to the bathroom. Your blood studies indicate that you have diabetes. Do you know anything about diabetes?

Patient: Yes, I do. I know what causes it because a close friend of mine has it. But I'd like to know what you are going to suggest to me in terms of correcting the situation. I think there's more than one way to treat it.

Health Professional: You are absolutely right. There are generally three ways that we treat diabetes—diet, exercise, and medication. Usually, however, we try diet and exercise before medication. Since there is a lot of information I could give you about all three of these today, I'd like to just focus on control of diabetes by diet and see if that seems like a reasonable initial approach to you. How does that sound?

Patient: OK, I'd rather not use the medicine if I don't have to. How does the diet work?

Health Professional: Essentially control by diet does three things. First, by controlling the diet so that only moderate amounts of carbohydrates are eaten, there is less requirement for insulin, and consequently the amount of insulin that the body produces helps to utilize the sugar that is eaten efficiently. Second, in order to level out some of the times during the day when levels of blood sugar are very high—for example, immediately after eating a meal—the amount of carbohydrate in each meal is restricted to some degree and spread throughout the waking hours. As a consequence, a bedtime snack is usually recommended so that, instead of dividing the day's carbohydrate intake into just the three meals, you divide it into four smaller meals. Third, we know that people who are overweight tend to utilize insulin much more inefficiently than those who are at recommended body weight. Consequently, it will be to your advantage to reduce your weight somewhat to the recommended body weight, which for you would be approximately 120 pounds. Does that make sense so far?

Patient: Yes, I think I see what you are driving at. However, I doubt that I can lose all that weight.

Health Professional: Well, it is not surprising that you should feel that way. It is certainly very difficult to lose weight. However, any efforts that you can make to reduce your weight by any degree will certainly contribute to your better health. What is your reaction now to this information?

Patient: I am a little shaken up by the whole thing—I guess the real impact of having diabetes has not yet really affected me.

Health Professional: You are probably right in the sense that it takes some time for the impact of any illness to sink in. However, you do seem very able to understand the concepts we have been discussing. In order to make things more clear to you and provide you with some references when you get home, I would like you to read these books and pamphlets about treatment of diabetes, and we'll discuss them at your next visit.

Patient: All right, I will be happy to read everything I can find about diabetes.

Health Professional: One other thing I would suggest to you. There are many references on diabetes in newspapers, magazines, and books. These may be quite bothersome to you if you read about some of the potential side effects and complications of diabetes. Consequently, if you should read anything that troubles you, please bring it in so that I can read it and discuss the problem with you. Although we cannot cure diabetes, we can certainly alleviate most of its symptoms by proper treatment.

Patient: All right, that sounds like a fair enough deal to me. Where should I start now?

Health Professional: Well, the first thing that we should do is get you to understand what is involved with a diabetic diet. So, let me provide you with the particulars of your diet, which I think should be a 1200 calorie American Diabetic Association diet. It is important that you begin the diet right away, and I will see you again in the office in two weeks. At that time we can assess the impact of the diet during that period and discuss any other concerns you may have.

Your assessment of the health professional's information giving (check the appropriate box):

1. Did the interviewer limit the amount of information given at one time?

   _____ Yes   _____ No

2. Did the interviewer use language that was easy for the patient to understand and avoid technical terms?

   _____ Yes   _____ No

3. Did the interviewer deliver the information in a sensitive and friendly manner?

   _____ Yes   _____ No

4. Did the interviewer present the information in a realistic yet nonthreatening way (no "scare tactics")?

   _____ Yes   _____ No

5. Did the interviewer ask for and discuss the patient's reaction to the information given?

   _____ Yes   _____ No

Feedback

1. Yes, the interviewer did a good job of limiting the amount of information given. The interviewer mentioned three available treatments but restricted the information to the treatment to be used initially. Other treatments can be discussed at future visits. The interviewer also gave the patient some information to read at home at her own pace.

2. Yes, the interviewer avoided technical terms and explained the concepts in language the patient seemed to understand.

3. Yes, the interviewer appeared to deliver the information in a sensitive and friendly manner.

4. Yes, the interviewer was realistic yet nonthreatening. One aspect of this was encouraging the patient to bring in any questions she had or readings she found about the effects of diabetes that worried her.

5. Yes, the interviewer asked for the patient's reaction to the information and acknowledged that it may take some time to sort out her feelings about having diabetes.

Simulation Activity

According to Chapter Objective 3, you will be able to give information about a particular syndrome to a hypothetical patient. Your delivery of the information should meet at least four out of five criteria listed in the checklist on "How to Give Information," found on p. 198. The following procedure is a suggested way for implementing this activity, which may be completed in dyads, triads, or small groups.

1. Study any standard textbook to determine the cardinal features of an illness. Consider the common cold, acute appendicitis, mononucleosis,

Graves disease (hyperthyroidism), otitis media (ear ache), acute chole-cystitis (gall bladder disease), and gastric or duodenal ulcer, as examples.

2. In the role of interviewer, give information to a partner (patient) about one of the chosen syndromes, following the guidelines for delivery of information listed on the checklist below.

3. In the role of patient, react to and ask questions about the information given by the interviewer. Also give feedback to the interviewer after the role play is completed about his or her delivery of the information.

4. Other persons in the group can act as observers using the "How to Give Information" checklist for assessment.

Checklist on How to Give Information

1. Did the interviewer limit the amount of information given at one time (about two items)?

   _____ Yes   _____ No

2. Did the interviewer use language that was easy for the patient to understand and avoid technical terms?

   _____ Yes   _____ No

3. Did the interviewer deliver the information in a sensitive and friendly manner?

   _____ Yes   _____ No

4. Did the interviewer present the information in a realistic yet nonthreatening (scare tactics) way?

   _____ Yes   _____ No

5. Did the interviewer ask for and discuss the patient's reactions to the information given?

   _____ Yes   _____ No

Observer Comments: _____

_____

_____

patient. Avoid jargon. According to Pratt, Seligmann, and Reader (1957), the language and concepts of health care are not widely understood by the lay public. Kirscht and Rosenstock (1979) suggest that "not only are many of the technical words not shared by patients but also many commonly used bits of advice do not convey meanings as intended—'reduce salt intake' or 'take the medicine on an empty stomach' may not be interpreted correctly" (p. 202). These authors also note that efforts on the part of the professional to promote patient comprehension result in better compliance (p. 207). An additional technique that may promote patient comprehension is to write an outline or a diagram of the problem or illness as the interview progresses. The patient can then take the outline or diagram home for later review.

Patient comprehension is to some degree related to their retention of the data. In two studies reported by Bernstein and Bernstein (1980), the more easily patients understood the information, the greater the amount of information they retained. Patients remember information best if they understand it when they hear it.

The third guideline for effective delivery of information is to present it in a sensitive and friendly manner. Patient satisfaction with the patient/professional relationship is important in recall and in compliance. According to Matthews and Hingson (1977), patients are less likely to comply if: (1) they feel they are not held in adequate esteem by the professional; (2) tension emerges during an interaction and is not addressed or resolved; and (3) they feel that the professional is not behaving in a friendly manner (p. 884). Clearly, the quality of the relationship is a major factor in determining whether the patient will remember and/or use the information.

When delivering unpleasant information, the interviewer must be especially careful to be friendly and sensitive to the patient's needs. Above all, the interviewer must not be abrupt but be willing to talk as openly and as directly as the patient desires and to provide emotional support as needed for the patient and/or the family (Bernstein & Bernstein, 1980). The facts should be presented from an optimistic point of view so that the patient does not lose all hope immediately. At the same time, it is also important that the interviewer be realistic and honest. However, the interviewer should not use scare tactics to facilitate patient recall or compliance. Matthews and Hingson (1977) note that "review articles on the use of fear arousal have reached the same fundamental conclusion: fear arousal is not consistently successful and, in some situations, may actually hinder compliance" (p. 885).

A fifth and final guideline for effective delivery is to ask for and discuss the patient's reactions to the information. Information that may seem relatively "cut and dried" to a professional can have a strong emotional impact on the patient. For example, a patient who has been healthy for 40 years and is suddenly told that she has a chronic illness such as hypertension or diabetes that will have to be "controlled" for the rest of her life is likely to have strong feelings upon hearing this information. Similarly, a patient who is informed about a poor prognosis may have very intense feelings. In such instances, the professional does the patient a disservice by delivering the information and then not spending time with the patient to process the emotional impact of the "bad news." In the case of unpleasant information, professionals can indicate their willingness to talk fully about patients' reactions and questions and then allow a patient to raise whatever issues he or she may choose. Taking the time to inquire about and listen to patient reactions also has the added benefit of strengthening the professional/patient relationship. (Now do learning activity on p. 195).

Chapter Summary

This chapter presented guidelines for the effective delivery of instructions and information giving in health care settings. It also discussed the role of these two skills in improving patient compliance with prescribed regimens.

Instructions are one or more verbal statements in which the interviewer instructs or directs a patient to perform a task or follow a treatment program. Instructions have both informational and influential effects. To be most effective, instructions must be specific, concise, and delivered as suggestions, not commands. The interviewer must confirm whether the patient has understood the directions and should give the patient clear written or typed instructions to take home. In some instances, oral instructions may need to be supplemented with demonstrations of a particular task or regimen. Compliance with instructions may increase if it is linked to positive or rewarding consequences, such as relief of symptoms, social support, or other positive reinforcing events. Giving instructions is not a one-time event. Adequate follow-up is essential.

Information giving is verbal communication of data to a patient. Information giving is used to inform a patient of possible options, to help a patient evaluate the options, and to correct inaccurate information. For each patient, health professionals must identify when to give information and what information to give. Effective delivery of infor- mation is extremely important because it is the cornerstone of patient education.

Interviewers should limit the amount of information given at any one time. They should relay information in a sensitive and friendly manner and avoid the use of scare tactics. It is important for professionals to take time to request and discuss patient reactions, as most information given in health care settings may have an emotional impact on the patient.

Suggested Readings _____

Bernstein, L., & Bernstein, R. *Interviewing: A guide for health professionals*. New York: Appleton-Century-Crofts, 1980. Chapter 3, "The Evaluative Response," contrasts the difference between advice giving and information giving and discusses the role of compliance in health care management.

Cormier, W. H., & Cormier, L. S. *Interviewing strategies for helpers: A guide to assessment, treatment, and evaluation*. Monterey, Calif.: Brooks/Cole, 1979. Chapter 7, "Sharing and Teaching Responses," describes the role and purposes of instructions and information giving in the interviewing process.

Epstein, L. H., & Masek, B. J. Behavioral control of medicine compliance. *Journal of Applied Behavior Analysis*, 1978, *11*, 1–10. This article discusses the effective use of patients' written recordings to monitor and improve compliance with prescribed medication.

Kirscht, J., & Rosenstock, I. Patients' problems in following recommendations of health experts. In G. C. Stone, F. Cohen, & N. E. Adler (Eds.), *Health psychology*. San Francisco: Jossey-Bass, 1979. The chapter by Kirscht and Rosenstock presents a number of factors related to patient compliance, including the role of instructions, information giving, and the patient/professional relationship.

Matthews, D., & Hingson, R. Improving patient compliance. *Medical Clinics of North America*, 1977, *61*, 879–889. This article very succinctly describes how professionals can maximize patient compliance to instructions and information given by professionals.

Melamed, B. G., & Siegel, L. J. *Behavioral medicine: Practical applications in health care*. New York: Springer, 1980. Chapter 4, "Patient Management," suggests a number of practical techniques the professional can use to increase patient compliance with treatment regimens.

Shulman, J. Current concepts of patient motivation toward long-term oral hygiene: A literature review. *Journal of American Society of Preventive Dentistry*, 1974, *4*, 7–15. The author has reviewed over 100 references and summarized practices that motivate patients to maintain effective oral hygiene procedures.

Zifferblatt, S. M. Increasing patient compliance through the applied analysis of behavior. *Preventative Medicine*, 1975, *4*, 173–182. This short article describes procedures designed to enhance patient compliance from a behavioral framework.

Dealing with Defensive Reactions

Objectives

After completing this chapter, you will be able to do the following:

1. Recognize an operating style of patient communication and identify in writing how that style of communication changes, given a written description of a patient/health professional interaction.

2. Identify in writing the implicit meaning of the patient's communication change, given a written description of a patient/health professional interaction.

3. Formulate in writing an example of a verbal response that an interviewer could use to respond to the patient's communication change.

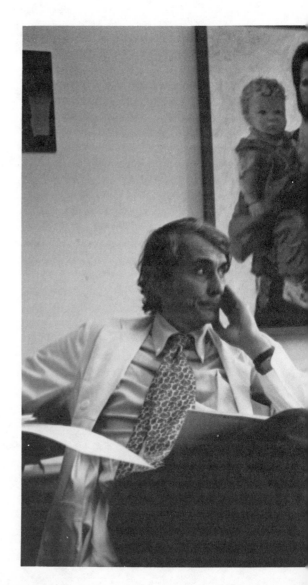

10

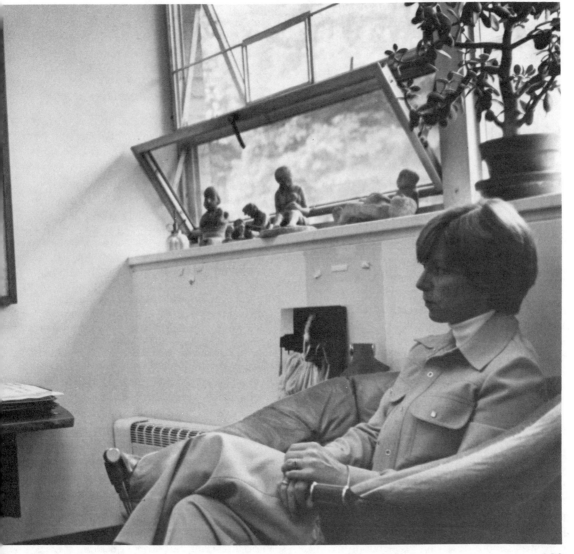

Encounters between health professionals and patients usually occur under adverse circumstances, especially from the patient's point of view. Not only are patients frequently physically ill, but they are also asked to reveal their most personal thoughts to a complete stranger and even asked to undress—the ultimate loss of their personal privacy. They find themselves in a vulnerable and frightening set of circumstances wherein they must relinquish control not only of their situation but also of their own bodies.

In defense, patients develop a number of strategies through which they try to manipulate and defy the situation and the interviewer. By so doing, they can maintain some measure of personal esteem and retain some control over their situation. They are then able to resume an offensive, rather than a totally defensive, personal posture.

This process is not always a conscious or deliberate one. In many instances, patients may not even be aware of their own discomfort or anxiety. They may be unaware of the defensive reactions they use to protect themselves from the perceived threat of the situation. Nevertheless, their ploys, feints, interruptions, and distractions may unnerve the unsuspecting interviewer. If the patient's plight is not overlooked, skillful interviewers can turn this situation to therapeutic advantage, verifying their professional credibility and cementing rapport with the patient.

Because patients seek to reduce their discomfort and increase their control, they often reveal significant feelings and concerns in an indirect rather than a direct manner. Such feelings and concerns frequently must be inferred from almost imperceptible and obtuse clues; skillful interviewers detect such clues in subtle changes in the patients' communication style.

These changes are frequently expressed through alterations in mood, changes in time orientation during conversation, shifts in subject matter, and modifications in body language. Patients may attempt to distract the interviewer away from painful or sensitive areas of inquiry or may focus the interviewer's attention on a problem area they perceive as more deserving of attention or con-

cern. Whatever the strategy, the end result assures them some small measure of control and satisfaction.

Although a specific issue that the patient brings up may seem relatively insignificant, the unspoken or implicit message may be of great importance in revealing the patient's ideas, thoughts, concerns, or feelings. Once the interviewer recognizes the implicit message or concern, he or she may respond in a variety of ways, ranging from total ignorance of the behavior to overt confrontation. This chapter will discuss changes in communication style that serve a defensive function for patients by reducing their anxiety and increasing their sense of control.

Recognizing Changes in Patient Communication

Consider the following vignette of a physician/patient interaction. Note any subtle shifts in the patient's verbal communication that may provide clues about feelings of anxiety or discomfort:

A 30-year-old female physician was interviewing a middle-aged male patient while obtaining the health history. The patient was very cooperative until he suddenly interrupted the physician to say:

> You know, Doctor, I really admire you young women who are willing to work so hard to become physicians. It has only been during the past few years that I have even been seen by a woman physician. Were there many other women in your medical school class?

In this example, there is a shift in content when the patient diverges from the health history to observe that it is only "during the past few years that I have even been seen by a woman physician" and then asks "Were there many other women in your medical school class?" The shift in communication may imply that the patient feels uncomfortable being examined by a female physician.

In response, the physician has three choices:

1. She may respond only to the superficial or obvious part of the patient's communication by simply answering the patient's questions at "face

value" and then proceeding with the health history. For example, the physician could agree "Yes, there are a number of women who are willing to work hard to become physicians. There were 31 other women in my medical school class," and then proceed to obtain the rest of the patient's medical history.

2. She may attempt to ignore the patient's shift in communication by breaking eye contact and responding briefly ("No, not too many") and then proceeding with the health history. For example, "Tell me more about the kinds of illnesses you had when you were a child."

3. She may respond to the concern implied by the patient's questions and recognize that he may feel uncomfortable being treated by a female physician. Because interviewers can never be certain that their interpretation of the communication shift is accurate, any verbal response should be phrased tentatively. For example, the physician could ask the patient "Have you ever been treated by a woman doctor before?" or "Could you tell me if you feel a little uncomfortable being seen by a woman doctor?" After responding to the patient's concern, the physician may choose to discuss the concern in some detail or simply proceed with obtaining the health history.

In this chapter we are concerned primarily with the third choice—formulating a verbal response to deal with the implied meaning of the change in the patient's communication style. Most interviewers have learned only too well how to respond to the obvious or superficial meaning of communication—as depicted in choice one—and additional reinforcement of that option is not necessary. It is important, however, to recognize the patient's concerns, although they may often remain implied or unspoken. Responding directly to the concern can facilitate communication between the two people, and, by contrast, communication may be impeded if covert concerns are neglected. Occasionally, however, responding or attending to a changed style of communication may reinforce inappropriate behavior, and it is desirable

to ignore the change. For example, during an interview with a hypertensive female who is also engaged in divorce litigation, she blurts out:

> It's no wonder my blood pressure is high. Do you know what my husband did last week? That S.O.B. took our new car and went joyriding with his new girlfriend.

In this situation, the interviewer may wish to ignore the comments about the husband and bring the focus back to the primary topic of the interview, which was hypertension.

It is not the intention of this chapter to provide an inventory of all the subtle meanings that may underlie changes in patients' verbal and nonverbal behaviors. However, this chapter will teach you how to recognize typical shifts in patient or colleague communication and provide suggestions on how to deal effectively with their implied meaning.

Four Changes in Verbal and Nonverbal Communication

In this section we describe and illustrate four ways in which patients may shift their communication style verbally or nonverbally. These communication shifts include alterations in mood, changes in time orientation, shifts in subject matter, and alterations in body language. We also present some examples of possible verbal responses that an interviewer could use in response to such shifts. Although these examples do not include all the possible responses, they do provide some suggestions for managing the four shifts and any other shifts in patient communication that may be encountered. Table 10-1 lists the four shifts in communication styles and suggestions for possible verbal responses.

Alterations in Mood

Patients can express a variety of feelings or emotions during an interview, but an abrupt shift in the manner in which the feelings are expressed may provide a clue that a significant issue has been touched on. For example, during a discussion of treatment alternatives with a hospitalized patient,

Table 10-1
Examples of Changes in Patient Communication Style and Suggested Verbal Responses

Shifts in Communication Style	Some Possible Verbal Responses
Alterations in mood	Silence (Chapter 5)
Changes in time orientation (past, present, future)	Clarification (Chapter 6)
	Paraphrase (Chapter 6)
	Reflection of feelings (Chapter 6)
Shifts in subject matter	Summarization (Chapter 6)
Alterations in body language	Questions (Chapter 7)
	Confrontation (Chapter 7)
	Instructions (Chapter 9)
	Information giving (Chapter 9)

the patient's overall emotional tone is pleasant. Suddenly the patient expresses feelings of disgust and hostility toward the hospital staff. The patient's abrupt shift in mood from pleasantness to anger and hostility may indicate that something has occurred that challenges the patient in some way or that an issue has been uncovered about which the patient has strong feelings.

Acceptance and support of feelings. Sierra-Franco (1978) recommends that in responding to emotions of any type, one should demonstrate the acceptance or recognition of the emotion either verbally, nonverbally, or both. For example, imagine a 31-year-old woman in her fourth month of pregnancy who is being evaluated for hyperthyroidism. On the verge of tears, she blurts out "I'm really scared—because I'm not sure what effect this thyroid problem will have on my baby." The interviewer could respond to her emotion by saying something like "You seem to feel apprehensive and uncertain about the effects your thyroid condition may have on your unborn baby."

At times patients want to cry but may not feel comfortable crying in the presence of another person. In such cases, the interviewer may give the patient "permission" to cry. Consider a parent who has just been informed that his seven-year-old son has acute leukemia. While discussing the prognosis of the disease, the interviewer notices that the father appears to be holding back tears. The interviewer may invite crying by saying "Please feel free to cry. It's OK." This kind of statement tells the patient that the health professional understands how difficult it is to maintain composure and also feels comfortable with the possibility the patient may lose composure (Hein, 1980, p. 91). Restraining emotions can sometimes impede the progress of the interview. An invitation to cry or express an emotion can have the effect of "clearing the air" in the interview.

Anger and hostility. One of the most difficult kinds of patient feeling to respond to effectively is anger. Anger is a very common defensive reaction; when an individual feels threatened or uncomfortable, this discomfort may be revealed more by anger or hostility than by anxiety or nervousness. For example, consider the anger expressed by a female patient with a severe drinking problem who has come to the hospital for her annual checkup. Upon entering the examining room, she is surprised to meet a stranger—a young male intern—who was scheduled to examine her. She says angrily "Listen, buster, I have always seen the chief before—he knows all about me! I don't know why I have to tell a twerp like you all the same stuff. I am not about to let you put a hand on me!"

The examiner could use one of the following responses:

I suspect you are upset because you expected to see the chief. [reflection] **Or** You appear to feel angry about not seeing the chief of the department today and are upset because I'm here instead. How would you feel if we talked about the situation? [reflection and open-ended question] **Or** Let's talk about your anger about the situation and how I feel when I am just trying to do my job. [reflection and instruction]

If the angry messages continue, the interviewer could reflect the message and instruct the patient to calm down:

> I know you are angry because you expected to see the chief. The chief and I work as a team. If I could examine you, it really would help me, the chief, and the team. I cannot examine you when you are angry and upset. If it is possible for you to relax, we can continue the interview. Otherwise, if you prefer, we can reschedule the examination.

Notice that in the last response, the interviewer has suggested or instructed the patient to engage in another behavior (to relax) and has indicated that the interview cannot continue while the patient remains angry.

The same principles for dealing with patient anger can apply to patients who disrupt the interview with excessive expressions of depression, sadness, or continual crying. It is sometimes easy for an interviewer to become "hooked" and spend a great deal of time during the interview responding to these emotions. The interviewer has to use his or her judgment about what is excessive in discussion of a patient's feelings. For some patients, a lengthy discussion can be therapeutic, but with other patients dwelling on emotions may reinforce inappropriate behavior.

Changes in Time Orientation

Another type of shift in a patient's communication style involves talking about the past or future when the interviewer is focused on the present. Reiser and Schroder (1980) say that "talking about the past as a way of communicating feelings and concerns in the present is an extremely common way for patients to express their concerns" (p. 115). Generally, patients who are experiencing a "serious" prognosis, illness, or treatment may adopt this form of communicating as a way to defend against true anxiety over their present circumstances. Passons (1975) maintains that dwelling on the past may be used "as a shield against suggestions for different patterns of behaving" (p. 161).

Other patients may avoid the present by focusing on the future. Imagine an interviewer discussing a chemotherapy treatment protocol with a patient. The patient talks about how terrible the treatment is going to be and speculates how long it will take until the treatments eventually kill him. Passons (1975) claims that anticipations in the form of "worrying, catastrophizing, scheming and rehearsing" are detriments for dealing with the present.

Frequently such a change in time orientation can be identified by a change in the verb tense the patient uses. For example, a patient may be talking about a current health problem (such as redness or swelling of the breast), using the present verb tense to describe this information. Abruptly, the patient may revert to the description of an incident that occurred in the past or may shift to the future by being excessively preoccupied with losing her good health. The patient's use of the present tense would probably change to use of the past or future tense and, thus, signal a change in time orientation. For example, the patient would say:

> Recently I became aware of this swelling in my right breast. It is swollen now, and it seems to be slightly red in color. I'm concerned about what is happening. [shift from present to past] You know, one of the most awful things that has ever happened to me was having my mother die when I was only 15. I was left all alone with only my sick father. I had to care for him—he was too weak to care for me. [shift from past to future] It's constantly on my mind that I will never have good health again. I always think about how I will probably end up either dying young or becoming an invalid.

The interviewer might determine that the patient is much more concerned about her symptoms than she has stated because she has linked them to a painful past event and to the prospect of an unhealthy future, similar to the fates of her mother and father. The interviewer could respond by saying:

> You seem to feel very concerned and upset about these symptoms. [reflection of feelings] **Or** You've noticed some symptoms with your

breast that bother you. Perhaps your concern about this is heightened by recalling the early death of your mother and the illness of your father. [summarization] **Or** How does the death of your mother relate to your present concern with these symptoms? [open-ended question]

The interviewer also may decide to pause and remain silent to see if the patient herself provides a link or a clue to the shift in her next messages.

Deliberate shifts in time orientation. Occasionally an interviewer may need to provoke or initiate a shift in time orientation if the patient focuses exclusively on the past or the future without talking about the present. Dwelling either on the past or on the future can contribute to the patient's denial and avoidance of present concerns or feelings. In such cases, the health professional should respond by attempting to refocus the interview on present concerns and feelings.

For example, the interviewer is discussing the pain a patient is experiencing with bowel cancer and massive liver metastases. Throughout the discussion, the interviewer noted that the patient was able to talk only about the anger and hostility she had toward her sister when they were growing up. The interviewer could paraphrase and question by saying "When I have attempted to discuss the pain you are experiencing, you talked about the anger and hostility you felt for your sister while growing up. Can you tell me how the anger and hostility you felt toward your sister are related to the pain you are experiencing right now?" In this example, the interviewer is attempting to clarify and deal with the present feelings and concerns of the patient.

We do not wish to convey the idea that talking about the past or future may not be helpful for a patient. A discussion of the past and/or future can be very therapeutic. However, dwelling on *just* the past and *just* the future, or shifting to the past or future, may be a way for the patient to avoid the anxiety associated with the present. In contrast, a patient may focus only on the immediate present without consideration of the past or the future.

For example, the mother of a severely retarded child with trisomy 21 (Down's syndrome) who dwells on the small accomplishments of her child without any consideration or admission of potential problems associated with educating the child should be encouraged by the interviewer to expand her focus on the child's problems and to include future educational considerations.

Shifts in Subject Matter

Topic shifts are another form of change in patients' communication patterns that may reveal clues about their feelings and concerns. Such shifts may take various forms. A patient may initiate discussion about another totally irrelevant subject or may talk about two unrelated topics or ideas as shown in the following vignette.

> Let me see, yes, my sister Bertha did have rheumatic fever. She was the only one of all us girls that was a good cook. Every summer she'd make quarts and quarts of tomatoes, pickles, and fried peppers. . . .

Other patients may make chatty asides, nervous jokes, trivial comments, or small talk. Frequent interruptions or long irrelevant monologues may distract interviewers and leave them scratching their heads in an attempt to reconstruct the chain of thought that prompted the patient's digression.

On occasion, patients may provide hints about significant concerns by asking questions. Frequently such questions are reserved until the end of an interview session and may be appended as apparent afterthoughts as posed in the following situation.

> *Health Practitioner:* Well, Ms. Jones, that should complete our interview for today. I expect that we can make the necessary child care arrangements that you have requested. Have you any other questions?

> *Ms. Jones:* Oh yes. I almost forgot. Is it true that you can get herpes or VD from a toilet seat?

Topic changes may occur during the course of one session or over the span of several interviews. The interviewer can recognize topic shifts typically by noticing the focus areas of the interview (physical, psychological, environmental) and comparing the topics or remarks initiated and discussed by the patient.

Irrelevant subject matter. Reiser and Schroder (1980) observe that patients may shift either away from or toward a particular topic of discussion. Some patients will shift away from a topic to avoid the problem of most concern. For example, after several conversations with a patient dying of amyotrophic lateral sclerosis ("Lou Gehrig's Disease"), the interviewer noted that when the topic of the illness was introduced, the patient responded with unrelated "chit chat" or by discussing non-health-related concerns such as friends, family, sports, and so on. Such a pattern of avoidance may suggest that the patient is uncomfortable discussing himself or herself and the illness and may be coping with the psychological pain by focusing on other topics, other people, or other situations. The avoidance of more personal and painful topics may or may not be a useful coping strategy to deal with the problem. The health professional may wish to respond to the patient's avoidance of the topic in one of several fashions. The interviewer could self-disclose by saying "When I have problems or feel pain, I don't like to talk about it with other people" or "I have trouble sometimes talking about the things that bother me." Alternatively, the interviewer could reflect the patient's feelings by saying "It seems difficult for you to talk about your illness" or "It appears difficult for you, but I think it would be helpful if we could talk about how you feel about your illness."

Other patients may change the topic by initiating a deliberate shift to a new subject, seemingly unrelated to the previous discussion (Reiser & Schroder, 1980). For example, during an initial interview a woman has been discussing her past medical history. Abruptly, she begins a lengthy discussion about her agitation over a recent crisis in her family. The interviewer must determine why the patient has deliberately shifted to the new topic at this particular time (Reiser & Schroder, 1980). In this example, the shift may indicate that the patient is seeking assistance or support more for emotional or psychological concerns than for physical ones. The interviewer could respond by asking "What is it about your family situation that bothers you?" or by confrontation—"For the past 30 minutes, your responses to my questions about your health have been rather vague. Now, all of a sudden, you are talking very specifically about a situation in your family." Or the interviewer could instruct the patient by saying "Right now I must get some specific information about your physical health. After I get that information, we can discuss the problem that is bothering you about the recent crisis in your family." In the last response, the interviewer attempts to bring the focus of the interview back to the patient's physical health (physical focus) and also indicates a willingness to discuss the family situation (environmental, psychological focus) at a later point in the interview.

Jokes, trivial remarks, and interruptions. Other topic shifts that patients may use are jokes, trivial comments, or frequent interruptions (Reiser & Schroder, 1980). For example, imagine a 52-year-old man who has had an acute myocardial infarction with successful convalescence. An interviewer is reviewing and discussing his diet and exercise programs on the day he is to be discharged from the hospital. While discussing the rehabilitation regimen, the patient makes jokes and trivial remarks about his condition, such as "Maybe I could try out for basketball on the local wheelchair team." At another time the patient states "Perhaps we ought to hire a cook to help my wife because she'll have to plan meals for her and a separate meal for me" or "When I go out to eat with someone, I can just 'brown bag' it—just bring my diet food and watch my friends eat and drink whatever they want."

This patient feels burdened and restricted by the requirements of the new diet and exercise program. The interviewer could respond by paraphrasing and asking a question such as "You mentioned trying out for the wheelchair team, employing a cook, bringing your diet food when going out with friends. I am wondering how these comments are related to your feelings about the diet and exercise program we have been discussing?" Remember that humor is frequently used as a disguise. The seemingly unrelated or unconnected topics may in reality be very relevant and important to the patient.

Questions. Another shift in subject matter can occur in the form of a question or a series of questions. An interviewer may be in the process of obtaining a past medical, family, or social history (see Chapter 8), and the patient interrupts or shifts the focus or content with a question or a series of questions. The question or questions may appear unrelated to the content of the interview, or "off the wall." Bernstein and Bernstein (1980) claim that a question "... may be either a request for information or the expression of a feeling or attitude" (p. 35). Sierra-Franco (1978) notes that questions are not always a request for information but may be a way of expressing concern and can provide clues to the patient's underlying thoughts and feelings.

For example, it is not uncommon to have a patient ask a question that seeks either information or the professional opinion of the interviewer. Here are some typical examples:

How do you treat ulcerative colitis?

What does a gastroenterologist do?

How long do people with my diagnosis usually live?

Will I have to have an operation to clear up my hemorrhoids?

How much penicillin will I take?

Which blood pressure is more important—systolic or diastolic?

When will you stop the chemotherapy?

What do you mean by "functional heart murmur"?

Do you think I am healthy?

Should I have this operation?

If you were in my place, would you have an abortion?

Is that the best treatment for me?

Generally, most health professionals agree that straightforward answers should be given to patient questions about health, illness, or treatment. In most cases, the patient has a right to have that information (refer to Chapter 14 on legal and ethical issues for a discussion of informed consent). Therefore, if the patient asks for information, the interviewer should provide an honest answer. If the interviewer does not know the answer, she or he should readily admit that fact and then attempt to find the answer or refer the patient to another information source. If, however, a patient requests information about subject matter outside the content of the interview, there is a shift in the topic. In such instances, the interviewer may wish to clarify what the patient is asking. Sierra-Franco (1978) believes that in such cases reflecting or paraphrasing the message may be more useful than giving a literal answer to the question (p. 357).

For example, imagine a professional taking the history of present illness from a patient when suddenly the patient asks "Do you think I'm healthy?" The interviewer could say "You seem concerned about your health" [reflection], "You want to know if I believe that you are well" [paraphrase], "What do you mean by healthy?" [probe], "For what reason do you ask that question?" [probe], or "Are you concerned about your own health or are you worried about the health of some member of your family?" [clarification]. After one of these responses, the interviewer may provide a more informed and specific answer to the question. Remember that when requests for information occur that are outside the focus or context of the interview, it is wise to determine why the patient is asking the question by using one or more of the suggested responses above. As Bernstein and Bernstein (1980) observe, out-of-context questions are indirect "expressions of a feeling or attitude" (p. 35). A literal answer to a question may miss the patient's concern or provide more or less information than the patient can process effectively.

Patients also may shift the topic by asking an interviewer personal questions that are unrelated to the focus of the interaction. For example, during the course of a dental examination, a patient may ask a dentist or a hygienist questions such as:

Are you married?

How old are you?

How did you vote in the last election?

Do you have any children?

Have you ever been divorced?

Have you ever had a root canal?

What kind of toothpaste do you use?

How much experience have you had in treating a patient with teeth like mine?

Generally personal questions represent a "relief measure" the patient uses to divert the focus of the interview from himself or herself to the interviewer (Hein, 1980, p. 92).

Many health professionals report extreme discomfort in handling personal questions from patients. Reiser and Schroder (1980) suggest that interviewers get trapped by personal questions and feel self-conscious when answering them. Because of this discomfort or embarrassment, the interviewer may respond with too much self-disclosure or defensively, thus deflecting the focus of the interaction even further.

According to Froelich and Bishop (1977), "the rule is to answer a patient's personal questions honestly and directly *only* when you understand clearly why they are asked and are confident that your reply will further the maintenance of a comfortable professional relationship" (p. 35). In other cases, the interviewer should clarify or probe to discover the reason the patient is asking the question.

For example, suppose a medical intern is conducting a physical examination on a patient with active tuberculosis when the patient asks "Have you ever treated tuberculosis before?" The interviewer could respond by asking "How would it help you to know my answer to that question?" or "What is the reason for your asking?" Each of these open-ended questions could be prefaced by "Yes, I have treated tuberculosis" or "No, I have not treated tuberculosis."

An interviewer might use a clarification in response to a personal question. Imagine a 35-year-old plumber with an inflamed appendix. The surgeon is explaining to the patient that she will be inserting an intravenous catheter through which fluids and antibiotics will be administered. Suddenly, the patient asks the surgeon "How old are you?" The surgeon may clarify by saying "Do you want to know how old I am, or are you asking how much experience I have had with inserting the catheter?" Or the surgeon could respond by asking "How will knowing my age help you?"

The primary aim in responding to any personal question is to redirect the interview by refocusing on the patient. According to Hein (1980), "refocusing can be done in a variety of ways, but the message should be the same: that the patient's question has been answered and now it is time to return to the patient's concerns" (p. 95).

Another shift in the subject matter can occur when a patient initiates a series of questions. Sierra-Franco (1978) claims that "sometimes a patient may ask a whole series of questions before he finally arrives at the one he really wants to ask" (p. 357). She asserts that "the earlier questions are pilot balloons, and as he receives answers to each one, he gathers a little more courage so that he can eventually ask what he really wants to know" (pp. 357–358).

For example, suppose a nurse is helping a patient with heart disease prepare for discharge from the hospital. The nurse, the patient, and the patient's spouse are engaged in amiable conversation related to packing, the results of recent diagnostic studies, and plans for readmission within the week for open-heart surgery. Suddenly, the patient interjects a series of questions about how a cardiac by-pass machine operates. The nurse answers all the questions about the machine. Then finally the patient blurts out "How long will I live after having this surgery?"

Under such circumstances, the attending professional must determine whether the questions posed by the patient are simply information seeking or are a true expression of significant anxiety. If the questions are unrelated to the focus or context of the interaction, more often than not a series of questions represents an important issue for the patient. If the interviewer determines that such questions do reflect significant patient concerns, clarification, open-ended questions, and reflections may be useful responses.

In the example above, the nurse could clarify by saying "You are asking a lot of questions about the cardiac by-pass machine. Are you concerned about the machine, or do you have some other worries?" Or the nurse could ask "How do you feel about having to trust your life to a machine during surgery?" These responses may help to focus on the concern or discomfort the patient is experiencing but is unable to express directly.

In summary, when confronted with patient questions that are outside the context of the interview, do not assume that the question has only its "face value" meaning. Rather, determine why the patient is asking the question or series of questions *now*. According to Reiser and Schroder (1980), "patients rarely ask questions that are not also important statements of what is on their minds" (p. 121). This is particularly true when the type of question represents a change in the patient's pattern of communication or is unrelated to the apparent focus of the interaction.

Alterations in Body Language

In addition to verbal behaviors, it can be useful to note patterns of nonverbal behavior, including changes or shifts in body language. According to Passons (1975), nonverbal behavior can change, disappear, or begin patterns over time (p. 104). For example, a patient may adopt a particular posture or exhibit a certain facial expression that differs from previous body language whenever the

health professional introduces a certain topic. Patients may also attempt to reduce discomfort or protect themselves by adopting a particular nonverbal posture during a medical interview. Shifts in body language may occur very abruptly and many times during a single interaction or may occur gradually during a series of patient contacts. Changes in nonverbal behavior patterns may be an index of the patient's feelings, comfort level, and accuracy in presenting information.

For example, while talking initially on the ward, a new male patient avoids eye contact, speaks in an almost inaudible voice, and leans back in bed. Later, after rapport has been established, the patient's nonverbal stance changes. Now when professionals appear in the room, the patient sits up and leans forward to greet them. He speaks clearly and audibly and maintains eye contact. In this example, the change in the nonverbal behavior probably indicates that the patient's comfort and confidence level have increased dramatically as he has come to know and trust the professionals.

In noting alterations in a patient's body language, the health professional should determine whether such alterations should be acknowledged or ignored. There are three ways to handle a patient's shift in body language: first, by noting the shift covertly or mentally, but without comment about the change to the patient; second, by describing the shift and interpreting its implied meaning to the patient; and, finally, by asking the patient about the intended meaning of the shift.

The health professional should use the latter two alternatives with discretion, however. It is perfectly appropriate for the interviewer to make a mental note about a nonverbal shift and a covert guess about its meaning. At the same time, the interviewer must remember that overt responses to changes in the patients' nonverbal behavior may be disturbing to patients who do not understand their own reasons for such shifts. Also, if the change in nonverbal behavior is irrelevant or unrelated to the focus of the interaction, responding to the shift can disrupt the flow of the interview and disrupt the patient's train of thought. As Passons (1975) observes, commenting on a single nonverbal behavior that appears out of phase with other expressions can result in resistance, confusion, or subsequent lack of cooperation by the patient (p. 105). Also, because the meaning of nonverbal behavior may vary extensively between patients, "care should be taken in imparting meaning to nonverbal behaviors" (Passons, 1975, p. 104). Passons (1975) suggests that the decision to respond overtly to a patient's nonverbal behavior depends on the interviewer's experience, intuition, and knowledge of the patient (p. 105).

An instance in which it may be very appropriate to comment on the patient's shift in nonverbal behavior is when this shift suggests some inaccuracy in the information the patient has given. For example, a 19-year-old mother brings her six-month-old daughter to the emergency room. The infant has a broken arm and multiple bruises. The mother claims "My baby leaned over in her high chair and then fell out on her arm" [verbal message]. At the same time, the mother is obviously nervous, frightened, and biting her fingernails [nonverbal message].

The interviewer might say "You say your daughter fell out of her high chair and landed on her arm, but you also appear very nervous and are biting your fingernails as you say this. Is it possible that she may have been hurt some other way?" or "Could you tell me what seems to be making you so nervous?"

The seductive patient.   Patients may also send nonverbal cues to the health professional through flirtatious or seductive actions. The overly affectionate or seductive patient can be extremely difficult to manage (Hainer, 1982). Patients may express intimacy, affection, or seductiveness with nonverbal behaviors such as smiles, longing and persistent glances, touching, and certain body postures and gestures. Sometimes the shift in body language is accompanied by excessive praise or compliments. Both verbal and nonverbal flirtations may represent genuine efforts on the patient's part to seduce or to establish an intimate relationship with the health professional. Other patients, however, may respond with behaviors that appear

on the surface to be flirtatious but that are in fact only nervous and unsuccessful attempts to show cooperation with the professional and to establish rapport. Many such behaviors may be extinguished if the professional resorts to silence or simply ignores them. However, if such behaviors persist throughout the interview, they may be very distracting and embarrassing, and the professional may need to resort to confrontation of the seductive or flirtatious behavior to regain control and correct the focus of the interview.

Consider the following example of an attractive woman who has been scheduled for a pre-employment physical examination with a male physician. As he walks into the examining room, he sees that she is sitting cross-legged on the examining table completely naked and reading a magazine. Her black lingerie is strewn carelessly on the writing desk.

M.D.: Good morning, Ms. Jones. I'm Doctor Brown. I've been scheduled to perform an insurance physical exam on you.

Ms. Jones: Good morning, Dr. Brown. I'm very pleased to meet you. [She stands up to shake his hand.] I've heard a lot about you from the other girls who work at the plant.

M.D.: Oh? Well, I hope what you heard was all good!

Ms. Jones: It sure was! You must be a fine physician, the way you impressed all the other girls.

M.D.: Well, thank you very much. Here is a gown that you can put on, and here is a sheet that you can throw across your lap. This will make you a bit more comfortable during this interview.

Ms. Jones: Oh, I don't mind. It's not often that I get to show off my suntan all over.

M.D.: Well, you certainly do have a nice tan. However, since it will take quite a while to complete this interview, I would appreciate it if you would put on the gown and drape so that we can proceed with the interview.

Ms. Jones: OK, if you insist. [She puts on the gown.]

He proceeds with the interview, and during the health history he asks:

M.D.: Do you take any medicines on a daily basis?

Ms. Jones: Just birth control pills. I'm not quite ready to settle down yet, so I want to be sure that I don't get pregnant. Are you married?

M.D.: No, I'm not married. Can you tell me exactly which birth control pills you take?

Ms. Jones: No, I can't recall the name, but I always carry the pack with me so that I'll be prepared if I stay somewhere overnight. If you'll hand me my purse, I'll get them for you. [He hands her the purse, and she rummages through it until she eventually finds the pills.]

Once again he proceeds with the interview. During the social history he asks:

M.D.: Are you married?

Ms. Jones: No, I'm too wild to settle down yet. Is that why you're still single? I've heard that doctors like to have a good time!

Dr. Brown ignores the last comment; he completes the interview and proceeds with the examination. She gazes longingly at him. As he begins to examine her breasts, she grasps his hand, directs it to a specific area of her left breast and asserts:

Ms. Jones: Sometimes I have pains right here, especially just before my periods. Could that be from the pills?

M.D.: Well, it is possible. However, it is more likely caused by the fact that your body

retains fluid just before your periods. That's when you are off the pills, right? [She nods in agreement.]

After answering her questions he proceeds with the examination. Again, she grasps his hand, directs it to the pelvic region, and states:

Ms. Jones: I also have very painful cramps during my period. Do you think that more intercourse would help relieve them?

M.D.: Again, that is a hard question to answer. However, I am becoming a bit flustered by your questions. Some are quite personal, and all of them have sexual overtones. I would appreciate it if you would reserve these questions until I have completed this examination. Then, we can discuss them in more detail in my office after you have dressed.

In order to deal appropriately with behavior such as that of Ms. Jones, health professionals must first determine the underlying causes and intentions of such behavior. If ignoring such actions fails to extinguish them, more overt action may be necessary. However, before resorting to overt confrontation, health professionals must be certain that the seductive message they are receiving is in fact the same message the patient is sending.

To help make such a critical distinction, health professionals should first describe the patient's verbal and nonverbal behavior. They must then reveal their own interpretations of the activity. If their suspicions are confirmed, they must instruct the patient that such behavior is detrimental to the professional relationship and to the patient's best interest.

On the other hand, if their suspicions of seductive behavior are not confirmed through confrontation with the patient, health professionals should advise the patient that other people may interpret such behaviors in a way that differs from the way the patient intended. Further, such behaviors may obscure the patient's real needs, desires, and intentions by crippling attempts to establish a productive professional/patient relationship.

LEARNING ACTIVITIES

Responding to Changes in Patient Communication Styles

This learning activity consists of seven descriptions of interactions between patients and health professionals. For each vignette or interaction:

1. Identify in writing how the style of patient communication has changed or shifted (Chapter Objective 1).

2. Identify in writing the implied meaning of the communication change (Chapter Objective 2).

3. Assuming that you would respond to the shift, formulate in writing an example of a verbal response that you might use to respond to the communication change (Chapter Objective 3).

The first vignette is completed as an example. Feedback follows the learning activity.

Patient 1

A very attractive model was injured in an automobile crash. Both her legs were heavily scarred as a result of her injuries, and she had little movement in her left leg. Whenever the physical therapist mentioned leg exercises, the patient avoided or ignored the subject and instead discussed her concern about the future, specifically whether she would ever be able to model again.

1. Identify how the style of communication has changed.

There has been a change in time orientation. During conversation, the patient shifts to her concern about the future whenever the therapist discusses present recuperative activities.

2. Identify the implied meaning of the change.

The implied meaning is that the woman feels so discouraged about her future as a model that she has given up hope. She sees no value in doing anything at present to help herself improve her condition.

3. Formulate a verbal response to the change.

You seem to be concerned about your future as a model because of your leg injuries. Possibly it seems so discouraging to you that you see no purpose to these activities. I think that it is important that we are at least able to talk about this treatment program so that you understand what it can do for you.

In this verbal response, the physical therapist reflected the patient's concern and feelings and instructed her to focus on talking about the treatment as an initial step in the overall treatment regimen.

Patient 2

A 59-year-old executive for a large corporation had a severe myocardial infarction one month ago but has recovered uneventfully. A nurse educator and the patient have been discussing his diet during an office visit, and he has been in a cheerful and pleasant mood. When the educator advises him that recent lab studies indicate an abnormally high cholesterol and triglyceride level, the patient angrily says:

> Don't give me any of that cholesterol stuff. I have only three years left before I can retire. My job is very important to me. I have to take my clients out for dinner, and I don't have time to watch everything I eat.

1. Identify how the style of communication has changed.

_____

_____

_____

2. Identify the implied meaning of the change.

_____

_____

_____

3. Formulate a verbal response to the change.

_____

_____

_____

Patient 3

   A 38-year-old male is hospitalized following gall bladder surgery. An attractive female L.P.N. enters his room for a routine check. He is very cooperative in talking with her and in allowing her to take his temperature and his blood pressure. As she starts to leave the bedside, the patient grabs her and attempts to kiss her.

1. Identify how the style of communication has changed.

_____

_____

2. Identify the implied meaning of the change.

_____

_____

_____

3. Formulate a verbal response to the change.

_____

_____

_____

Patient 4

A cancer patient is discussing with an X-ray technician the effects of radiation therapy. During their discussion, the patient interrupts and says:

> I am getting bald. But do you know that could really be dangerous and worse than my cancer. They say that some women prefer bald men—they're sexy. I guess I'll have to hire a bodyguard, or I might be smothered by all that attention.

1. Identify how the style of communication has changed.

_____

_____

_____

2. Identify the implied meaning of the change.

_____

_____

_____

3. Formulate a verbal response to the change.

_____

_____

_____

Patient 5

A 28-year-old woman is fearful of an additional pregnancy as a result of multiple complications with a previous delivery. While discussing birth control methods with her physician, she says:

> I don't know what method I should use. I have a real bad reaction to those pills. I don't want any more kids. How many kids do you have? What kind of contraceptives do you use?

1. Identify how the style of communication has changed.

_____

_____

_____

2. Identify the implied meaning of the change.

_____

_____

_____

3. Formulate a verbal response to the change.

_____

_____

_____

Patient 6

A dentist is talking with a 75-year-old patient about the importance of dental hygiene and the need for regular checkups in order to avoid periodontal (gum) disease. The patient constantly interrupts the dentist to discuss his wife, who died three years earlier, and to lament his loneliness.

1. Identify how the style of communication has changed.

_____

_____

_____

2. Identify the implied meaning of the change.

_____

_____

_____

3. Formulate a verbal response to the change.

_____

_____

_____

Patient 7

A nurse practitioner was talking with a female patient who had had a coronary by-pass six months previously. The nurse asked the patient about her return to sexual activity. The patient replied:

> My doctor said I could resume normal activity and everything has been just fine.

While saying this, she had a furrow in her brow, broke eye contact, and developed a slight tremor in her hands.

1. Identify how the style of communication has changed.

_____

_____

_____

2. Identify the implied meaning of the change.

_____

_____

_____

3. Formulate a verbal response to the change.

_____

_____

_____

Feedback

The following examples are suggested interpretations and responses—yours may be somewhat different.

Patient 2

1. There is an alteration in mood, from cheerfulness to direct expression of anger.
2. The patient feels upset about having to adhere to a restricted diet as he feels it may interfere with his lifestyle, in light of only several remaining years of an active work life. He also may resent the nurse's implication that because of his abnormal lab reports, he is not being a "good" patient. He also may feel anxious about his cardiovascular condition.

3. "I can see that you feel angry about this. Do you think it will be impossible to stay on this restricted diet while trying to fulfill your job responsibilities at the same time?" This response both reflects his anger and asks him to discuss more openly the problems he anticipates in remaining on the diet while working.

Patient 3

1. There is an alteration in the patient's body language—from cooperating with the temperature and blood pressure to becoming openly seductive and intimate in his nonverbal behavior.
2. The meaning is rather obvious in this case—the patient would like to distract the nurse from her job and have her respond to him in like fashion!
3. Removing herself from his grasp, leaving his bedside, and instructing the patient: "The next time I come in to take your temperature and blood pressure, I'd appreciate it if you wouldn't try to kiss me. It interferes with my getting my job done properly."

Patient 4

1. There is a shift in subject matter during the conversation. The patient attempts to disguise his concern about chemotherapy with humorous remarks.
2. Humor may simply provide the patient with a means to cope with or defend against illness and treatment; or it could be a reflection of underlying concern and anxiety about his illness and treatment.
3. "How do you really feel about the chemotherapy and the fact that you are getting bald?" The open-endedness of this question lets the patient inform you whether the humor does reflect a significant concern or whether it is a coping strategy for the patient.

Patient 5

1. There is a shift in the subject matter during the conversation. The patient shifts from discussing a particular topic (birth control) to asking the physician two personal questions.
2. The reason for this shift is unclear. The patient may be expressing anxiety, may be avoiding the topic, or may simply want to hear how the physician handles this situation.
3. "How will knowing how many children I have and what method of contraception my spouse and I use help you?" or "What are your reasons for asking?" These open-ended questions will help clarify the meaning of the personal questions. Then the physician may decide to supply the answers or change the focus.

Patient 6

1. There is a change in time orientation—the patient refers to the past whenever the dentist talks about the present and the future care of his teeth.

2. Possible sadness, regret, and loneliness, as well as avoidance or discomfort in discussing gum disease.
3. "You have talked about how much you miss your wife. How is that related to the importance of taking care of your teeth?" This question asks the patient to "connect the shift," to explain how the discussion of his wife is related to his dental care. An alternative response might be to simply instruct the patient to focus on the present topic: "I would like us to spend a few minutes before you leave, discussing the importance of these aspects of your dental care."

Patient 7

1. There is a shift in body language or nonverbal behavior. When the topic of sexual activity is introduced, the patient breaks eye contact and furrows her brow, and her hands tremble.
2. The shift in nonverbal behavior suggests inaccuracy in her verbal account that resumption of sexual activity has been fine. There is reason to suspect some problems with her sexual adjustment and a reluctance to discuss possible solutions.
3. Assuming you decide to respond to this shift at this time, you could reflect her discomfort or nonverbal messages as in the following two responses: "You seem to feel a little uncomfortable talking about this topic." Or "I'm confused. I realize you said everything is fine, but I also notice that you look differently now as we're talking about this." The first response involves a reflection of the patient's feelings. The second response is a confrontation.

Chapter Summary

In patient/interviewer interactions, patients will shift or change their communication style to reveal a significant, although often unspoken, concern or feeling and to defend themselves against the anxiety created by the interaction. The interviewer's ability to recognize such shifts is important to respond to patient concerns effectively and to avoid getting trapped by difficult or manipulative patient communication. The interviewer must recognize that a communication shift has occurred and decide whether to respond verbally or to ignore the shift. A variety of verbal responses can be used to respond effectively to communication shifts, including clarification, open-ended questions, paraphrase, reflection of feelings, confrontation, instructions, and information giving. If health professionals decide to acknowledge the shift in patient communication with appropriate verbal responses, they must also be willing to take the time to stay and discuss the patient's concerns or feelings.

The most common communication shifts occur in four different patterns. These include *alterations in mood, changes in time orientations, shifts in subject matter,* and *alterations in body language.* One common shift involves the manner in which the patients express their emotions. Intensely felt emotions, such as extreme sadness and hostility, are often especially difficult for health professionals to handle. A second shift involves changes in time orientation. Patients may constantly shift focus to the past or the future and avoid the present. Shifts in subject matter are a common way in which patients reveal concerns. Patients may shift away from or toward a very significant topic during the course of one or more interactions. Patients may also change the topic by the use of jokes, casual remarks, or irrelevant comments.

The type or number of questions the patient asks also reveals patient concerns or discomfort. A request for information or for the professional's opinion may actually be a statement of an important patient concern. Aspects of patient concerns are also disclosed when patients ask the interviewer personal questions. At times a patient may flood the interviewer with a series of questions that gradually reveal what the patient is really thinking or wanting to know.

In addition to changes in verbal communication, alterations may occur in body language. In such cases the interviewer might choose more often than not to ignore shifts to avoid making the patient self-conscious or unwilling to continue the interaction. At times, however, shifts in patients' body language may require a verbal response, as when the nonverbal shift reflects inaccurate verbal information or flirtatious or seductive behavior.

Although the focus of this chapter has been recognizing and responding to shifts in patient communication styles, these same changes frequently occur in communications between health professionals and their colleagues, as well as patient family members. For example, colleagues may disrupt a patient/professional relationship by expressing strong, inappropriate feelings or by obscuring important topics with jokes, trivial remarks, or irrelevant comments. Likewise, family members, under the strain of illness in a loved one, may experience intense feelings of rage or anger and may express or repress such feelings by joking, changing the topic, rambling, or asking excessively detailed questions.

Health professionals may succumb to the distractions these defensive reactions create. Awareness of such communication shifts may help prevent such distractions and be rewarded by savings in time, accurate diagnoses, and increased rapport with patients and other members of the health care team.

Suggested Readings _____

Elder, J. *Transactional analysis in health care*. Menlo Park, Calif.: Addison-Wesley, 1978. Chapter 10, "Permission, Protection and Potency," describes the role of these "three P's" in health care. The author suggests how the health professional may use the three P's to give patients permission to express themselves and their feelings in a direct way.

Froelich, R., & Bishop, F. *Clinical interviewing skills*. St. Louis, Mo.: Mosby, 1977. Chapter 5, "Specific Interview Problems," discusses possible meanings of patient questions and ways of responding to these direct or implied meanings.

Hainer, B. L. Recognition and management of the overly affectionate patient. *The Journal of Family Practice*, 1982, *14*, 47–49. This article describes succinctly ways in which patients can express affection and seductiveness or can be overly solicitous toward health professionals.

Hein, E. C. *Communication in nursing practice*. Boston: Little, Brown, 1980. Chapter 8, "Defensive Behaviors in Interviewing," discusses a variety of ways in which both health professional and patient may react defensively during an interview to guard against feeling emotionally unprotected and vulnerable.

Passons, W. R. *Gestalt approaches in counseling*. New York: Holt, Rinehart & Winston, 1975. Chapter 6, "Nonverbal Awareness," describes the meaning of changes in nonverbal communication patterns and possible ways of responding to such changes.

Reiser, D. E., & Schroder, A. K. *Patient interviewing: The human dimension*. Baltimore, Md.: Williams & Wilkins, 1980. Chapter 6, "The Interview Process," describes a number of communication patterns used by patients that these authors refer to as "process tracks."

Dealing with Patients' Emotional Reactions

Objectives

After mastering the material presented in this chapter, you will be able to:

1. Identify, when given a written case history, the eight emotional reactions of an ill patient.

2. Identify, when given a written case history, five helpful ways of responding to emotional reactions to illness.

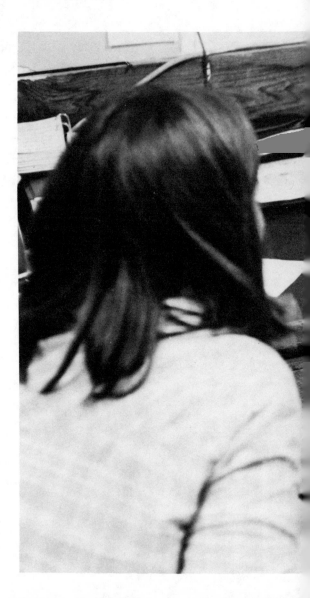

11

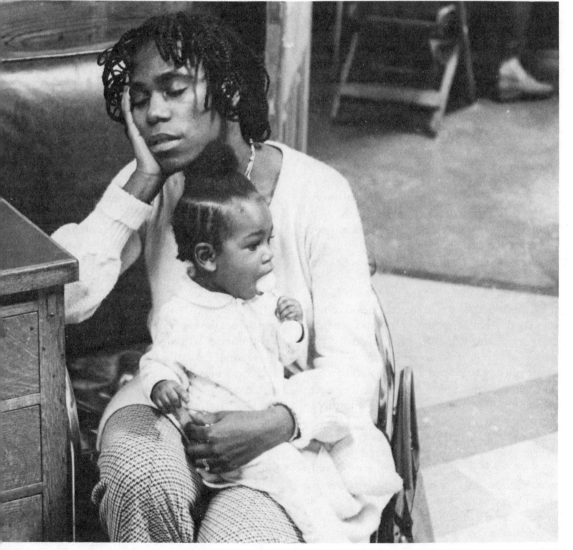

The ability to recognize, understand, and deal with the ways in which patients react emotionally to illness is the hallmark of a successful health professional. In contrast to the physical manifestations of disease that can be objectively observed, measured, tested, and defined, the emotional responses remain subjective, unmeasurable, and obscure. Whereas physical problems can be actively treated, emotional wounds usually cannot be medicated, excised, splinted, rested, or bandaged.

It is impossible, however, to separate the emotional aspects of an illness from the physical aspects. Whether physical illness occurs as a result of emotional pain and stress or vice-versa is a moot argument. Each patient is a complete package containing both mind (emotion) and body, and the two are inseparable.

Most physicians agree that between 70 and 80 percent of the patients who visit their offices suffer from emotional and stress-related diseases (Fisher, 1978). Human beings have only a limited amount of emotional energy, and when life becomes too hectic or coping mechanisms fail, illness may be the result. The degree of incapacitation may be largely independent of the amount of actual organic pathology present (Bernstein & Bernstein, 1980). If health professionals are to deal effectively with the ill, they must first learn to detect and respect emotional complaints as a significant part of a health problem.

Several factors inhibit the professionals' ability to deal effectively with the emotional components of illness. Perhaps the most significant factor is the emphasis on the organic (physical) aspect of disease during professional education. Diseases are frequently presented via mechanical models with "mechanical failures." Cures are thought to result from careful "trouble-shooting" that reveals the site of the failure.

Another factor concerns the ability of professionals to deal with their own emotions. Professionals who grew up in families where emotions were subdued may have negative responses to a patient's emotional outburst and may not be able to understand and help the patient deal with the problem. On the other hand, professionals who were raised in families where emotions were freely and honestly expressed may be able to deal very well with a hysterical patient response.

Another limiting factor for most health professionals is lack of time. Heavy patient loads put very real limits on the time available for therapeutic listening and, as a result, snap judgments may be made, which can be counterproductive and even traumatic for patients. It is not difficult, therefore, to understand why health professionals do not always deal with emotional reactions in a satisfactory manner.

This chapter has two sections. The first section describes some typical emotional reactions that patients express toward illness and presents some brief suggestions for dealing with these reactions. The second section describes in more detail some general methods for handling the emotional reactions of patients.

Typical Emotional Reactions to Illness

The emotional reaction to illness begins before individuals become fully aware of their illness, continues in a sporadic and disorganized manner during the acute phases of the illness, and progresses through an integrating stage as the individual either becomes well (returns to *pre-illness homeostasis*), develops a permanent handicap or chronic illness (a *nonfunctional equilibrium*), or learns from the experience in a growth producing way (Reiser & Schroder, 1980).

During the earliest stage, that of beginning awareness, the patient faces the dilemma of denying the existence of the illness and wanting to learn about it at the same time. Consequently, his or her internal dialogue and overt behaviors swing back and forth between these opposite poles. The process advances into a period of disorganization where the person loses a sense of connection, control, and even identity. The mind turns inward, reason fails to operate, and the patient may rebel against measures that would ease or cure the distress. The outcome depends on the patient's ways of handling problems, the nature of the illness, the availability of support, and the quality of care given by health professionals (Bernstein & Bernstein, 1980).

Ambivalence about Knowing

The onset of illness is characterized by both denial and the need to know. Initially patients notice a lump, an ache, a pain, or the inability to perform a task that had previously been easy. Their first impulse is to ignore the symptom: "It will go away," or "It's nothing, I'll go to bed and take aspirin, or get busy to keep my mind occupied. I'll be OK tomorrow." If the problem resolves (which it often does), the process stops at this point. If it recurs, the process may recur, with added thoughts: "I wonder what it is?" "If it isn't gone by tomorrow, maybe I should call a doctor."

It is not unusual for people to arrive in the emergency room late at night or on weekends with an illness that has been present for several days. For example, a person may come to the emergency room on Christmas Eve after having had severe abdominal pain for three days. In another instance, a mother may bring her four-month-old baby to the hospital at midnight after the child has had a cough for several weeks. Or a patient who has been having asthma attacks periodically for several months may present at the emergency room at 3 A.M. in a panic. Such patients are no longer able to deny their illness and feel an immediate need to know.

In this period of ambivalence about knowing, ill people may be unable to accept warm and tender caring from family, friends, or professionals. They may see this concern as indicating a degree of seriousness that they are not ready to accept. They may feel threatened or may feel that their privacy has been invaded. Consequently, they may respond with irritation (Enelow & Swisher, 1979).

Fear and Anxiety

Fear and anxiety are common reactions to illness. These emotions strain controls and defenses, use up energy needed for recuperation, and contrib-ute to continuing disorganization. Fear is seldom expressed directly. More often it is recognized as the force behind constant pleas for reassurance, repetition of the same question, and demands for frequent attention (Bernstein & Bernstein, 1980).

Physically, fear may cause pallor, restlessness, muscular tension, headaches, diarrhea, or consti-pation, thus obscuring the true symptoms of an illness (Bernstein & Bernstein, 1980). For exam-ple, if a woman who is three months pregnant slips and falls, she may be extremely afraid of los-ing or hurting her baby. It may be difficult to dif-ferentiate between a genuine complication of her pregnancy and basic fear if she develops pallor, restlessness, or muscle tension.

Overhearing conversations among medical personnel may greatly increase fear in some patients even though the conversations do not apply to the patients who overhear them. An unusual example follows.

After the uncomplicated removal of her gall bladder, a middle-aged woman believed she was dying. She failed to regain her strength, was un-able to eat, moved very little, and was seriously depressed. Her incision healed on schedule, and after a week of no emotional improvement and with no organic explanation, a psychiatric consul-tant was called in to see her. Under hypnosis, she recalled hearing her surgeon say, "I'm sorry, you're not going to make it" as she was going into anes-thesia. When the situation was later reconstructed, it was determined that the surgeon had spoken these words when talking with the operating room nurse who was forced to miss a social engagement due to the late hour of the surgery. Once the patient understood, the idea of dying was immediately dispelled and she promptly recovered.

Anxiety is a more diffuse, less specific emo-tion than fear. It is associated with feelings of uncertainty and helplessness and is sometimes described as free, floating dread with no known cause. A low to medium level of anxiety may be useful in motivation. An illustration of this is study-ing for a test or seeing a physician about a physical symptom. A high level of anxiety, however, may cause panic and immobility. One manifestation of anxiety in illness is a paradoxical dilemma. In this situation, a person may experience a strong desire for something simultaneously with a strong repulsion to the same thing. Some examples expressed by patients are "I'm afraid to be alone, but I don't want to be bothered" or "Stay with me, I need you, but having you around is hard for me."

Supportive listening is usually effective in reducing anxiety. Occasional comments that the worries and concerns are reasonable and understandable give patients permission to voice their fears and overcome them. Careful explanations of what is actually happening now, what the test will be like, what the medicine will do, what will happen tomorrow, or what will occur after the operation may also allay fears and anxieties. (The importance of preparatory information is discussed in more detail in Chapter 13.)

Anger

Anger is another typical emotional reaction to illness. It is both appropriate and understandable given the turmoil and disruption that illness causes. At least temporarily, goals must be altered, dependency becomes necessary, and privacy is invaded.

Anger may be useful in helping provide the emotional energy to fight disease. However, some patients react angrily to nearly everything, and others cover up fear with anger and use it as a defense against intimacy or a denial of dependency. They may respond with helpless rage, lashing out at everyone and everything. They may get in the way of their own recovery by refusing medication, failing to cooperate with rehabilitation efforts, not adhering to their diets, or smoking heavily. They may also physically attack other people or objects.

Suspicion and lack of trust are also manifestations of anger. Health professionals need to view these responses as symptoms and combat them with patience, consistency, realism, and firmness. For example, a belligerent young man has been subdued and handcuffed. He continues to fight, struggle, and plead to have the cuffs removed. The nurse says firmly and calmly "I will listen to you. Tell me about it." She listens to him for a few minutes and then continues "I have listened to you. Now you listen to me. The cuffs are there for your safety and our protection. If you continue to fight and struggle it will be impossible for us to help you. If you calm down and remain quiet, we will loosen the cuffs in a little while."

People bring to illness patterns of behavior and emotional response that they have learned and developed over their entire lives. They react to illness according to these personal patterns. Such patterns ordinarily help people maintain their equilibrium; however, during illness they may be more vulnerable, and many of their usual coping methods may not be readily available. For example, a man who vents his feelings through jogging may not be able to express those same feelings when he has a broken hip. He will need to learn an alternate way of coping.

Feelings need to be accepted and respected, whether they belong to the patient or to the health professional, and the manner of expressing those feelings is a matter of individual choice. Feeling angry is human, and it is often difficult not to retaliate after being the target of a patient's displaced anger. However, retaliation is not useful for either party. What may be useful is to acknowledge *internally* the desire to strike back or swear at a patient, then decide to express it later in a more acceptable way. Having a friend or colleague as a listener may be helpful.

It is important to let patients know that their feelings are acknowledged and respected, even if they have to alter their usual ways of expressing them. Sometimes a simple discussion of what they are angry about will prevent a tantrum.

Guilt and Shame

Guilt is another typical way of reacting to illness. Some persons see illness as a punishment for sin (Reiser & Schroder, 1980), to be tolerated passively as penance. A patient may think "I must have done something terribly wrong for God to have done this to me." Others may imagine themselves as "psychosomatic" and actually causing their own illness. In this situation, they might consider the mind/body connection but envision themselves as able to retain more control. Still others may project their guilt as blame and become chronically quarrelsome and dissatisfied with treatment and attention from family and health care personnel (Enelow & Swisher, 1979).

Shame is closely allied to guilt; it is a painful feeling of being exposed and ridiculed, to a degree that brings disgrace or dishonor to one's self and family. Feelings of guilt and shame are usually unrelated to any actual sin or dishonor, but to the person experiencing such feelings, they are painful. It is sometimes helpful to be gently realistic. For example, the health professional might say "Marie, I'm sorry that you feel so ashamed about having contracted gonorrhea. However, gonorrhea is an infectious disease which is very common and easily treated. There is no reason why you should feel that you have disgraced your entire family."

Excessive Compliance or Noncompliance

Some people who are ill regress to a child-like state. One characteristic of small children who are sick is that they vigorously express all of their feelings. They kick, scream, and fight when they are angry; they cry, hide, and try to run away when they are scared. Children also express positive emotions; they sit up, play and giggle, and happily greet their parents, or they tease and hug their nurses. Children heal and recover from illnesses much more rapidly than adults. Although they do seem to heal more rapidly in the physical sense, part of their rapid healing is related to their ability to express themselves spontaneously. Most adults, on the other hand, have learned a set of behaviors about "how to be ill," which seldom includes the free expression of feelings. They rarely react in the natural way children do but switch to the adaptive behaviors they have learned to use in unfamiliar and frightening situations. Most hospitalized patients adapt rapidly to meet the expectations of the institution. They feel helpless and at the mercy of the staff. Many will complain to their friends, relatives, or to a sympathetic aide that they are afraid to ask for what they want, or complain

about things they don't like, for fear of reprisals. Others may rebel and refuse to follow orders; they may be constantly angry, uncooperative, and demanding when they don't immediately get attention. Some may behave "very well," act overly friendly or cheerful, or be very cooperative and anxious to please. Still others may overcomply and try to please by hiding pain and withholding information.

Superstitious or Egocentric Thinking

Most patients secretly believe that illness can't happen to them. During the shock of discovering that illness has, in fact, happened, disorganization progresses. One of the early reactions to the onset of illness is egocentricity. As one patient described it, "I see the world only in terms of me, like a two-year-old who hides under a blanket and can't figure out how his mother knows he is there." Consider the executive with a massive coronary who says "I'll go to the hospital tomorrow. I have important appointments today."

Some people become concerned with limitations: "Do I have enough medicine?" "Are there steps to climb?" "How long do I have?" "Am I a burden?" "Must I stay here alone?" "Does anyone care?" "If only someone cared, I wouldn't have to ask." "What's the use anyway?" Other people believe in magic remedies at this stage. "The doctor knows everything." "The nurse can fix it if she wants to." "If only I can get enough exercise, eat health food, and take vitamins, then I'll be OK." These superstitious or egocentric ways of thinking may interfere with the patient's acceptance of the real issues. The professional may answer the patient's questions honestly and accurately and then reinforce the true nature of the illness. For example:

> Mrs. Rockford, some people do claim that bee pollen has a beneficial effect on multiple sclerosis. However, there is not much good evidence to support that contention at this time. So, since the pollen will probably not hurt you, feel free to continue to use it. But at the same time, don't neglect your visits to physical therapy.

Loss of Autonomy;
Dependence; Helplessness

In our culture, people who are ill receive sympathy from relatives and friends. The seriously ill depend on health professionals for their survival. For passive people who normally rely on others, this adjustment is not difficult. However, for those who are usually independent, autonomous, and self-reliant, dependence and helplessness are a serious threat to which they may respond with anger, stubborn rebellion, or panic (Enelow & Swisher, 1979).

Health professionals may help to alleviate these feelings by speaking gently but frankly with patients. For example:

> Tom, since your accident in the coal mines, it has been necessary to help you breathe with the use of this respirator. From the way that you are breathing and from the look in your eyes, I get the feeling that you are panic stricken by your dependence on the machine. So far your recovery has been progressing very well. So well that now we must think about weaning you off the respirator. You may find that to be very scary. However, if you will try not to panic and trust that I will not let you down, I think we can manage it together, one day at a time.

In the following instance, the health professional must deal with a rebellious patient.

> Mr. Hall, I need to talk very seriously with you for a couple of minutes. Your asthma has been very easily and well controlled ever since you were placed on that new medication. However, despite the new medicine, this is now the third time that you've been hospitalized for the asthma in six months, and each time your blood studies show that you have not taken the medicine. Now I know that you pride yourself on being a "self-made man," and I suspect that the need for medicine implies to you that you are weak and unable to control the asthma on your own. Is it possible that you can consider the *taking* of the medicine the manner in which you can control the asthma on your own so that you will not end up in the hospital again?

Conversely, as recovery or convalescence begins, the situation is reversed. Independent people may quickly respond to opportunities for self-care and overexert themselves, while dependent people may have difficulty in resuming responsibility for their own care. For example, Mr. Hilling, a successful stock broker, was a hard-driving, competitive individual. After a myocardial infarct he was intent on returning to work the day of his discharge. It was necessary to encourage him not to overexert himself.

> Well, Mr. Hilling, today is your day to go home. I am a bit concerned that you will attempt to do too much too fast and hinder your recovery. Therefore, I have had this exercise protocol set up for you. Please follow it very carefully and do not proceed to the next exercise level until you have completed all the previous requirements for seven days each.

Notice that the use of a protocol, or treatment regimen, has a limiting effect by prescribing that the patient must repeat the lower exercise level for seven days before progressing to the next step. The hard-driving individual has daily goals to meet before progress can be claimed.

Loss of Identity and
Self-Esteem

Frequently, illness threatens a person's self-esteem and sense of identity.

> My body is failing me, limits my activity, and has almost become my prison. My heart doesn't work well, my hip is fractured, and I have pneumonia. I'm sure not the man I used to be. What will become of me?

When illness strikes it may take some time before the patient's mental image becomes congruent with the reality of the body's problems. In the interim, the self-image is disorganized, which in turn contributes to feelings of low self-esteem. Low self-esteem decreases the patient's ability to understand a treatment program and to carry it out (Bernstein & Bernstein, 1980), to understand directions, and to think clearly. It also inhibits permission to ask clarifying questions. A patient may assume "They will think I'm stupid if I ask about that."

Patients with long-term chronic illnesses may begin to equate themselves with their particular disease and believe: "I'm a diabetic, arthritic, alcoholic," and so on. Their symptoms become the focus of their thoughts and conversations. Health professionals may inadvertently encourage this equating of self with disease through their own conversations and writings. Many professional conferences and journal articles are introduced by such statements as "J. R. is a 58-year-old white, male, diabetic alcoholic." Also, hospitalized patients may overhear conversations like "This is Mrs. Smith, the rheumatic heart that I consulted you about." It is imperative that health professionals continue to respect patients as people—not as convenient disease entities. In order to prevent this occur-

rence, it may be useful to advise patients to interrupt anytime they feel that they are being overlooked and talked about—for example:

> Mr. Grey, this is Doctor Smith, the heart specialist I told you about the other day. During the course of this consultation, we will be concentrating our efforts on establishing an appropriate diagnosis and treatment plan for you. While we are doing this, it may appear that we are discussing only the disease process and totally forgetting about you. If you begin to feel that way, please don't hesitate to interrupt so that you will personally better understand what is going on.

By using this tactic, the patient is given permission to interrupt and, at the same time, becomes personally involved in his or her own treatment program.

◯

================ *LEARNING ACTIVITIES* ================

Emotional Reactions to Illness

In this learning activity we present the written case history of Paula. Following the narrative, the eight emotional reactions to illness are tabulated. You are to match the appropriate emotional reaction with the underlined section of the narrative that best depicts that reaction (Chapter Objective 1). Feedback follows the learning activity. The first item is completed as an example.

The case of Paula

Paula was an energetic, ambitious, 32-year-old college English teacher. She had recently been granted a sabbatical year to complete her doctorate. While driving home from a party in her honor on a rain-slicked road, she was involved in a collision. Her new car was demolished, and she was hospitalized in critical condition suffering from a broken arm, thigh, shoulder, and jaw, and a fractured skull.

After weeks in the intensive care unit she became alert and realized that her head had been shaved, her jaws had been wired, several teeth were missing, and her right arm and left leg were totally encased in casts. (1) Despite the obvious extent of her injuries, she asked no questions about her condition and remained virtually motionless in bed. (2)

Her best friend and roommate had been involved in the same accident and had sustained a broken back. Recently she had been discharged from the hospital in a full body cast and had returned to her parents' home to recover. A mutual friend had informed Paula that her roommate blamed her for the accident. (3) Paula's boyfriend had visited her on one occasion, had been aghast at the extent of her injuries, and had never returned.

Paula was angry and irritable, snapped sarcastically at the nursing staff, and screamed whenever members of the staff attempted to work with her. (4) Her actions made it necessary to use four attendants any time she was moved. The staff of the intensive care unit was happy to see her transferred to the orthopedic ward for further recovery. By the end of the first week on the ward, Paula had earned the dislike of all who cared for her. She viciously and loudly berated and abused the staff each time they attempted to move her from bed to chair, screaming "Stop it! You'll drop me!" She also objected to every aspect of her treatment plan, claiming "I can't stand the pain!" or "You're trying to kill me. You're going to drop me!" (5) She refused to bathe, refused to take her medication on schedule, and refused physical therapy. (6)

The orthopedic surgeon in charge of her care lost all patience and scolded her as being "thoughtless, selfish, and unfair to the staff who were trying to help." The oral surgeon, who had repaired her original facial trauma, removed the wires from her jaws and was able to advance her from a liquid to a soft diet. Once her diet was altered, it also became impossible to please her with food. She insisted on a diet consisting of yogurt, wheat germ, large quantities of vitamins, and other health foods that were not readily available in the hospital kitchen. She insisted the health foods "will help me heal." (7)

The oral surgeon approached her one day and discussed plans for further reconstructive surgery to correct her shattered teeth and jaws and to revise several scars involving her lips and left cheek. He placed a mirror in front of her to better describe the anticipated surgery. She screamed, refused to look at herself, closed her eyes, and remarked matter-of-factly "That's not really me." (8)

Emotional reactions	Excessive compliance or noncompliance	6
	Superstitious or egocentric thinking	___
	Guilt and/or shame	___
	Loss of autonomy; dependency; helplessness	___
	Anger	___
	Loss of identity and self-esteem	___
	Fear and anxiety	___
	Ambivalence about knowing	___

Feedback	1. 6	3. 3	5. 4	7. 5
	2. 7	4. 1	6. 8	8. 2

General Methods for Dealing with the Emotional Reactions of Patients

An ill person surrenders a certain amount of self-control and, with it, self-esteem. In a health care environment, the patient is a victim at the mercy of strangers who have the power to be kind or unkind, to relieve or not relieve pain, to listen or ignore. Under such conditions, patients may behave passively and fail to make their feelings and concerns known. An astute interviewer is able to identify significant feelings and deal with them constructively. In recognizing and responding to a patient's emotional reactions, an interviewer can (1) provide psychological protection, (2) encourage expression of feelings, (3) offer support, (4) express understanding of the negative realities of illness, and (5) provide reinforcement of self-care.

Provide Psychological Protection

In most health care environments, patients need some time to adjust and also need encouragement to ask for what they want and to express how they feel. Whether or not they will respond to such encouragement depends on how secure they feel. Do they feel vulnerable or protected?

Protecting the patient means indicating in nonverbal ways that you will remain and listen with concern. This can be done by being calm, quiet, and attentive. This simple approach is often all that is needed to elicit a direct response to questions. However, sometimes it becomes necessary to observe, intuit, and deduce what kind of encouragement and protection are needed (Elder, 1978).

One way to establish such an interaction follows.

> Ms. Davis, you've been here in the hospital for three days, and you've barely spoken to me even though I've spent several hours in your room making beds and passing medicine. I have a feeling that I may have done something to offend you, and I'd like to have a chance to make it right.

Such an encounter requires an honest response. If the patient has been offended, the problem can be discussed and possibly resolved. More often the patient will respond "Oh, no. I just don't have much to talk about." Now the professional has an opportunity to ask "Don't you have any close friends, or hobbies, or pets. . . ." and so on. By opening in an apologetic tone, the professional has taken a personal risk. Such a tone communicates to the patient that the health professional is aware of the patient's vulnerability and is genuinely interested in protecting the patient.

Encourage Patient Expression of Feelings

The most helpful thing a health professional can do is to respect the right of patients to react and to feel, regardless of how they choose to express themselves. Encouraging patients to express whatever feelings they have about the situation is a very useful thing to do. To "cry it out," "cuss it out," or admit to fear may release pent-up tensions and help the patient progress. However, such encouragement must be done very carefully and with the following four guidelines in mind:

1. The health professional must be comfortable in the presence of strong emotion. Encouraging the expression of deep, personal feelings and then exhibiting embarrassment and discomfort is counterproductive.

2. The health professional must have adequate time to stay with patients during their expression of strong feelings. To invite patients to "let it all out" and then to leave the room or change the subject before they are finished may leave patients traumatized and psychologically defenseless.

3. The health professional must determine how patients really feel and must not project his or her own feelings. Anxiety is contagious. The health professional who senses a feeling of anxiety in the presence of a patient should examine his or her own feelings about the situation. Only after ruling out personal sources of anx-

iety should the professional inquire "Are you feeling anxious?" Frequently, the patient will respond in the affirmative.

4. Health professionals must ensure that patients are temporarily willing and able to express themselves or reveal their feelings. Questions that are currently inappropriate may be very appropriate at some later time. However, the patient alone may know the "right" time.

When a patient obviously is on the verge of tears, the health professional may give permission to cry nonverbally with an arm around the patient's shoulders or a gentle touch. Verbally, the same message can be related by a simple statement such as "It's OK to cry if you feel like it" or "I'd probably cry too if I was in your position!" Sit quietly without interruption until the patient stops crying, and then respond with sincere validation of the feeling (Enelow & Swisher, 1979). Say, for example, "Those tears needed to come out," or "It's normal to be sad about . . ." (the situation), or let them see your concern in your expression. It may be appropriate to gently hug the patient. Do not rush patients by exclaiming "Well, now that's over, you'll feel better" and hurriedly leaving.

When patients are angry, it is often useful to invite them to tell you about it, if you are able to consider angry responses without getting defensive or angry in return. Many patients are impatient and may be angry about unrealistic expectations that are not being met.

Some patients may use profanity when expressing anger. If you are offended or uncomfortable with profanity, say that you will find someone else to whom they can talk and do not encourage them to ventilate to you. It would not be unreasonable to say "Fred, I have a problem hearing so much profanity. I'm not sure that I can help. But, if you would like, I will find someone else here on the staff with whom you can talk this matter out to your heart's content!" Such a statement allows the patient the option of "cleaning up" the profanity or discussing the matter with another professional who can better deal with it.

Offer Support

One important task of the health professional is to counteract the depersonalization of the health care system by treating the patient as a person. This process begins by getting to know the patient. Who is the patient? What does she or he do? How did she or he handle illness in the past? What is his or her culture like? Is there someone on the staff who has a similar culture? What does this particular illness mean to the patient? What kind of support system does the patient have? Are the supporters family, friends, colleagues, pets? Can they be contacted?

For example, a man who had fallen from a roof at work, sustaining multiple fractures, was depressed and unable to eat. A friend contacted the nursing supervisor and explained that the man had a beautiful, devoted German shepherd who was also not eating, losing weight, and lying on the doorstep awaiting his master's return. Due to the anticipated length of the hospitalization, the friend explained that the dog would probably die before his master returned. The patient was equally concerned about his dog but had said nothing. Although animals in the hospital were strictly forbidden, the supervisor arranged for the friend to bring the dog in late at night so he could see that his master was alive. The dog recovered, and so did the patient.

Understand Negative Realities of Illness

In addition to the symptoms and dangers of a particular illness, patients must deal with many other negative realities. One of them is nakedness in the presence of strangers. Physical examinations require undressing and exposing the body for inspection. For some people nakedness means defenselessness, vulnerability, and, in the presence of others who are fully clothed, embarrassment. Health professionals can minimize such embarrassment by ensuring that patients are carefully draped, that the room is warm, and that the examination is done politely, in a businesslike manner, and as quickly as possible. It is most respectful to have the post-examination discussion after the patient is dressed again.

An additional consideration for the patient is to provide seating that is at eye level with the professional. Such seating places patient and professional on an "equal footing" and minimizes feelings of intimidation.

Another negative reality facing patients is removal from their usual sources of satisfaction. Their schedule is disrupted. Their time no longer has value. They must go to the office or laboratory at a time that is convenient for the professionals. They must leave their jobs, their homes, their familiar places, possessions, and faces. Often patients must wait for seemingly interminable amounts of time to be seen and to get their questions answered.

If patients are hospitalized, they are expected to eat, sleep, bathe, dress, and amuse themselves on a schedule that is arranged for the convenience of the staff. Patients have few choices about what they will eat, wear, do, or be. They also know that their care is costing a great deal of money. If they were staying in a luxury hotel, a similar amount of money would bring luxurious accommodations, gourmet food that they could select when hungry, and many other services. They could watch television all night if they chose, and their privacy would not be invaded.

In the hospital, patients often must share a room with strangers, turn off lights and television at a specified hour, and show consideration for the staff and other patients. They must also tolerate multiple interruptions and intrusions by maids, nurses, doctors, technicians, and ministers who feel free to enter their rooms at will and engage in conversation. Business office personnel may come at odd hours to question them about their finances. Their wine, their before-dinner cocktail, and their cigarettes are either forbidden or carefully monitored. The health professional who is understanding and tolerant of this displacement may help to alleviate some of the patient's frustrations.

Another negative reality of illness is that patients are expected to wait for someone to bring them food, medicine, and water. They are expected to stay in their rooms and are encouraged in subtle ways not to do anything for themselves or even to think for themselves. It is small wonder, then, that during the course of a serious illness patients begin to define themselves in terms of their illness and lose touch with their identity as people. For example, instead of thinking "I'm Mary, a teacher, wife, and mother who is loving and kind," the patient may think "I'm a diabetic" or "I'm an epileptic."

Patients who are offered choices, no matter how small, keep their identities intact better than most. For example, a person who watches daytime television might be given a choice about having a bath or doing exercises before or after a favorite program. Does the patient have a radio? What does he or she listen to? Are there flowers in the room? Did the patient grow them? Who sent them? Noticing and commenting on such small details may help the patient feel less displaced.

Provide Reinforcement of Self-care

People get well faster when they help themselves. Self-care for some may mean the ability to get themselves fed, dressed, and out of the house to keep an appointment. For people hospitalized with an acute illness, self-care begins with getting themselves to the bathroom, brushing their own teeth, and combing their own hair. It proceeds to making decisions and beginning to take responsibility for their own recovery.

Before expecting patients to participate in planning and carrying out treatment programs, it is important that you find out what they can do and how much they know about the process. The usual assumption that patients know nothing and that a complete explanation is necessary may be a "put-down" for some people. Others may simply tune out the information. Conversely, it is not useful to assume that patients are well informed simply because they have had a similar illness before or are health professionals themselves. Careful inquiry will reveal how much information they need.

It is also important to determine whether patients are emotionally ready to participate in their own recovery. The health professional can deduce this by observing patients' general grooming and alertness and the interest they show in response to questions and information.

Helping patients develop a problem-solving attitude is essential. Positive reinforcement begins the process. Listen carefully to what patients tell you about their perception of the problem and give them feedback that clarifies the issues. (See also Chapters 5 and 6.)

Whenever patients do something for themselves, they are likely to continue it if their actions are noticed and rewarded. It is important to notice what the patient does or says in a matter-of-fact partnership style, rather than in a parental fashion. Say, for example, "I see that you are doing your exercises without help today. How does that feel?" rather than "Oh, I'm so proud of you. You did your exercises all by yourself!"

Another aspect of helping people resume responsibility for themselves is to allow them to do as much as they are able to do for themselves and to help only when necessary. There is a fine line between useful assistance and dependence-inducing "rescuing."

To clarify whether the health professional is helping or rescuing, he or she must ask the following questions: (1) Is this person unable to do it without my help? (2) Will what I am doing contribute to independence? (3) Did this person ask me for help or accept my offer of help? (4) Is there a clear understanding between us about the nature of my help?

For example, George is recovering from a broken hip. He weighs 285 pounds. Every morning two orderlies lift him into a wheelchair, which is a difficult task. The orderlies come from different parts of the hospital. The same scene recurs when he is ready to go back to bed. Both orderlies and George become disgruntled and irascible in this situation each day. By asking themselves questions 1 and 2, the orderlies might be able to determine whether or not George could learn to get himself into the wheelchair by pivoting on his good leg (Elder, 1978, pp. 103–104).

Consulting the patient about changes in his or her plan for care is also useful. Describe what needs to be done, and offer choices—for example, "These exercises will strengthen your muscles so you will be able to walk without help. It looks like you are ready to do them twice each day. When do you think would be a good time to do them?"

Patients begin to exchange self-pity for acceptance of their new self-image at some point. Carefully mentioning small specific changes is important (Bernstein & Bernstein, 1980)—for example, "I see you have put on your make-up this morning. Does that mean you are feeling better and beginning to be interested in your appearance again?"

When the new self-image incorporates a loss of a body part, a sense, or an ability, the patient will need to grieve for the loss. Sometimes an explanation of the grieving process may be helpful, or a simple statement such as "It's difficult to accept losing a breast, and it will take a while to get over those feelings of disfigurement, but you can do it."

○

=========== *LEARNING ACTIVITIES* ===========

Helpful Ways of Responding to Emotional Reactions to Illness

In this learning activity, Paula's story continues. Following the description, you are to match the five helpful responses of the health professionals with the appropriate sections of the description (Chapter Objective 2). Feedback follows the learning activity. The first item is completed as an example.

The case of Paula   While seeking support systems for Paula, it was discovered that her only relatives were her elderly parents who lived in a retirement home almost 3000 miles away. Two or three of Paula's colleagues called occasionally, but none visited regularly due to the distance involved. Paula did not belong to a church and had had a disagreement with the hospital chaplain. She resented "do-gooders." Neither would she consider a psychiatric consultant. "Psychiatrists," said Paula, "are for crazy people."

After diligent searching, the supervisor of student nurses at Paula's hospital was identified as a possible source of support. The nursing instructor visited Paula to talk with her and to assess her situation. Paula responded well to the contact with another "teacher." The nursing instructor assigned a student to work with Paula for a few days weekly and visited personally as well. (1) The student spent some time initially just quietly sitting and listening to Paula as she related her story. (2)

Soon Paula was discussing her fears and anxieties about the long time it would require for recuperation before she could proceed to work on her doctorate. (3) Her real concerns began to emerge. "Will I ever be pretty again?" "Will anyone ever like me?" "How are my mom and dad managing since I have not been able to visit them?" The nursing student attempted to understand how Paula was trying to adjust to the problems she faced as a result of her accident. (4)

The nurse instructor also heard of Paula's "bad reputation" among the nursing staff. Paula's notion that the staff didn't like her was not unfounded. The instructor and Paula identified the bed-to-chair transfers as Paula's most hated activity and devised a new plan for them. With much apprehension, Paula agreed to attempt getting into the chair with just one assistant instead of the previously required four. The instructor, whom she had grown to trust, supported her cast left leg. Paula used her good left arm and her right leg and positioned the cast right arm across her chest. She was surprised to discover that she was able to transfer to the wheelchair without difficulty. Once she was successful she agreed to stop her complaining if the staff would allow her to take control of the transfer process.

Once the transfer problem was resolved, staff members became more sympathetic to Paula's plight. They began to spend more time with her and encouraged her to bathe, groom herself, apply make-up, and so on. She soon realized that she was able to use cosmetics effectively to hide her scars and accepted suggestions to consider future surgery. (5) At about this same time, a child who had also been involved in an accident was admitted to the orthopedic service. Paula "adopted" the child and began to encourage her, making suggestions for easier transfers and encouraging physical therapy.

Once she began to channel her energy into the recovery process, she progressed rapidly, and by the time of her discharge, the staff was genuinely sorry to see her go.

Helpful responses   1. Understand negative realities of illness.   _____

                                    2. Offer support.   _____

3. Reinforce self-care and problem solving.   _____

4. Encourage patient expression of feelings.   _____

5. Provide psychological protection.   _____

Feedback
1. 4	4. 3
2. 1	5. 2
3. 5	

Chapter Summary

Health care is more effective and more comfortable for both patients and professionals when emotional reactions are understood, accepted, and confronted openly.

Typical reactions to illness include ambivalence; fear and anxiety; anger; guilt and shame; excessive compliance or noncompliance; superstitious or egocentric thinking; loss of autonomy; and loss of identity.

Health professionals are encouraged to accept their own feelings and to encourage acceptance and expression of feelings by patients. Ways to assist patients with emotional reactions include providing psychological protection; encouraging expression of feeling, understanding the negative realities of illness, providing reinforcement of self-care, and offering support.

Suggested Readings

Bernstein, L., & Bernstein, R. *Interviewing: A guide for health professionals.* New York: Appleton Century Crofts, 1980. Chapter 10, "Emotions in Illness and Treatment," provides a helpful description of some typical emotional reactions to illness.

Enelow, A. J., & Swisher, S. N. *Interviewing and patient care.* New York: Oxford University Press, 1979. Chapter 9, "Emotional and Behavioral Responses to Illness and to the Interviewer," describes ways in which patients react emotionally to illness.

Fisher, D. *I know you hurt, but there's nothing to bandage.* Beaverton, Ore.: Touchstone Press, 1978. This book provides a description of many cases of stress-induced illness.

Reiser, D. E., & Schroder, A. K. *Patient interviewing: The human dimension.* Baltimore: Williams & Wilkins, 1980. Chapter 4, "Reactions to Illness," discusses a variety of emotional reactions to illness.

Helping Patients in Crisis___

Objectives

After studying this chapter, you will be able to do the following:

1. Identify the six characteristics of a crisis, given a written patient case report.

2. Identify the six principles of crisis intervention, given descriptions of them from a patient case report.

3. Identify the six steps of crisis intervention, given descriptions of them from a patient case report.

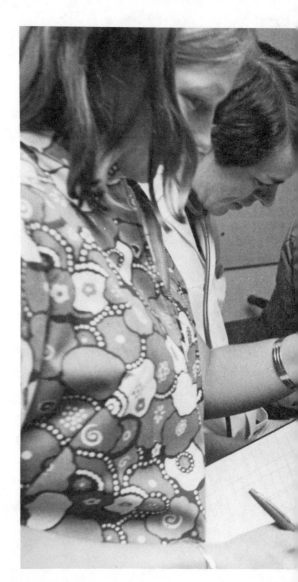

12

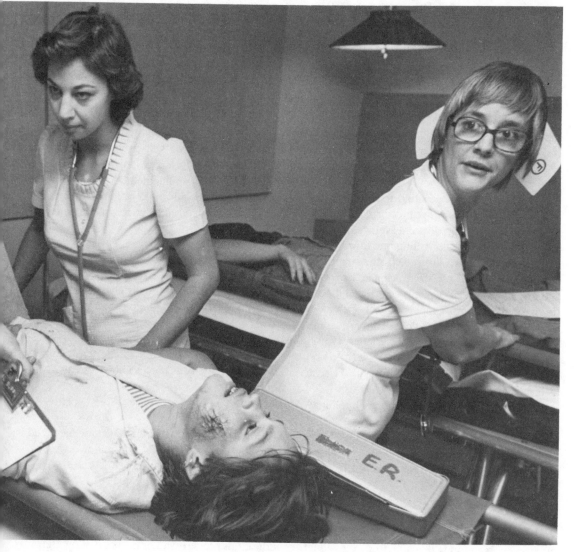

A crisis is a situation in which a person's usual coping methods have failed and the person is overwhelmed and immobilized. A crisis usually occurs in response to a sudden event that disturbs a person's equilibrium. If this event is not resolved within a few hours by whatever means the person usually uses to solve problems, the disruption is called a crisis (Puryear, 1979). The three main signs of a crisis are: (1) a heightened feeling of stress; (2) an inability to function normally; and (3) intense, unpleasant feelings. These result in a temporary inability to cope (Whitlock, 1978).

A crisis may be developmental (internal) or situational (external). Developmental crises occur during times of major life changes. For example, a 19-year-old young woman begins to have panic attacks when she rents an apartment and plans to move away from her parents, or an 80-year-old woman experiences severe anxiety as she makes arrangements to sell her house and move to a retirement home. A situational crisis occurs in response to specific external events. For example, a 50-year-old man with a middle management job goes on a "weekend bender" and fails to return to work after he has been told to "shape up or else" by his boss. Or a 22-year-old college senior who has a very high grade-point average becomes seriously depressed after failing one quiz.

Crises are not usually predictable or expected (Okun, 1982). They can be precipitated by such occurrences as the discovery of a terminal illness, death, suicide attempts, rape, physical abuse, loss of job, and so on. The usual types of crises encountered by health professionals are grief crisis, critical illness, terminal illness, loss of loved one, and chronic illnesses requiring life-long treatment, such as diabetes, arthritis, or multiple sclerosis.

Crisis intervention is a "temporary but immediate relief for an emergency situation" presented by a person in distress (Belkin, 1980, p. 329). The purpose of this chapter is to describe the characteristics, principles, and steps involved in crisis intervention, so that health professionals will understand the process and recognize possible crisis situations during their encounters with patients. Understanding the principles and steps of crisis intervention will enable the professional

to: (1) refrain from acting in ways that interfere with crisis intervention; (2) refrain from reacting in ways that exacerbate the crisis; and (3) possibly avert a crisis by making helpful interventions or by referring the patient to another helping professional.

Characteristics of a Crisis

Health professionals need to be able to recognize a crisis, because many patients are unaware that their situation has become so intense or overpowering. Other patients realize that they are in an intolerable situation but feel hesitant to ask for help. Health care settings have some responsibility for helping patients avert or resolve a crisis situation. In some settings there is a crisis team that is available to see patients in crisis. In other settings, when such a team is unavailable, the health professional may be the only person available to intervene in the crisis. This section describes six characteristics that will help professionals identify a crisis situation. These six characteristics include failure of usual coping methods, symptoms of stress, feelings of panic or defeat, an intense desire for relief, reduced efficiency, and decreased concentration.

Failure of Usual Coping Methods

The onset of a crisis is usually characterized by a period of overwhelming helplessness. In a crisis, usual coping methods have failed, and patients are unable to devise new or alternate methods. Additionally, in a crisis, patients usually sense vulnerability and fragility as they acknowledge their inability to cope.

Symptoms of Stress

Physiological symptoms of stress include increased heart and respiratory rate, skin pallor, excessive sweating, nausea and diarrhea, and increased frequency of urination (Kozier & Erb, 1979). Since these symptoms also may be signs of particular illnesses, the health professional must evaluate whether these symptoms suggest disease or are indications of a stressful or crisis situation. Behavioral stress reactions include restlessness, impatience, circular thinking, inappropriate tears or laughter, and generally a noticeable change in the individual's typical way of responding.

Feelings of Panic or Defeat

Emotional reactions to a crisis include feelings of panic or defeat. Nonverbal clues such as posture, voice tone, extreme restlessness, lethargy, and inappropriate responses to minor stimuli suggest the presence of such feelings.

Intense Desire for Relief

Another characteristic of a crisis is an intense desire for relief. Persons in crisis constantly talk, think about, and dream about the crisis. They are intensely preoccupied with themselves and the crisis situation. They are unable to focus on anything other than the crisis, yet they wish very much for their pain and anxiety to be alleviated.

Reduction in Efficiency

An individual's efficiency decreases during a crisis. Usual work habits are disrupted, and the person tries harder and accomplishes less. For example, Mary, an extremely competent secretary, has just learned that budget cuts will mean the elimination of her job at the end of the month. She begins to forget where things are and takes longer to find them. Her typing speed decreases, and her errors increase. The volume of work not yet done piles up on her desk. She used to have time to talk with people in the office and also get the work done, but now, because of the crisis, she spends every minute working and accomplishes less.

Decreased Concentration

The sixth characteristic of a crisis is diminished power to concentrate. A patient may read the same pages of a book over and over and yet not really understand the meaning. Another person may read directions carefully and then be unable to follow them. In conversation, such people may exhibit flight of ideas, switching topics suddenly and unrelatedly in the middle of a sentence. They may tend to dwell on one topic of conversation even when a new subject is raised. Patients in crisis have dif-

ficulty focusing on conversation or instructions, especially if these are unrelated to the crisis situation.

Principles of Crisis Intervention

Crisis intervention has six main characteristics:

1. immediacy

2. limited goal

3. time-limited process

4. support

5. patient's responsibility for action

6. calm atmosphere

These principles set the guidelines for all the help a professional offers during the crisis intervention process.

Immediacy

During a crisis, it is important to intervene promptly and to focus on the current situation. If a patient recognizes the beginning of a crisis and seeks help promptly, the crisis may be averted. If the situation can be identified and acted on before total deterioration, the odds are high for a successful solution. The outcome in the following example might have been very different if the man had been seen immediately.

A 35-year-old man presented to a county mental health clinic claiming that he needed help because he was afraid he was going to kill someone. He was given an appointment for the next day. Later that evening, he murdered eight people in his family. People need to be listened to and seen immediately when they are in crisis. If the crisis is not dealt with promptly, inappropriate patterns of behavior may evolve (Puryear, 1979).

Limited Goal

The goal of crisis intervention is to help patients return to pre-crisis levels of functioning (Aguilera & Messick, 1974) through resolution of the crisis and prevention of a catastrophe. Crisis intervention is not synonymous with therapy, although therapeutic techniques may be used. In crisis intervention, the interaction focuses only on material that is directly related to the crisis. It is inappropriate to deal with past experiences or even other current experiences that are unrelated to the crisis situation. Along with restoring equilibrium, appropriate intervention also may prevent the development of neurotic or psychotic symptoms following catastrophes. Whitlock (1978) believes that a person who resolves a crisis successfully will tend to be more healthy emotionally than before the crisis occurred.

Time-Limited Process

Most crisis theorists believe that six weeks is a maximum period for the duration of a crisis. If the crisis is not resolved within that time, the patient integrates the dysfunction and regains equilibrium, *including* the dysfunction. For example, if a man loses his job, he may react with a feeling of failure and inadequacy. The obvious solution is to find another job. However, his reaction (feelings of failure and inadequacy) may influence his behavior during job interviews, and he may not succeed in finding new employment. Without dealing with his feelings of failure, he may integrate a new self-image that includes "I'm a failure" or "There isn't any hope for me to ever find a job," and he stops looking for work. Because a crisis is of limited duration, any intervention must also be short-term. A health professional may have only one chance or a few chances to intervene with a patient in crisis.

Support

According to Puryear (1979), the lack of an adequate social network that provides support from "significant others" is one of the factors that determines if a particular problem develops into a crisis. To intervene effectively with patients in crisis, the health care worker needs to provide support while also encouraging patient self-reliance. Support is essential in helping the patient to feel secure and relieved and can be offered by being available and reliable. Patients must be allowed to relate their story in their own way and at their own speed,

and the professional must respond with an accepting and nonjudgmental attitude. Responses of the health professional need to convey hope, expectation of resolution, and confidence in the patient's ability to resolve the crisis. It is important to avoid any implication that someone else will take care of the problem or that it will go away by itself.

Support from significant others is also critical. The health professional needs to encourage patients to enlarge and strengthen their own social network (Puryear, 1979). Support may be available through others who have assumed importance in the patient's life, such as friends, family, or church groups.

There are some community groups that provide support to patients in crisis. "Reach for Recovery" provides counseling and comfort for mastectomy patients. The American Diabetes Association has local chapters that hold group meetings for diabetic patients. The "Ostomates" is a society for those who have had colostomies, ileostomies, and so on ("ostomies"). Other people who have had the same physical problems and have grown beyond the crisis can give comfort, hope, and important information to patients.

Patients' Responsibility for Action

A person in crisis usually feels helpless and desperate. Consequently, when help becomes available, the patient "may be tempted to let go and just fall in your lap" (Puryear, 1979, p. 47). Puryear observes that the health professional must combat from the start the patient's tendency to abdicate all responsibility for resolution of the situation.

It is helpful to patients to take prompt action on their requests and to give help with things that they cannot do unaided. At the same time, it is necessary to encourage patients to be active, to participate in physical care, to make decisions, and to voice their concerns. The health professional needs to avoid doing anything for the patient that he or she can successfully do alone (Puryear, 1979). Another way to encourage patients to take responsibility for resolving the crisis is to make it clear that the professional doesn't have all the answers and expects some effort from the patient (Puryear,

1979). Patients must also be encouraged to be actively involved in developing their own plan of action. Solutions developed by professionals for patients rarely alleviate a crisis; the patient is far more likely to take action if it is his or her own choice. Sometimes it is difficult to stimulate an immobilized person to take any action at all. In such instances, even a small action such as "deciding not to decide" can be significant and should be commended. Such small steps gradually develop into self-reliance.

A Calm Atmosphere

The nature and intensity of a crisis situation can sometimes arouse anxiety in health professionals. Intense feelings on the part of the patient may be "contagious," and the health professional may begin to experience parallel feelings (Belkin, 1980). The professional who "catches" the patient's feelings is usually too frightened and defensive to be of help.

It is important to be aware of this possibility to function more comfortably and calmly. Such awareness will help avoid giving the patient meaningless reassurances that in reality are intended to reassure the professional. The professional can leave the situation, and "everything will be all right" at the end of the work day, but the patient is not guaranteed such a neat outcome. If the health professional remains calm, poised, and self-confident, the patient will usually also gain greater confidence. The calmness of the health professional is "an emotional tranquilizer," subtly helping patients pull themselves together (Belkin, 1980, p. 335).

Techniques of Crisis Intervention

There is no one interviewing or counseling technique that is specific to crisis intervention. The techniques need to be varied and depend on the skills of the person using them, the situation, the time available, and the needs of the patient (Whitlock, 1978). Listening skills form the basis of patient support. Information giving may help to avert or alleviate a crisis. Constructive confrontation is also useful to help the patient face "dis-

crepancies or ramifications of the crisis situation in order to stimulate action of some kind" (Okun, 1982, p. 222). In using confrontation with a patient in crisis, it is essential that the confrontation be designed for the patient's benefit and not to express the professional's own frustration. It is also important to remember that a constructive confrontation is not just negative. As Okun (1982) observes, it includes acknowledgment of the person's strengths and ability to choose a particular course of action (p. 223).

Role playing is often part of crisis intervention. Role playing promotes change through simulation or re-enactment of a particular situation. Role playing can be used for a variety of purposes, including helping the patient to express feelings, promoting attitudinal and behavior change, and resolving conflicts.

A final technique that can be a very important part of crisis intervention is use of a contract. The health professional may help the patient write down some guidelines or actions to follow, as well as some actions to avoid in resolving the crisis. Sometimes significant others may be included in developing the contract. It is important to make the terms of the contract as specific as possible and to make the contract renegotiable if necessary (Puryear, 1979). A contract can be short and simple—such as "I (patient's name) agree to call you whenever I feel so terrible I have to take a lot of medicine"—or it can be more elaborate and lengthy.

Regardless of whatever techniques are used in crisis intervention, it is extremely important to be realistic and to focus on what is true. An accident or death cannot be reversed, but the feelings associated with those events can be dealt with and changed.

Steps in Crisis Intervention

Steps in crisis intervention include the following:

1. establish rapport

2. identify the problem

3. identify the patient's resources, strengths, and coping methods

4. decide on an action plan

5. terminate

6. follow-up

Because the time involved in crisis intervention is so brief, the first four of these steps occur simultaneously and continuously during the crisis intervention process.

1. Establish Rapport

The establishment of rapport is the sine qua non of helping people in crisis. The health professional must always remember that two people— the professional and the patient—participate in the health care relationship. When rapport exists, the patient perceives the health professional as a person who cares and does not act judgmentally.

Rapport is established through the communication of trust, respect, and caring. The health professional's reliability is essential (trust); casual promises that cannot be kept should not be made. When faced with false promises, patients may withdraw from participating in their own care, passively accept whatever suggestions are offered, or become angered and make impossible demands (Elder, 1978).

2. Identify the Problem

The next step in crisis intervention is to identify the problem. To solve a problem, it is essential to assess it clearly, and identification of the problem often leads directly to a solution. According to the philosopher Ludwig Wittgenstein (1958), if a problem is identified clearly enough, it tends to disappear. Occasionally a previously hidden problem emerges.

Problem identification is usually done most successfully with the participation of the patient. Sometimes the patient can immediately define the problem. Other times he or she may need to explore a variety of feelings in order to identify the problem. While listening to the patient, the health professional should be alert for: (1) the immediate situational concern; (2) the sequence of events that led up to the current situation; and (3) a specific event, problem, or person that pre-

cipitated the crisis (Puryear, 1979, p. 106). Often what the professional expects will be the major problem is not a problem at all. For example, you might assume that a patient who has just been diagnosed as having tuberculosis is most disturbed about the illness. In fact, the patient may be worrying about who is going to feed her dog. That problem is the crisis of the moment.

3. Identify the Patient's Resources, Strengths, and Coping Methods

As patients relate their story, it is possible to note their strengths and resources and the extent to which these are being used to cope with the crisis. The health professional can help the patient make a list of resources and coping methods. Ask the patient to describe how he or she usually copes with problems, and point out the patient's particular strengths that you notice. In addition, you should assess your own resources and strengths and not offer to do more than you realistically can. Know what other professionals or agencies are available, and tell the patient about them.

As the patient continues his or her story, listen for clues indicating other important people whom he or she might use as a support system; ask the patient about these people. A person in crisis often feels alone and may find strength and hope in the support of others. Patients may, however, need encouragement to let family and friends know that their support is needed.

4. Decide on an Action Plan

After assessing the crisis (problem) and the patient's strengths, your next step is to decide on a plan of action. The action plan should contain one or more tasks that the patient can do today, tomorrow, and this week to begin to resolve the crisis. Although the health professional can collaborate with the patient in formulating the plan, the action plan will be more successful if the patient helps to develop it. The tasks selected should also be major enough to be significant, yet not too difficult to achieve (Puryear, 1979). The patient is more likely to carry out the task if he or she knows that the health professional will follow up on whether the task was actually completed. The plan of action also needs to be very specific and should include time frames for completing certain tasks. The action plan can be developed in terms of what, when, where, how, and with whom the patient will carry out the appointed tasks.

The action plan may include helping patients find practical ways of expressing feelings of anger or sadness or helping them gather information to allay their fears. For example, a 52-year-old woman was in crisis. Her 55-year-old husband became psychotic and was committed to an institution. Her friends criticized her severely for "putting him away." She felt guilty because of the relief she felt at his absence. The crisis worker helped her decide to visit her husband, to take her son along for emotional support, and to set a specific date for the visit. After taking that action, she felt much better and said "I'm so glad I saw him. He's crazy as hell, and there is no way I could have handled him. I've not done anything to be ashamed of!"

5. Terminate

The next step in crisis resolution is closure or termination. The health professional needs to talk about "closing" in the first session, by discussing the time limit and asking the patient to set a goal. A helpful goal-setting question is "How will your situation be different after our sixth (or last) session?" Termination can be gradual, by decreasing the frequency and length of contacts with the patient. At the final meeting it is important for the patient to review his or her progress and to go over post-crisis intervention plans and tasks.

In some hospital situations, a formalized termination does not occur. Termination may be the patient's discharge, transfer, or death. It is useful to say goodbye to patients and to give them an opportunity to close out this period of their lives with a ritualized goodbye. Ritual goodbyes are particularly important in intensive and chronic care units.

6. Follow-Up

The final step in crisis intervention is follow-up. Follow-up care and evaluation of the success or failure of the crisis intervention is important. Such an assessment includes written notation of the situation, the patient's response, the techniques used for crisis intervention, and the results or outcomes. This review is useful to health professionals because it helps them to critique their own actions. Follow-up is also useful to patients, who can report on their progress and request additional counseling or intervention.

The health professional can also contact the patient by telephone several weeks after the last session to provide support and to assess the patient's continuing progress. If the health professional has referred the patient to another professional, then the call can be used to follow up on the referral as well.

LEARNING ACTIVITIES

Helping a Patient in Crisis

In this learning activity we present a patient case report that illustrates the content of this chapter. After reading the case, you are to respond to some questions that reflect the content of the three chapter objectives. Feedback follows the questions.

The case of Diane

Diane has been teaching psychology at a university for 20 years. She is married and has three teen-age daughters. She is devoted to her family and her students.

For the past 15 years, she has been supervised and constantly criticized by her department chairperson. Her ways of coping have been to avoid thinking about the criticism, to try to please everyone, to work harder, and to reward herself frequently with candy bars.

Five years ago her family physician began to treat her for hypertension, and three years ago she developed diabetes mellitus. She has gained weight steadily since.

During these years she has managed to cope by dealing with one semester at a time and counting the weeks until the next university recess when she can rest. In the summers, she has worked hard at home trying to make up to her family for her absence during the school year. About six months ago, her oldest daughter, who is 17, was sent by the court to an institution for juvenile offenders after several arrests for drug abuse and petty theft.

Diane coped with this situation in the same ways, escalating her overeating, avoiding the issue, and working harder (1). At the same time, her personal appearance has deteriorated, she has been very irritable and short-tempered with her colleagues, and she has developed recurrent headaches (2). Recently Diane has been having problems concentrating at work, and the criticism from her supervisor has increased in frequency and intensity (3). She has been having increased difficulty in meeting with her classes on time, has failed to turn in her mid-semester grade reports, and failed to attend the annual department banquet (4). She has been told to either "shape up or ship out." She applied for a sabbatical leave to go back to school and update her knowledge. Her supervisor returned her application with the curt message, "I'm not recommending you for this. You haven't done your work well enough to deserve it."

Diane went home, ate a box of candy bars, and ended up in the hospital in a diabetic coma. After a few days of treatment, her laboratory findings stabilized, but she continued to perspire profusely and urinate frequently—symptoms typical of uncontrolled diabetes. She appeared sad and moved and talked slowly in a very low voice. She responded with sudden tears to questions and statements (5). She repeated over and over again "I've got to have that sabbatical, I've got to" and then cried "I hurt so bad, there is so much pain."(6)

Her physician and the head nurse discussed her symptoms and decided that she was probably in a crisis. Because of the seriousness of her diabetes and hypertension, as well as her previous history of unsuccessful resolution of her problems, her physician recommended that she consult a crisis counselor for the emotional component of her problem and a dietitian to help her lose 50 pounds. He also told her frankly "I don't have the time to counsel you about your work and family problems, and the dietitian will be able to help you better with your diet. I will continue to see you about your medical problems and will monitor your progress."

Working with the crisis counselor, Diane was able to identify the cause of the crisis as her inability to perform well on her job and her lack of success in obtaining the sabbatical leave that would educate her to perform better at her job.

After assessing her resources, she realized that she had accumulated about eight months of sick leave and decided to take it. She also had the support of her husband. Another problem that she discovered was that she thought she had to do everything alone and unaided. She envisioned herself as a "superwoman" and then was disappointed when she failed to meet her own unattainable expectations. She agreed to accept support and specific help from the counselor and the dietitian. The crisis resolved and she was discharged from the hospital. She then implemented a diet plan, remained on the diet, and agreed to bring her emotional concerns with her to weekly therapy sessions instead of eating candy bars.

Activities

1. Match the six characteristics of a crisis with the underlined sections of Diane's case report that best demonstrate that characteristic (Chapter Objective 1). The first one is completed as an example.

___1___ Failure of usual coping methods

_____ Symptoms of stress

_____ Feelings of panic or defeat

_____ Intense desire for relief

_____ Reduction in efficiency

_____ Decreased concentration

2. Match the six principles of crisis intervention with the paragraph that best illustrates how that principle applies to Diane (Chapter Objective 2). The first one is completed as an example.

___d___ Immediacy

a. There is the need to focus concurrently on her emotional dilemma and her medical problem. She has constantly repeated that she needs to get away from the situation at work and has been denied the opportunity to do so by the same supervisor she sees as the cause of her stress.

_____ Limited goal

b. Diane needs encouragement to resolve her crisis from her family, colleagues, her physician, dietitian, and counselor. She might also gain support by participation in the American Diabetes Association.

_____ Time-limited process

c. Diane needs encouragement to discover her own means of resolving her dilemma. Solutions suggested or imposed by others are not likely to be successful.

_____ Support

d. Diane needs to have prompt relief from her emotional pain, or the situation will degenerate to include more dysfunction.

_____ Patient responsibility

e. The staff concerned with Diane's care must determine how their own prejudices about diabetes, candy binges, and so forth may interfere with their ability to provide support for Diane. Above all, they must maintain a nonstressful, calm atmosphere and avoid meaningless reassurance that "everything will be all right."

_____ Calm atmosphere

f. Because this crisis had evolved over several years, immediate intervention must be oriented toward resolving the crisis in three to six weeks.

3. Match the six steps of crisis intervention with the paragraph that describes how that step was accomplished during Diane's crisis (Chapter Objective 3). The first one is completed as an example.

__f__ Establish rapport

a. Diane continues to see the physician and dietitian and the counselor periodically. She believes that she keeps herself on the "straight and narrow" by continuing to get support. Since she was formerly a "superwoman," this is a significant change.

_____ Assess the problem

b. Diane decided to take the sick leave, to get beyond the crisis, and to work with the counselor to develop alternative coping methods. She decided to lose 50 pounds to improve her diabetes, to accept the help of the dietitian, and to seek the counselor's help for her feelings of stress. She also considered volunteering at the American Diabetes Association to whatever degree her physical condition would permit.

_____ Assess patient resources and strengths

c. The physician identified Diane's problem physically as diabetes and hypertension and advised her to lose weight. He also recognized her acute anxiety and recommended outside support. With the counselor, Diane identified the crisis problem and the double bind—that is, her need to get away and the denial of that need.

_____ Decide on a plan

d. Diane's crisis was terminated by leaving the hospital, although she continued to have weekly conferences with the counselor after her discharge.

_____ Terminate

e. Diane's eight months of sick leave proved to be a valuable resource. Her husband was supportive of her need to stop working. Another strength was her background as a psychology teacher. She had a warm, caring personality. Her family and friends were also available to give her continued support.

_____ Follow-up

f. Diane and her physician already knew each other well, so he was able to be direct and active in his advice. Had he not known her, he might have needed to take time to listen for half an hour and then deliver the same advice in a gentler manner. (A hospital-based nurse could establish rapport well by spending time with Diane listening, touching, and quietly being with her, and could offer positive reinforcement whenever she was in Diane's room. However, for her to be the primary helper in this situation might be unrealistic. Referral to a crisis worker is a good step in this situation.)

Feedback

Activity 1

Failure of usual coping methods—1
Symptoms of stress—2
Feelings of panic or defeat—5
Intense desire for relief—6
Reduction in efficiency—4
Decreased concentration—3

Activity 2

Immediacy—d
Limited goal—a
Time-limited process—f
Support—b
Patient responsibility—c
Calm atmosphere—e

Activity 3

Establish rapport—f
Assess the problem—c
Assess patient's resources and strengths—e
Decide on a plan—b
Terminate—d
Follow-up—a

Chapter Summary

A crisis is a situation in which a person's usual coping methods have failed, leaving the person overwhelmed and immobilized. The characteristics of a crisis include failure of usual coping methods, signs of stress, feelings of panic and defeat, an intense desire for relief, decreased efficiency, and lowered concentration.

Health professionals can help patients in crisis by using the principles of crisis intervention. Understanding these principles helps professionals determine when they should intervene and when referral to a crisis counselor is warranted. The six principles of crisis intervention are (1) intervening immediately; (2) limiting the goal to resolution of the current problem; (3) keeping the intervention brief and time limited; (4) being supportive; (5) encouraging patients to take action; and (6) providing a calm atmosphere.

Steps in crisis intervention are (1) establishment of rapport; (2) identification of the problem and (3) of the patient's resources and strengths; (4) development and implementation of an action plan; (5) termination; and (6) follow-up.

Suggested Readings

Aguilera, D., & Messick, J. *Crisis intervention: Theory and methodology.* St. Louis: Mosby, 1974. This book discusses crisis intervention and gives examples of various kinds of crises.

Elder, J. *Transactional analysis in health care.* Menlo Park, Calif.: Addison-Wesley, 1978. Chapter 12, "Problem Solving," presents concepts useful for helping patients in crisis to resolve their problems.

Kozier, B., & Erb, G. *Fundamentals of nursing.* Menlo Park, Calif.: Addison-Wesley, 1979. This general nursing textbook has an excellent section on crisis intervention.

Okun, B. *Effective helping.* Monterey, Calif.: Brooks/Cole, 1982. Chapter 8, "Crisis Theory and Crisis Intervention," discusses the principles of crisis intervention.

Puryear, D. *Helping people in crisis.* San Francisco, Calif.: Jossey-Bass, 1979. This book gives many excellent examples of crisis intervention.

Whitlock, G. *Understanding and coping with real life crises.* Monterey, Calif.: Brooks/Cole, 1979. This book emphasizes the practice and stages of crisis intervention and examines different types of crises.

Intervention Strategies_____

Objectives

After completing this chapter, you will be able to do the following:

1. Given a written description of a hypothetical patient situation, write an example of preparatory information to acquaint the patient with the procedure and sensations associated with proctosigmoidoscopy.

2. Given written instructions for the use of muscle relaxation, use the muscle relaxation procedure with yourself.

3. Given written instructions for respiratory or clinically standardized meditation, use the meditation procedure with yourself.

4. Given a role-play patient situation, explain and apply the procedure of emotive imagery.

5. Given two hypothetical written patient descriptions, write three coping statements that patients could use to cope before, during, and after a painful or discomforting experience.

6. Given a hypothetical patient description, identify in writing at least four stimulus-control techniques the patient could use to decrease two undesirable health-related behaviors.

7. Define a health-related behavior of your own that you want to increase or decrease. Write a plan for using self-monitoring to change the target behavior, specifying the timing, method, and device for self-recording.

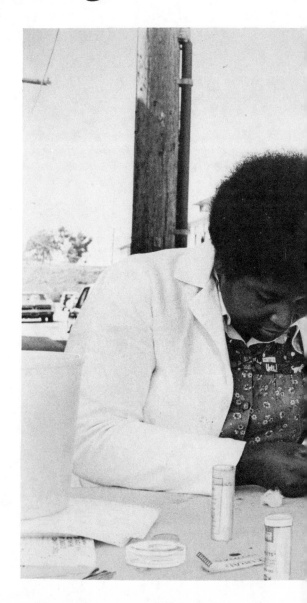

13

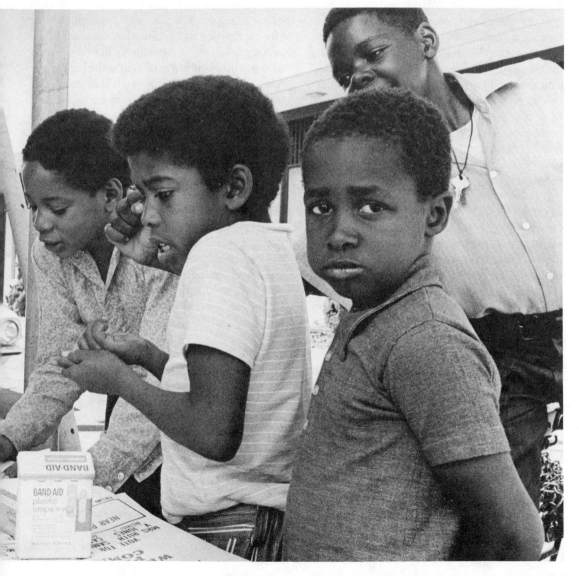

According to Jonsen, Siegler, and Winslade (1982), patients fall into three different categories: (1) those with acute, critical, unexpected, responsive, and easily diagnosed and treated illnesses, such as acute meningitis (acronym—ACURE); (2) those with critical, active, recalcitrant, and eventual illnesses, such as multiple sclerosis (acronym—CARE); and (3) out-patients with chronic, palliative, and efficacious illnesses, such as diabetes and hypertension (acronym—COPE). There is also one more category—patients with no evident illness who visit health professionals for periodic routine examinations that are preventive in nature (acronym—PREP).

This chapter describes seven nonmedical intervention strategies that patients in these four categories can use to maintain health, prevent disease, cope with a chronic condition, or reduce the severity of their illness. These seven strategies are preparatory information, muscle relaxation, meditation, emotive and guided imagery, stress inoculation training, stimulus control, and self-monitoring.

Patients with no evident illness, for example, can maintain their health and prevent disease by increasing desirable health behaviors, such as exercise and dental hygiene, and decreasing unhealthy behaviors or risk factors, such as smoking and intake of saturated fat, salt, or excess calories. These patients can use stimulus control (also known as environmental planning) and self-monitoring strategies to enhance healthy behaviors. Patients with chronic conditions such as hypertension can use strategies such as muscle relaxation, meditation, and stress inoculation as a nonmedical adjunct or, in some cases, as an alternative to the medical treatment. Preparatory information, relaxation, and emotive and guided imagery can be used as an adjunct to the health care regimen for patients with severe illnesses.

Patient adherence means the extent to which the patient's behavior follows or coincides with the health care prescription. Adherence to a medical or nonmedical treatment program can be a problem for many patients. There are four guidelines that health professionals can follow to increase patient adherence to the strategies we describe in this chapter.

First, educate patients about their illness and about their responsibility for maintaining wellness and for helping to manage chronic or critical illness. Second, present any nonmedical intervention strategy as part of the overall health care treatment program. If the patient perceives that the intervention strategy is an integral part of treatment, it is more likely that he or she will follow it. Third, train the patient to use the strategy. For most patients, the behaviors associated with each strategy are new ones. As with anything new or foreign, practice and information about use of the strategy are essential ingredients in following the strategy successfully. Finally, enlist the help of significant others who can support and encourage patient efforts at compliance with the treatment.

A word of caution is necessary before you undertake any of these strategies with a patient. Some patients may not wish to use a nonmedical strategy on a daily basis. They may find it easier to take daily medication. On the other hand, some patients dislike the side effects of their medication and welcome the opportunity to substitute a nonmedical intervention that may produce the same outcome. For example, a male patient with essential hypertension may prefer to decrease his salt intake and engage in daily exercise rather than live with possible side effects of antihypertensive medication. However, another patient who is extremely busy may find the medication easier.

Preparatory Information

Information about a new experience can help prepare patients to cope with an impending stressful event. How does information help reduce stress? One explanation is that preparatory information about an impending event reduces stress because the patient knows specifically what to expect (Johnson & Leventhal, 1974). For example, consider a person who will have a root canal procedure in the near future. Information about the procedures and techniques involved and the sensations commonly experienced before and after the procedure can decrease the negative expectations or misconceptions the patient might have. The informed patient is also able to use familiar coping responses to control his or her emotional reactions (Leventhal & Johnson, 1981). The patient who knows what to expect from a forthcoming operation or a "painful" examination will feel more in control of the situation, which in turn may increase the ability to cope and facilitate recovery.

Giving preparatory information consists of instructing or providing a person with specific knowledge about an anticipated process or procedure. It is an integral part of an overall patient education program. There are three types of preparatory information: procedural, factual, and sensory. *Procedural information* tells patients what they will be doing, what will be done to them by the attending professional, the sequence of events in the procedure, the time involved, the equipment, instruments, and medication used, and possible ways in which they can help the procedure go more smoothly. *Factual information* tells patients about body functions, disease processes, treatment alternatives, and so forth. *Sensory information* tells patients about the sounds, tastes, smells, sights, and kinesthetic and psychological feelings commonly experienced by patients who have had the same experience.

Guidelines for Using Preparatory Information

Preparatory information is used with patients in a variety of ways. For example, it has been used to reduce stress and anxiety in children about to undergo cast removal or tonsillectomies and also with children with insulin-dependent diabetes. Adult patients undergoing uncomfortable examinations and procedures also have received preparatory information as a way to anticipate and cope with various sensations. Finally, it has been used to reduce anxiety about and to facilitate recovery from surgery.

Preparatory information can be delivered to patients verbally during an interview or through an established commercial or professionally prepared informational program. Regardless of how it is delivered, it is important that the information be standardized for consistency and accuracy. Standardization is more likely to occur if the following five factors are considered: (1) purpose of the information; (2) type of information; (3) patient characteristics; (4) medium selection; and (5) content. We discuss these five components in the following section (refer also to Table 13-1).

Purpose of information. The first step is to determine the purpose of the information to be provided. In general, the information provided pertains to a specific situation, operation, examination, illness, dental procedure, diet, exercise, medication, or coping strategy. Table 13-1 lists situations and events where information may be needed by patients.

Type of information. After determining its purpose, health providers must decide what type of information (that is, procedural, sensory, or factual) to give to the patient. In some situations, procedural information about being admitted to a hospital or about a medical procedure may be sufficient to help the patient cope with the impending event. For example, patients about to undergo nasogastric intubation saw a film depicting the actual tube insertion procedures "showing first, the preparation of the nasogastric tube for insertion into the nasal cavity of the sitting patient, the patient then swallowing to pass the tube into the stomach, the nurse's check of the tube position, and finally, the securing of the tube to the patient's face and clothing" (Padilla, Grant, Rains, Hansen, Bergstrom, Wong, Hanson, & Kubo, 1981, p. 377).

Johnson, Rice, Fuller, and Endress (1978) presented procedural information to cholecystectomy patients about the things the staff could do for and to the patient, such as "skin preparation, physicians' visits, intravenous infusion, location and transfer to operating room and recovery rooms, and postoperative diet progression . . . Patients were told they probably would have pain and to ask the nurse for pain medication if they needed it" (p. 9).

Table 13-1
Guidelines for Using Preparatory Information

Purpose of Information	Type of Information	Patient Characteristics	Medium Selection	Content
Prehospital admission	Procedural (e.g., vasectomy)	Mental ability, background experiences, and education	Photographs or illustrations	Overview of purpose for information
Preoperative	Sensory (e.g., pelvic, endoscopic sensations during examination)	Age	Audiotape	Nontechnical language and no medical jargon
Postoperative		Sex	Videotape	
Examination (e.g., pelvic or breast)		Ethnic origin or cultural practices	Filmstrip	
Illness (e.g., diabetes or cancer)	Factual (e.g., chemistry, physiology, anatomy, or pathology)	Fluent in what language	Written self-instructional modules	Personal pronouns used
Dental procedure (e.g., root canal)		How frequently will the patient use the information	Hand puppets	Integration of photos or illustrations
Medication regimen				Common references used (e.g., "tube is about the size of a pencil")
Diet				
Exercise				
Coping strategy (e.g., medication, imagery, or relaxation)				Summary of presentation

Sensory as well as procedural information may be required for patients about to undergo certain procedures, such as proctosigmoidoscopy or renal biopsy, for the first time. For example, patients scheduled for abdominal surgery received the following sensory information prior to the operation on an audiotape. They were told:

> ... that the preoperative medications would make them sleepy, light-headed, relaxed, free from worry, and not bothered by most things. The sensations in the incision were described as tenderness, sensitivity, pressure, pulling, smarting, or burning, and the message stated that sensations might become sharp and seem to travel along the incision when the patient moved. The message instructed patients to request pain medication, if needed, and told them that the arm with the intravenous would seem awkward and restricted but there would be no discomfort or pain associated with the intravenous. Other sensations described were dryness of the mouth, tiredness after physical effort, bloating of the abdomen and cramping with gas pains, and pulling and pinching when stitches are removed (Johnson et al., 1978, p. 9).

Sensory information was also given to children before cast removal. The children were told:

> When the cast was cut she/he would feel vibrations or tingling, feel warmth, and see chalky dust fly; that her/his skin under the cast would be scaly and look dirty; and her/his arm or leg might be a little stiff when she/he first tried to move it, and that the arm or leg would seem light because the cast was heavy (Johnson, Kirchhoff, & Endress, 1975, p. 407).

Other patients may require factual information regarding the effects of cancer cells on the body, as well as sensory information concerning the sensations commonly experienced by cancer patients. (See Chapter 9 for further discussion on factual information.)

When you are providing factual information, remember to provide enough specific information but not so much that the patient is overwhelmed. After determining the general purpose and the type of information needed, consider the characteristics of the patients who will use the information.

Patient characteristics. The most important patient characteristics to be considered are his or her mental abilities and background experiences. Often the patient's educational level may be an indicator of his or her ability to comprehend information presented at a particular level. Unless information is provided by means of comprehensible words, drawings, and so on, all efforts may be wasted. Other important patient characteristics are listed in Table 13-1. The terms used to describe certain procedures and sensations may vary greatly with consideration of the age and sex of patients. The primary language used in the home and ethnic origin are additional important patient characteristics. For example, some patients may converse generally in Spanish; or older patients from some backgrounds may be especially reluctant to disrobe for an examination. Ethnic origins and/or religious practices may also be important where dietary information is concerned.

In general, most information can be given to both females and males. Many medical procedures and examinations, however, pertain to one sex and not the other. For example, information about the prostate gland is generally developed for a male audience. Fuller, Endress, & Johnson (1978) have described a procedure to help women cope with pelvic examinations.

The frequency with which the patient will use or need the information is another important patient characteristic and is determined by the purpose of the information. For example, a patient awaiting surgery may have procedural and sensory information presented only once or a few times before the operation. In contrast, patients who are using a particular diet, exercise program, or coping strategy may need to have the information presented daily, weekly, or monthly for reinforcement. The frequency with which the patient will use the information in turn influences the method used to present the information.

Medium selection. The purpose, type of information, and relevant patient characteristics will influence the medium selected to present preparatory information. Because it is often very time consuming to present information to patients verbally, other modes of presentation must be considered, such as audio- and videotapes, filmstrips, photographs, and instruction booklets.

Content of preparatory information. The final consideration for delivery of preparatory information involves its specific content. First, consider the duration of the presentation. The shorter the presentation, the better it will be received, assuming that all of the relevant information is included. For example, Johnson, Morrissey, and Leventhal (1973) developed a seven-and-a-half minute audiotape recording with 11 photographs to present sensory and procedural information. Another presentation to children about impending hospitalization and surgery was 15 minutes long (Peterson & Shigetomi, 1981).

Preparatory information should include the following elements: a brief overview of the purpose of the information, nontechnical language, personal pronouns, appropriate descriptions if illustrations or photographs are included, common references or analogies, and a short summary.

The overview describes to the patient what the information is about and what its value may be for the patient. It may be very brief, consisting of only a few sentences. For example, Johnson, Rice, Fuller, and Endress (1978) introduced their tape recording to cholecystectomy patients by saying that the information included in the recording "should answer many of their questions and should help them to know what to expect following an abdominal operation" (p. 8).

The language should be nontechnical and free of jargon. If technical language is necessary, define terms in everyday language or analogies that the patient can understand.

All information presented should be "personalized" for the patient. One of the best ways to personalize the information-giving process is to use personal pronouns. For example, for patients undergoing nasogastric intubation for gastric analysis, the information could be written as follows:

> Most patients experience similar uncomfortable sensations when the nasogastric tube is introduced. First, you may notice a sensation of fullness and discomfort as the tube passes through your nose. When the tube reaches the back of your throat, you may gag, choke, and feel discomfort in the nose and throat areas. Your eyes will water profusely. Remember to continue to swallow using small sips of water, if necessary, and to breathe mostly through your mouth, as if you were panting like a dog. Concentrate on panting and swallowing, and the tube will quickly be in place.

If visual materials are used in a presentation, ensure that the verbal information corresponds with and is synchronized with the illustrations. Illustrations or photographs create a more vivid image of what is going to happen. Detailed imagery about what is occurring in a patient's body or what is going to occur (during an operation, for example) enhances the patient's ability to cope.

On the other hand, if illustrations or photography are not used, it is helpful to describe unfamiliar objects in terms of their similarity to common or familiar objects. For example, Johnson, Morrissey, and Leventhal (1973) described the tube used in an endoscopic examination as being like a thimble and a pencil. These health professionals also used photographs of the tubes that included a ruler in the picture, while telling the patient the diameter and length of the tubes.

The final component of preparatory information is a brief summary or a reiteration of its purpose. An appropriate ending might be: "The information presented should have answered most of your questions about the procedure (or operation). The sensations described are perfectly normal and can be expected by most patients."

Developing and using preparatory information may be a lengthy and time-consuming process. However, Padilla et al. (1981) maintain that despite the time-consuming preparation, once the informational program has been developed, cost factors decrease as less staff is needed to provide maximum benefit to a large number of patients. Informational programs can be developed for a variety of health maintenance concerns. These should be supplemented with one or more of the intervention and coping strategies discussed in the next six sections of this chapter.

=== *LEARNING ACTIVITIES* ===

Preparatory Information

You have been asked to provide both procedural and sensory preparatory information for patients about to undergo proctosigmoidoscopy. Given the following information about the purpose and type of information, the patient, and duration of the presentation, write an example of preparatory information that might be used to describe this procedure to a patient (Chapter Objective 1).

> Purpose of information: To help patients about to undergo proctosigmoidoscopy cope and relax during the procedure
>
> Type of information: Procedural and sensory
>
> Background and educational level: High-school graduate, currently employed as a sales clerk

Age of patient: Adult

Sex: Male or female

Ethnic origin: Anglo-Saxon

Preferred language: English

Frequency of use of information by patient: Once or twice immediately prior to the procedure

Medium selection: Written or audiotape

Duration of presentation: Five minutes

You may have to look up the essential features of this examination in a textbook. Be sure to include information about the procedure itself and commonly experienced sensations during the procedure. Begin your example with a brief overview of the purpose of the information and end with a brief summary. Avoid jargon, and explain any technical terms in everyday language. Use personal pronouns throughout, and provide references of commonly known objects to illustrate medical equipment or tools used during the proctosigmoidoscopy.

Check your example with the one provided in the feedback section that follows to determine if your presentation contains essential and accurate procedural and sensory information.

Feedback

Proctosigmoidoscopy is an examination that allows the health professional to actually look inside your body to examine the rectum and sigmoid areas of the large intestine.

The proctosigmoidoscope is a slender steel tube, about one-half inch in diameter and ten inches long. A light shines through the tube so that the inside of your intestine can be seen.

When the examination is performed, you will be asked to kneel down and rest your chest on a special adjustable examination table. Cross your arms in front of you and place them under your head, so that you will be as comfortable as possible. (Note: Other postures may also be assumed, depending on the preference of the examiner.) The table will then be raised and tilted so that you will be leaning forward with your weight supported by your thighs and your arms.

The health professional will first inspect your anus (the opening from the rectum) and insert one finger into your rectum. She or he will then move the examining finger around inside the rectum to ensure that there is no mass or stool present. If all is well, the examiner will next insert a small device called an anoscope, which is about one-half inch in diameter and four inches long. Through this instrument he or she will be able to look for hemorrhoids and other problems that may occur in the region of the anus. You will probably have only a little discomfort during this part of the examination. It will feel as if the anus is stretched, and you may have a desire to move your bowels.

When this portion of the exam has been completed, the examiner will withdraw the anoscope and insert the proctosigmoidoscope. As the instrument is inserted further into the bowel, you may experience an increasingly uncomfortable cramping sensation in the abdomen. These cramps may come and go as the examination proceeds. They are very normal.

Sometimes the bowel collapses in front of the proctosigmoidoscope and it becomes necessary for the health professional to pump air into the bowel to expand it. This is done with a small rubber pump, like the one used to inflate the blood pressure cuff. When the air is pumped into the bowel, you may again experience severe cramping. However, the cramps will quickly subside.

Another instrument, a suction machine, may also be used during the exam. This device attaches to the proctosigmoidoscope through a rubber tube and is used to remove any leftover stool from the bowel. The bowel cannot be properly inspected if it is not clean. Except for the unfamiliar noise, the use of this machine should not bother you or cause pain.

So, in conclusion, proctosigmoidoscopy allows health professionals to look inside your body to determine the condition of the large bowel. Although it may be embarrassing to your ego and may cause cramps in your abdomen, all the discomfort will subside soon after the examination, and you will probably be able to return directly to your job or home. More important, your health care provider will know much more about the condition of your bowel without having to operate to look inside.

Muscle Relaxation Training

Teaching patients to relax their muscles can be used as an intervention or as a health-promoting technique. Tension and relaxation can alter blood pressure, heart rate, and respiration rate and may influence a patient's behavior and thinking. The rationale for muscle relaxation training is that a person cannot be tense and relaxed at the same time. For example, if you clench your fist tightly, you can feel the tension in your forearm. Then, when you relax your fist, the tension in your forearm is removed. Patients can be taught to discriminate between tension and relaxation for different muscle groups in their bodies. After training, patients can "tell" or "instruct" a particular muscle group to relax when they feel tension.

Progressive relaxation training was described formally as early as 1929. More recently, Bernstein and Borkovec (1973) wrote a manual entitled *Progressive Relaxation Training*. Relaxation training has been used with patients who have insomnia or high blood pressure, as a health-promoting technique with older persons, and as a postoperative pain-reduction technique for cholecystectomy patients. Muscle relaxation also has been used to decrease tension and migraine headaches and to facilitate less painful childbirth.

There are two precautions to take in using muscle relaxation. First, make sure the patient is medically cleared to use this technique. For example, tensing a particular muscle group may be detrimental for some patients with certain types of organic illness, such as arthritis. Second, determine if a patient is taking medication that is incompatible with the purpose of muscle relaxation.

Four Preparatory Steps

There are four preparatory steps for muscle relaxation. These steps are the same for both "live" and audiotaped presentations of muscle relaxation.

These steps are (1) to provide information about the procedure, (2) to instruct patients in appropriate dress, (3) to provide a conducive environment, and (4) to describe or model the procedure.

Information about muscle relaxation. Patients can be told that this procedure can help them manage stress, reduce hypertension, or relieve insomnia and tension headaches if it is used regularly. The procedure entails learning to tense and relax different muscle groups. Contrasting tenseness and relaxation enables patients to recognize tension so that they can eventually instruct themselves to relax. Muscle relaxation can augment the perception of being in control of a situation and can increase patients' awareness of arousal cues.

Appropriate dress. Patients should be instructed to wear comfortable and loose-fitting clothes and not to wear contact lenses or regular glasses during the training.

Conducive environment. The setting for relaxation training should be quiet and free of distracting noises. Patients should be as physically comfortable as possible. A recliner chair, the floor with blankets and pillows, or a bed can be used. Muscle relaxation training can be applied to an individual patient or a group of patients (Nath & Rinehart, 1979).

Describe or model the relaxation exercises. To influence patient expectations, describe or model some of the exercises. If the presentation is "live," the health professional can model several exercises. If the training is presented on audiotape, he or she can describe several of the exercises—for example, "You will do exercises like these. Make a fist, then relax the hand by opening the fingers. Bend the wrists of both arms and relax them. Shrug your shoulders and relax them." The patient should be told "When you clench your biceps, you feel the tension in your biceps muscles, and when you relax and drop your arm to your side, you notice the difference between tension that was in your biceps and the relative relax-

ation you feel." Use these comparisons to help the patient discriminate between tension and relaxation.

The following example illustrates these four preparatory steps.

> The name of the strategy that I believe will be helpful is *muscle relaxation*. Muscle relaxation has been used very effectively to benefit people who have a variety of conditions like insomnia, high blood pressure, anxiety, or stress, and people who are bothered by everyday tension. Muscle relaxation may be helpful in decreasing your tension, managing your illness, and promoting good health.
>
> I will ask you to tense and relax various muscle groups. All of us have some tensions in our bodies—otherwise we could not stand, sit, or move around. Sometimes we have too much tension. By tensing and relaxing, you will become aware of and contrast the feelings of tension and relaxation. Later I will train you to send a message to a particular muscle group to relax when nonessential tension creeps in. You will learn to control your tension and relax when you feel tension.
>
> Muscle relaxation is a skill. Like learning any skill, it will take a lot of practice to learn it well. A lot of repetition and training are needed to acquire the muscle-relaxation skill.
>
> At times during the training and muscle exercises, you may want to move while you are on your back on the floor (or on the recliner). Just feel free to do this so that you can get more comfortable. Also, you may feel "heady" sensations as we go through the exercise. These sensations are not unusual.
>
> During training, I'd like you to sit (or lie) comfortably. Also, remove your glasses or contact lenses.
>
> I would like to show you (some of) the exercises we will use in muscle relaxation. First, I make a fist to create tension in my right hand and forearm and then relax it. . . .
>
> Now, get as comfortable as you can, close your eyes, and listen to what I'm going to be telling you. I'm going to make you aware of certain sensations in your body and then show you how you can reduce these sensations to increase feelings of relaxation.

Instructions for Muscle Relaxation

In delivering instructions for relaxation-training exercises, the health professional's voice should be conversational, not dramatic. The muscles used for relaxation training can be divided into three sets, consisting of 17 groups, 7 groups, or 4 groups. (These sets of muscle groups are listed in Table 13-2 and are adapted from Bernstein and Borkovec, 1973.) After the patient has learned to alternately tense and relax each of the 17 muscle groups, the 7 or 4 muscle groups listed in Table 13-2 are brief enough for patients to use without inter-viewer or audiotaped instructions. Prior to administering muscle relaxation training, tell the patient to *listen* and to *focus* on the instructions. When presenting instructions for each muscle group, direct the patient's attention to the tension, which is held for five to seven seconds, and then to the feelings of relaxation that follow when the patient is instructed to relax. Allow approximately ten seconds for the patient to enjoy the relaxation associated with each muscle group before delivering another instruction. Intermittently throughout the instructions, make muscle-group comparisons—for example, "Is your forehead as relaxed as your

Table 13-2
Relaxation Exercises for 17, 7, and 4 Muscle Groups

17 Muscle Groups	7 Muscle Groups	4 Muscle Groups
1. Clench *fist* of dominant *hand.* 2. Clench *fist* of nondominant *hand.* 3. Bend *wrist* of one or both arms. 4. Clench *biceps* (one at a time or together). 5. Shrug *shoulders* (one at a time or together). 6. Wrinkle *forehead.* 7. Close *eyes* tightly. 8. Press *tongue* or clench *jaw.* 9. Press *lips* together. 10. Press *head* back (on chair or pillow). 11. Push *chin* into chest. 12. Arch *back.* 13. Inhale and hold *chest muscles.* 14. Tighten *stomach muscles.* 15. Contract *buttocks.** 16. Stretch *legs.* 17. Point *toes* toward head.	1. Hold *dominant arm* in front with elbow bent at about 45-degree angle while making a fist (hand, lower arm, and biceps muscles). 2. Same exercise with *non-dominant arm.* 3. Facial muscle groups. Wrinkle *forehead* (or frown), squint *eyes,* wrinkle up *nose,* clench *jaws* or press *tongue* on roof of mouth, press *lips* or pull *corners of mouth* back. 4. Press or bury *chin* in chest (neck and throat). 5. *Chest, shoulders, upper back,* and *abdomen.* Take deep breath, hold it, pull shoulder blades back and together, while making stomach hard (pulling in). 6. *Dominant thigh, calf,* and *foot.* Lift foot off chair or floor slightly while pointing toes and turning foot inward. 7. Same as 6, with *nondominant thigh, calf,* and *foot.*	1. Right and left *arms, hands,* and *biceps* (same as 1 and 2 in 7-muscle group). 2. *Face* and *neck* muscles. Tense all *face* muscles (same as 3 and 4 in the 7-muscle group). 3. Chest, shoulders, back, and stomach muscles (same as 5 in 7-muscle group). 4. Both left and right upper *leg, calf,* and *foot* (combines 6 and 7 in 7-muscle group).

*Use of this muscle group is optional.

biceps?" While delivering the instructions, gradually lower your voice and slow the pace of delivery. The actual instructions for training in relaxation, using 17 muscle groups, are as follows:

First study your right arm, your right hand in particular. Clench your right fist. Clench it tightly and study the tension in the hand and in the forearm. Study those sensations of tension. [Pause]

And now let go. Just relax the right hand and let it rest on the arm of the chair. [Pause] And note the difference between the tension and the relaxation. [10-second pause]

Now we'll do the same with your left hand. Clench your left fist. Notice the tension [5-second pause] and now relax. Enjoy the difference between the tension and the relaxation. [10-second pause]

Now bend both hands back at the wrists so that you can tense the muscles in the back of the hand and in the forearm. Point your fingers toward the ceiling. Study the tension, and now relax. [Pause] Study the difference between tension and relaxation. [10-second pause]

Now clench both your hands into fists and bring them toward your shoulders. As you do this, tighten your biceps muscles, the ones in the upper right part of your arm. Feel the tension in these muscles. [Pause] Now relax. Let your arms drop down again to your sides. See the difference between the tension and the relaxation. [10-second pause]

Now we'll move to the shoulder area. Shrug your shoulders. Bring them up to your ears. Feel and hold the tension in your shoulders. Now, let both shoulders relax. Note the contrast between the tension and the relaxation that's now in your shoulders.

We'll work on relaxing the various muscles of the face. First, wrinkle up your forehead and brow. Do this until you feel your brow furrow. [Pause] Now relax. Smoothe out the forehead. Let it loosen up. [10-second pause]

Now close your eyes tightly. Can you feel tension all around your eyes? [5-second pause] Now relax those muscles, noting the difference between the tension and the relaxation. [10-second pause]

Now clench your jaws by biting your teeth together. Pull the corners of your mouth back. Study the tension in the jaws. [5-second pause] Relax your jaws now. Can you tell the difference between tension and relaxation in your jaw area? [10-second pause]

Now, press your lips together. As you do this, notice the tension all around the mouth. [Pause] Now relax those muscles around the mouth. Just enjoy the relaxation in your mouth area and your entire face. [Pause] Is your face as relaxed as your biceps? [Muscle group comparison]

Now we'll move to the neck muscles. Press your head back against your chair. Can you feel the tension in the back of your neck and in the upper back? Hold the tension. Now let your head rest comfortably. Notice the difference. Keep on relaxing. [Pause]

Now continue to concentrate on the neck area. See if you can bury your chin into your chest. Note the tension in the front of your neck. Now relax and let go.

Now direct your attention to your upper back area. Arch your back like you're sticking out your chest and stomach. Can you feel tension in your back? Study that tension. [Pause] Now relax. Note the difference between the tension and the relaxation.

Now take a deep breath, filling your lungs, and hold it. See the tension all through your chest and into your stomach area. Hold that tension. [Pause] Now relax and let go. Let your breath out naturally. Enjoy the pleasant sensations. [10-second pause]

Now think about your stomach. Tighten the abdominal muscles. Hold this tension. Make your stomach like a knot. Now relax. Loosen these muscles now. [10-second pause] Is your stomach as relaxed as your back and chest? [Muscle group comparison]

Focus now on your buttocks. Tense your buttocks by holding them in or contracting them. Note the tension that is there. Now relax—let go. [10-second pause]

I'd like you now to focus on your legs. Stretch both legs. Feel tension in the thighs. [5-second pause] Now relax. Study the difference again between the tension in the thighs and the relaxation you feel now. [10-second pause]

Now concentrate on your lower legs and feet. Tighten both calf muscles by pointing your toes toward your head. Pretend a string is pulling your toes up. Can you feel the pulling and the tension? Note that tension. [Pause] Now relax. Let your legs relax deeply. Enjoy the difference between tension and relaxation. [10-second pause]

Now, I'm going to go over again the different muscle groups that we've covered. As I name each group, try to notice whether there is any tension in those muscles. If there is any, try to concentrate on those muscles and tell them to relax. Think of draining any residual tension out of your body. Relax the muscles in your feet, ankles, and calves. [Pause] Let go of your knee and thigh muscles. [Pause] Loosen your hips. [Pause] Loosen the muscles of your lower body. [Pause] Relax all the muscles of your stomach, waist, lower back. [Pause] Drain any tension from your upper back, chest, and shoulders. [Pause] Relax your upper arms, forearms, and hands. [Pause] Relax your face. [Pause] Let all the muscles of your body become loose. Drain all the tension from your body. [Pause] Now sit quietly with your eyes closed.

Now I'd like you to think of a scale from 0 to 5, where 0 is complete relaxation and 5 is extreme tension. Tell me where you would place yourself on that scale now.*

Variations of Muscle Relaxation

Recall. There are four shortened variations of the muscle-relaxation procedure just described. A *recall* procedure follows the relaxation exercises for the four muscle groups (Table 13-2) without muscular tension. First ask the patients to focus on each muscle group. Then instruct patients to focus on one of the four muscle groups (arms; face and neck; chest, shoulders, back, and stom-

ach; legs and feet) and to relax and recall what it was like when they released the tension (in previous muscle relaxation sessions) for that particular muscle group.

Counting. Another variation is called the *counting* procedure. The health professional says that she or he will count from one to ten and that after each number, the patient will become more relaxed. You might say slowly:

One—you are becoming more relaxed; two—notice that your arms and hands are becoming more and more relaxed; three—feel your face and neck becoming more relaxed; four, five—more and more relaxed are your chest and shoulders; six—further and further relaxed; seven—back and stomach feel deeply relaxed; eight—further and further relaxed; nine—your legs and feet are more and more relaxed; ten—just continue to relax like you are—relax more and more (Cormier & Cormier, 1979, p. 415).

You can combine this counting procedure with recall. Counting also can be used during actual situations that provoke tension.

Differential relaxation. A third variation can help the patient generalize the relaxation training from practice sessions to the everyday world. The procedure is called *differential relaxation*. For example, you might have a patient sit down in an ordinary chair and ask him or her to identify which muscles are used and which are not used when sitting. If he or she feels tension in muscles that are not used (face, legs, and stomach), the patient is instructed to relax and to maintain relaxation in the muscles not required for sitting. A patient can be instructed to engage in different levels of the differential-relaxation procedure—for example, sitting or standing up (Cormier & Cormier, 1979, p. 416). A patient also can be instructed to practice differential relaxation in a quiet restaurant, sitting in a noisy cafeteria while eating, waiting in line, or walking in a noisy and busy shopping center. The basic idea is to have the patient identify those

---

*Adapted from *Interviewing strategies for helpers* by W. H. Cormier and L. S. Cormier. © 1979 by Wadsworth, Inc. This and all other quotations from the same source are reprinted by permission of Brooks/Cole Publishing Company, Monterey, California.

muscles that are tense and those that are relaxed in various situations.

Cue-controlled relaxation. A final variation of muscle relaxation procedure is called *cue-controlled relaxation*. First, patients learn and practice the muscle relaxation procedure. Then they learn to say a "specific self-produced cue word such as calm or control while relaxed" (Russell & Sipich, 1974, p. 674). The cue word becomes paired or associated with relaxation. Also, patients are instructed to note their breathing patterns while relaxed and to repeat the cue word silently with each exhalation (p. 674).

It is very important that patients monitor themselves or maintain logs of their practice sessions on application of a specific intervention strategy. Self-monitoring or keeping a training log involves the patient in the intervention process more extensively than does mere practice of the muscle relaxation exercises. It also promotes

adherence to the procedure. The patient keeps the log as "homework" and records specific information relating to the practice sessions. The log should be arranged so that the patient can record the date of practice session, the number of practice sessions on each date, the location of the practice session, and the number of muscle groups exercised. In addition, the patient should record an estimate of the level of tension before and after the practice session, using a scale where 1 = little or no tension; 2 = some tension; 3 = moderate tension; 4 = marked tension; and 5 = extreme tension.

It is difficult for patients to learn and apply any intervention or coping strategy to promote health or manage illness unless they can relax. Acquiring skills associated with the muscle relaxation procedure is necessary for the health professional who hopes to successfully apply the other intervention strategies discussed in this chapter.

LEARNING ACTIVITIES

Muscle Relaxation   By yourself, tape record the instructions for muscle relaxation on pages 265–266. Select a quiet place and a time that will be free from interruptions, and go through the muscle relaxation exercises using the tape-recorded instructions. If you don't have a tape recorder, you can have a friend read the instructions to you. For maximum benefit, practice the muscle relaxation exercises once or twice daily for at least a week. After practicing for a week, you may then try one of the shorter variations, such as recall, counting, differential relaxation, or cue-controlled relaxation.

Meditation

Meditation is a mental exercise that is conducted in a quiet, calm environment. J. C. Smith (1975) states that the "term meditation refers to a family of mental exercises that generally involve calmly limiting thought and attention. Such exercises vary

widely and can involve sitting still and counting breaths, attending to a repeated thought, or focusing on virtually any simple external or internal stimulus" (p. 558). Benson (1974, 1976) has described meditation, or the relaxation response, as a counterbalancing technique for alleviating the effects of stress. According to Benson, four basic elements are needed to elicit the relaxation response: a quiet environment, a mental device, a passive attitude, and a comfortable position. In this section, two different meditation procedures will be described: Benson's (1974, 1976) relaxation response and Carrington's (1978) clinically standardized meditation. Although these two procedures are similar, the relaxation response described by Benson is a more structured meditation experience than clinically standardized meditation.

As a health-maintenance procedure, meditation has been used to treat insomnia, to decrease systolic and diastolic blood pressure of hypertensive patients, and to decrease stress.

Relaxation Response

Table 13-3 outlines the steps involved in developing the relaxation response (sometimes called *respiratory meditation*). The first step is to provide the patient with a rationale and overview of the procedure. Here is an example of a rationale for meditation used by D. H. Shapiro (1978):

> Meditation is nothing magical. It takes patience and practice; you have to work at it; and, just by meditating, all life's problems will not be solved. On the other hand, meditation is potentially a very powerful tool, and it is equally important to suggest what you might be able to expect from meditation the first month you practice it. Studies have shown that Zen meditation can have a strong effect within the first two to four weeks. Some of these effects can be measured physiologically—e.g., brain wave states, slower breathing, slower heart rate. These all contribute to a state of relaxation and inner calm. Meditation may

help you become more aware, both of what is going on outside you, and what is happening within you—your thoughts, feelings, hopes, fears. Thus, although meditation won't solve all your problems, it can give you the calmness, the awareness, and the self-control to actively work on solving these problems.*

Here is an illustration of an overview of the relaxation response procedure.

> What we will do first is select a focusing or mental device. You will then get in a relaxed and comfortable position. Afterward, I will instruct you about focusing on your breathing and using your mental device. We will talk about a passive attitude while meditating. You will meditate about 10 to 20 minutes. Then we will talk about the experience (Cormier & Cormier, 1979, p. 403).

The next step in the procedure is to select a mental device or sound that can be used during meditation. A mental device helps clear one's mind of intruding thoughts by helping the meditator to focus for a time on a word, sound, or phrase.

Repetition of the mental device assists in breaking the stream of distracting thoughts (Benson, 1976) and also helps patients focus on breathing. Benson (1974) suggests the use of the word "one" or any other simple and neutral word, sound, or phrase. The health professional may designate

---

*From "Instructions for a training package combining formal and informal Zen Meditation with behavioral self-control strategies," by D. H. Shapiro, *Psychologia*, 1978, *31*, 70–76. Copyright © 1978 by Kyoto University. Reprinted by permission.

Table 13-3
Steps for Relaxation Response and Clinically Standardized Meditation (CSM)

Relaxation Response (Respiratory Meditation)	Clinically Standardized Meditation (CSM)

1. Information about the procedure.
   a. Rationale.
   b. Overview of procedure.
	1. Information about the procedure.
	   a. Rationale.
	   b. Overview of procedure.

Table 13-3 *(continued)*

Relaxation Response (Respiratory Meditation)	Clinically Standardized Meditation (CSM)

2. Select a mental device.
  a. Provide rationale for mental device.
  b. Provide examples of mental device.
3. Instructions to patient.
  a. Get in quiet environment.
  b. Relax all muscles in body and keep them relaxed.
  c. Close eyes and assume comfortable body position.
4. Instructions about breathing and use of mental device. Breathe through your nose and focus on your breathing. Let the air come to you. As you do this, say the mental device for each inhalation and exhalation . . . "breathe in . . . out 'one,' in . . . out, 'one.' " Breathe in and out while saying your mental device silently to yourself. Try to achieve effortless breathing.
5. Instructions about passive attitude. When distracting thoughts occur, let them pass. Keep your mind open and return to your mental device.
6. Meditate for 10 to 20 minutes. Instruct the patient to meditate 10 minutes at first. Later, the time can be extended.
7. Probe about meditative experience.
  a. How does it feel?
  b. How did you handle distracting thoughts?
8. Instruct patient to meditate daily.
  a. Don't meditate within one hour after eating.
  b. Meditate in quiet environment.
  c. Meditate several hours before bedtime.
  d. Meditate twice daily.
	2. Select a mantra or sound.
	  a. Instruct patient to select a mantra.
	  b. Choose or make up a meaningless sound or word that has few associations and is not emotionally charged.
	3. Preparation for meditation.
	  a. Select a quiet environment free from distractions (such as the telephone)
	  b. Should not be interrupted while meditating.
	  c. Should not take any alcoholic beverages or nonprescription drugs at least 24 hours before meditation.
	  d. Should not drink any beverages containing caffeine one hour before meditation.
	  e. Should not eat any food one hour before. Do not smoke for half an hour before meditation. No chewing gum while meditating.
	  f. Select a comfortable straight-back chair in a room free of clutter. Face away from direct light in dimly lit room.
	  g. Loosen tight clothing and shoes.
	4. Instructions to meditate.
	  a. Sit quietly for about a half-minute before you say your mantra. Be relaxed and quiet.
	  b. First, close your eyes and say aloud your mantra, say it more softly, whisper, think the mantra to yourself without moving your lips or tongue. After the first session, hear or think your mantra.
	  c. CSM is not an exercise in discipline—it is a quiet peaceful time with yourself. It requires no effort.
	  d. Allow distracting thoughts to flow. Flow with the process—allow memories, images, thoughts to occur. Don't try to influence these. Your mantra will return to you.
	  e. Meditate 5 to 10 minutes. You can open your eyes to look at a watch periodically.
	  f. Come out of meditation slowly. Sit with your eyes closed for two minutes—take time to absorb what is happening. Get up slowly and open eyes slowly.
	5. Discuss patient's reaction to first meditation.
	6. Decide how often and when to meditate.
	  a. Meditate for three weeks, twice a day.
	  b. Meditate first thing in the morning after arising and during late afternoon or early evening.

other mental devices that are nonsense syllables, such as "zum" or "shyam" (Seer & Raeburn, 1980).

Patients are instructed to establish a quiet environment, to relax all their body muscles, to assume a comfortable position, and to close their eyes. They are then instructed to breathe through the nose and to concentrate on their breathing. While concentrating on breathing, the patients repeat the mental device silently to themselves. For example, after each inspiration/expiration cycle, each patient would repeat "zum" or "one."

Patients are instructed to maintain a passive attitude. For example, if attention wanders and distracting images or thoughts occur, the patient is instructed not to dwell on them and to return to repeating the mental device or word. As Benson (1974) states, "the purpose of the response is to help one rest and relax, and this requires a completely passive attitude. One should not scrutinize his (her) performance or try to force the response, because this may well prevent the response from occurring. When distracting thoughts enter the mind, they should simply be disregarded" (p. 54).

Initially patients are instructed to meditate for about 10 minutes. They may open their eyes to check the time. Later, patients can meditate longer—up to 20 minutes. The length of time varies with how satisfied the patient feels with this form of cognitive relaxation. After the first meditative experience, the health professional probes or asks "how the patient felt, how the mental device was used, what happened to any distracting thoughts, and whether the patient was able to maintain a passive attitude" (Cormier & Cormier, 1979, p. 405).

As with all strategies presented in this chapter, the patient must practice meditation for at least a two- or three-week period to feel or observe its possible beneficial effects.

Clinically Standardized Meditation (CSM)

Carrington (1978) has developed a very thorough instructional package with self-instructional audiotapes and a work booklet to teach Clinically Standardized Meditation (CSM). She defines meditation as a systematic way to get back to the quiet center of yourself. She observes that meditation requires no effort because it is not an exercise in discipline.

A health provider might give the following overview and rationale (adapted from Carrington) as the first step:

> The procedure called Clinically Standardized Meditation is a simple relaxation exercise. A variety of different positive effects can come from meditating. For example, meditation has benefitted people by reducing tension and stress, headaches, anxiety, and the time it takes to fall asleep. It has also been reported to increase athletic performance and energy. People who meditate report that they are more alert, are closer to their feelings, and have clearer thinking. Meditation may provide an alternative to tranquilizers and other drugs. If you choose to try meditation as a relaxation technique, you will be asked to select a sound mantra that you will use while you are relaxed and comfortable in a quiet environment. You can allow images and thoughts to flow freely. You will not have to concentrate, and meditation will require no effort. In fact, you will learn not to make any effort. Let your thoughts or feelings come and go. Your mantra will come back to you. Meditate for five or ten minutes at first. Then we will assess your reaction to this quiet and peaceful experience.

After the patient has received information about CSM, the next step is to select a mantra or sound. In Carrington's course workbook (*Learning to Meditate*), there is a list of 16 Sanskrit and various other sounds from which patients may choose (p. 10). Alternately, patients can create a meaningless sound or word with few associations that is not emotionally charged. "Grik" "shahm," and "rama" are examples of mantras.

Carrington provides extensive instruction on preparing to meditate (see Table 13-3). First, patients should select a quiet, uncluttered environment, free from interruption and distractions. They should not consume any alcoholic beverages for at least 24 hours before meditation. They should not meditate within one hour after consuming solid food or caffeine-containing beverages. Smoking is discouraged for at least a half-hour before meditation.

Patients should be instructed to loosen tight-fitting clothing or shoes, select a comfortable straight-back chair, and face away from direct light. These instructions are provided to ensure that meditation will occur and to enhance the quality of that meditation.

After patients have made these preparations for meditation, they should be instructed on how to meditate. It is important that they know how to relax their muscles before beginning. Carrington (1978) recommends sitting quietly for about half a minute before saying the mantra. After this brief period of quiet relaxation, patients are to close their eyes and focus on the mantra. At first they pronounce the mantra aloud. Gradually, they begin to say it more softly, whisper, and finally think or hear the mantra without moving their lips or tongue. Patients should be reminded that meditation is not an exercise in discipline but a quiet,

peaceful time alone, requiring no effort or concentration. Patients should allow distracting thoughts and feelings to flow, as if they were clouds floating by. They should not actively try to influence distracting thoughts or feelings but allow their mantra to return to them. They should meditate for five to ten minutes, opening their eyes occasionally to peek at a watch or clock.

Finally, patients should end each meditative session slowly. Carrington advises that they sit with closed eyes for about two minutes and take time to absorb what is happening at that moment.

Step 5 in Table 13-3 recommends that health professionals discuss or probe the patient's reaction to the meditation. People experience a variety of reactions toward meditation; no two meditative experiences are alike. They may feel unsure of themselves when meditating, possibly because there are no rules for the process. The last step in CSM is to instruct patients when and how frequently to meditate. Novices should practice twice daily for at least the initial three-week period. Car-

LEARNING ACTIVITIES

Meditation

Select one of the meditation procedures (respiratory meditation or CSM) and try it out. Do this in a quiet, restful place where you will not be interrupted for 20 minutes. Do not meditate within one hour after a meal or within two hours of going to sleep. It is a good idea not to have any caffeine-containing beverage for an hour before meditating.

1. Get in a comfortable sitting position and close your eyes.

2. Relax the muscles in your body.

3. Meditate for about five to ten minutes.

4. After meditating, assess your reactions to the experience. How do you feel?

5. If your meditative experience was a good one, you may wish to practice twice daily for two weeks.

rington suggests that people should regularly meditate in the morning after arising and during late afternoon or early evening.

Carrington (1978) advises that patients also under medical treatment, particularly those who are receiving medication for endocrine or metabolic control, or for the control of pain or of psychiatric symptoms, should have their meditation experience supervised by a health professional familiar with the effects of profound relaxation on medical conditions and on drug therapy (p. 11). Persons using insulin, thyroxin, or antihypertensive drugs *may* need to have their dosages decreased while they are regularly practicing CSM. (See learning activity on page 271.)

Imagery

Two types of imagery can help patients deal with chronic illness or maintain health. The first type is called *emotive imagery*. In this technique, a person focuses on positive thoughts or images while in an uncomfortable or anxiety-arousing situation (Cormier & Cormier, 1979). The images are pleasant ones, such as sailing on a sunny bay.

The second type of imagery is called *guided imagery*. Patients visualize their bodies performing particular desirable functions. For example, cancer patients might imagine their white blood cells aggressively and eagerly seeking, attacking, and destroying cancer cells (Simonton, Matthews-Simonton, & Creighton, 1980).

Emotive imagery may be used with patients experiencing chronic pain, having a stressful examination or operation, or receiving an injection. The patients' efforts to imagine a pleasant, tranquil scene while listening to a description of an uncomfortable or threatening situation tend to distract them from the anxiety-arousing circumstance. In training patients to imagine that healthy

Table 13-4
Steps for Emotive Imagery and Guided Imagery

Emotive Imagery	Guided Imagery
1. Purpose and overview: Information depicting how the procedure might help the patient.	1. Purpose and overview: Information depicting how the procedure might help the patient.
2. Assessment of patient's imagery potential. a. Instruct patient to engage in imagery that elicits good feelings and calmness. b. After 20 seconds, probe to ascertain the sensory vividness of patient's imagined scene. c. Decision to continue with procedure.	2. Assessment of patient's imagery. a. Determine patient's images of illness, body defense systems, organs associated with illness, and treatment. b. Instruct patient to describe or draw each one of the four elements.
3. Development of emotive imagery scenes. a. Scenes promote calmness, tranquility, and enjoyment for patient. b. Much sensory detail, so that patient experiences color, smell, temperature, touch, sound, and motion.	3. Develop guided imagery scenes. a. Use elements described on page 276 for cancer patients. b. Use elements described on page 277 for pain and other illnesses.
4. Practice using emotive imagery scenes. a. Patient uses scenes for 30 seconds. b. Assess how scenes will handle discomfort.	4. Practice using the guided imagery scene. Instruct patient to practice three or four times daily while relaxed and in a quiet place.
5. Application of emotive imagery. Instruct patient to use the scenes in distressful or discomforting situations.	

bodily processes are working to alleviate their cancer, diabetes, hypertension, heart disease, arthritis, or other illnesses, guided imagery capitalizes on the concept of positive thinking. According to Simonton et al. (1980), guided imagery plays a pivotal role in recovery from cancer.

In the following sections we present steps for introducing patients to the process involved in these two types of imagery.

Emotive Imagery

There are five steps in training patients to use emotive therapy (see Table 13-4). The first step is to provide patients with information about its purpose and overview.

Purpose and overview. The following illustration of the purpose and overview of emotive imagery has been used with pregnant women to reduce childbirth anxiety and to relieve discomfort during labor (Horan, 1976).

> Here is how *in vivo* emotive imagery works: In this culture women often learn to expect excruciating pain in childbirth. Even intelligent, sophisticated women have a hard time shaking this belief. Consequently, the prospect of childbirth is often fraught with considerable anxiety. In the labor room, early contractions are seen as signals for unbearable pain to follow. The result is that even more anxiety occurs. Now, since anxiety has a magnifying effect on childbirth discomfort, the more anxious you become the more actual pain you will probably experience. This "vicious circle" happens all too frequently.
>
> The process of *in vivo* emotive imagery involves having you focus on scenes or events which please you or make you feel relaxed, while the contractions are occurring. You simply cannot feel calm, happy, secure—or whatever other emotion the scenes engender—and anxious at the same time. These opposing emotions are incompatible with each other. So, *in vivo* emotive imagery blocks the anxiety which leads to increased childbirth discomfort. There is also some

> evidence which suggests that the holding of certain images can raise your pain threshold. Thus, *in vivo* emotive imagery not only eliminates anxiety-related discomfort, but it also has a dulling effect on what might be called real pain! (pp. 317–318)*

Imagery potential. If patients wish to try emotive imagery, the next step is to assess their imagery potential. Patients are instructed to imagine a scene that elicits good feelings and calmness and to hold on to this image for about 20 to 30 seconds. After this time (20 to 30 seconds) has elapsed, the health professional determines how vividly the patient imagined the scene. The health professional asks the patient to describe the scene in detail. The health professional then determines whether a variety of sensory experiences—color, sound, smell—is represented in the patient's imagery. If so, the decision is made to proceed to the third step of the procedure. If not, the interviewer may use another strategy that is not as dependent on detailed imagery for its success, such as muscle relaxation or stress inoculation training.

Development of imagery. The next step involves development of at least two imagery scenes for the patient to use in practical and real-life situations. There are two important ingredients for developing a scene. First, the scene should promote calmness, tranquility, and enjoyment for the patient. Appropriate scenes include hiking on a trail in the mountains, walking on a beach, listening to a symphony orchestra perform a favorite composition, or watching an athletic event (Cormier & Cormier, 1979). Pain patients are often instructed to imagine that they are floating on a cloud or in a hot air balloon.

---

*From "Coping with inescapable discomfort through in vivo emotive imagery," by John J. Horan in *Counseling methods*, edited by John D. Krumboltz and Carl E. Thorsen. Copyright © 1976 by Holt, Rinehart and Winston. This and all other quotations from the same source are reprinted by permission of Holt, Rinehart and Winston, CBS College Publishing.

Second, the imagery must include as much sensory detail as possible—sound, color, temperature, smell, touch, and motion. The more sensations a scene can elicit, the greater the intensity of pleasure and enjoyment the patient experiences. For example, consider the following emotive scene used by Horan (1976) for people who experience discomfort while having their teeth cleaned.

> Now close your eyes, sit back, and relax. Eyes closed, sitting back in the chair, relaxing. Now visualize yourself standing by the shore of a large lake, looking out across an expanse of blue water and beyond to the far shore. Immediately in front of you stretches a small beach, and behind you a grassy meadow. The sun is bright and warm. The air is fresh and clean. It's a gorgeous summer day. The sky is pale blue with great billowy clouds drifting by. The wind is blowing gently, just enough to make the trees sway and make gentle ripples in the grass. It's a perfect day. And you have it entirely to yourself, with nothing to do, nowhere to go. You take from your car a blanket, towel, and swimsuit, and walk off through the meadow. You find a spot, spread the blanket, and lie down on it. It's so warm and quiet. It's such a treat to have the day to yourself to just relax and take it easy. Keep your eyes closed, thinking about the warm, beautiful day. You're in your suit now, walking toward the water, feeling the soft, lush grass under your feet. You reach the beach and start across it. Now you can feel the warm sand underfoot. Very warm and very nice. Now visualize yourself walking out into the water up to your ankles; out farther, up to your knees. The water's so warm it's almost like a bath. Now you're moving faster out into the lake, up to your waist, up to your chest. The water's so warm, so comfortable. You take a deep breath and glide a few feet forward down into the water. You surface and feel the water run down your back. You look around; you're still all alone. You still have this lovely spot to yourself. Far across the lake you can see a sailboat, tiny in the distance. It's so far away you can just make out the white sail jutting up from the blue water. You take

another breath and kick off this time toward the shore swimming with long easy strokes. Kicking with your feet, pulling through with your arms and hands. You swim so far that when you stop and stand the water's only up to your waist, and you begin walking toward the beach, across the warm sand to the grass. Now you're feeling again the grass beneath your feet. Deep, soft, lush. You reach your blanket and pick up the towel, and begin to dry yourself. You dry your hair, your face, your neck. You stretch the towel across your shoulders, dry your back, your legs. You can feel the warm sun on your skin. It must be ninety degrees, but it's clear and dry. The heat isn't oppressive; it's just nice and warm and comfortable. You lie down on the blanket and feel the deep, soft grass under your head. You're looking up at the sky, seeing those great billowy clouds floating by, far, far, above (p. 319).

Practice. Once the imagery scenes have been developed, patients are instructed to practice using them. At this stage, the health professional slowly describes a scene to the patient in a low-pitched voice. Describing the scene slowly and quietly may elicit a feeling of tranquility from the patient. The health professional instructs the patient to close his or her eyes and imagine the scene as intensely as possible while listening to the description. The patient continues to imagine the scene for about 30 seconds following the end of the description. Then the health professional terminates the patient's imagery by saying something like "You may open your eyes as I count backward from five to one." Next the health professional queries the patient about the vividness of the imagery. This process is repeated for each scene. The health professional instructs the patient to practice imagining the scenes several times a day.

Application. The final step is for patients to apply the emotive imagery in actual distressful or discomforting situations. Remember that before applying emotive imagery, the patient should be in a relaxed state.

Guided Imagery

There are four steps in helping patients use guided imagery (see Table 13-4). The first step is to provide patients with information about the purpose and overview of the process.

Purpose and overview. First, information about the purpose and overview of guided imagery is given to patients. The health professional might give the following information to a cancer patient (adapted from Simonton, Matthews-Simonton, & Creighton, 1980).

> In addition to learning how to relax your body muscles, it is important that you be able to visualize your own recovery. Relaxation and mental imagery may facilitate the attaining of health and give you a feeling of being in control. Visualizing wellness can affect physical changes, enhance your body defense system, alter the course of malignancy, and change your thought patterns about your illness. For example, thinking of or visualizing your body cells (or organs) functioning in a positive way can influence how you cope with your illness and in turn can affect your progress toward health. The procedure is called guided imagery because it instructs you about how and what to visualize. We want to ensure that your mental images are positive. Some patients, for example, view their cancer or illness as strong and powerful and their own body defense systems as passive and immobile. The purpose of guided imagery is to reverse your visualization of the cancer and your body defense systems. Specifically, you will learn how to visualize the invading cancer cells being opposed by the effects of your treatment and your strong body defense systems. These will contribute to the destruction of the cancer cells and will promote your return to better health, while restoring your ability to engage in activities that make you happy.

The health professional might emphasize that guided imagery does not cure cancer or other illnesses, but the procedure may influence patient expectations about health, which may in turn enhance recovery or remission. Specifically, guided imagery seems to create positive beliefs that help to activate the body's defenses against disease. Benefits resulting from regular use of guided imagery include reduction of fear, tension, and stress, strengthening of the will to live, and enhancement of the immune system through modification of thoughts and beliefs (Simonton et al., 1980).

Assessment of patient's imagery. The next step in the use of guided imagery is an assessment of the patient's current visualization or perception of the illness. The health professional needs to find out how the patient imagines his or her illness and treatment and the body organs or systems involved in the illness. For example, Simonton, Matthews-Simonton, and Creighton (1980) found that patients' initial images of their illness and treatment were "negative." Some patients imagined their illness as "a big black rat," "a rock which is strong and impregnable," or "little gremlins." They saw the treatment as passive and the body defenses as submissive and inactive. The health professional may wish to explore the content of these images by instructing patients to draw their images of the illness, the body organs involved, body systems, and effects of treatment. Or patients may describe these images verbally. Assessment of these images is important for developing effective imagery.

Development of imagery. The next step is to help patients develop positive mental images that are personalized, or represented by their own symbolic language. Simonton et al. (1980) have recommended that effective visual images for cancer patients depict the following features. The cancer cells are imagined as relatively few in number, weak, and disorganized. When confronted by the vast army of aggressive, healthy body cells, acting in concert with effective treatment, they are readily overwhelmed. Other normal body cells and organs then quickly repair any damage resulting from the treatment and totally eliminate the dead cancer cells from the body. Eventually the body regains its health, and patients once again begin to pursue their personal goals and fulfill their destiny (pp. 130–132).

These images for combatting cancer may apply to other illnesses as well. For example, patients with endocarditis can imagine the disease as weak and their bodies and the treatment as very powerful. They may picture their bodies growing progressively stronger as the infection is eradicated.

The instruction for guided imagery that Simonton et al. provide the cancer patient is as follows. (Remember that most patients are first given muscle relaxation exercises.)

> Mentally picture the cancer in either realistic or symbolic terms. Think of the cancer as consisting of very weak, confused cells. Remember that our bodies destroy cancerous cells thousands of times during a normal lifetime. As you picture your cancer, realize that your recovery requires that your body's own defenses return to a natural, healthy state.
>
> If you are now receiving treatment, picture your treatment coming into your body in a way that you understand. If you are receiving radiation treatment, picture it as a beam of millions of bullets of energy hitting any cells in its path. The normal cells are able to repair any damage that is done, but the cancerous cells cannot because they are weak. (This is one of the basic facts upon which radiation therapy is built.) If you are receiving chemotherapy, picture that drug coming into your body and entering the bloodstream. Picture the drug acting like a poison. The normal cells are intelligent and strong and don't take up the poison so readily. But the cancer cell is a weak cell, so it takes very little to kill it. It absorbs the poison, dies, and is flushed out of your body.
>
> Picture your body's own white blood cells coming into the area where the cancer is, recognizing the abnormal cells, and destroying them. There is a vast army of white blood cells. They are strong and very aggressive. They are also very smart. There is no contest between them and the cancer cells; they will win the battle.

> Picture the cancer shrinking. See the dead cells being carried away by the white blood cells and being flushed from your body through the liver and kidneys and eliminated in the urine and stool.
> - This is your expectancy of what you want to happen.
> - Continue to see the cancer shrinking, until it is all gone.
> - See yourself having more energy and a better appetite and being able to feel comfortable and loved in your family as the cancer shrinks and finally disappears.
>
> If you are experiencing pain anywhere in your body, picture the army of white blood cells flowing into the area and soothing the pain. Whatever the problem, give your body the command to heal itself. Visualize your body becoming well.
>
> Imagine yourself well, free of disease, full of energy.
>
> Picture yourself reaching your goals in life. See your purpose in life being fulfilled, the members of your family doing well, your relationships with people around you becoming more meaningful. Remember that having strong reasons for being well will help you get well, so use this time to focus clearly on your priorities in life.
>
> Give yourself a mental pat on the back for participating in your recovery. See yourself doing this mental imagery exercise three times a day, staying awake and alert as you do it.
>
> Then let the muscles in your eyelids lighten up, become ready to open your eyes, and become aware of the room. Now let your eyes open, and you are ready to resume your usual activities.*

These clinicians have also used a guided imagery scene for pain management and reduction, as follows:

---

*From *Getting well again,* by O. C. Simonton, S. Matthews-Simonton, and James L. Creighton. Copyright © 1980 by O. Carl Simonton and Stephanie Matthews-Simonton. This and all other quotations from the same source are reprinted by permission of Bantam Books, Inc. All rights reserved.

1. Focus on the pain. What color is it? See its color and shape and size clearly. It may be a bright red ball. It may be the size of a tennis ball or a grapefruit or basketball.

2. Mentally project the ball out into space, maybe ten feet away from your body.

3. Make the ball bigger, about the size of a basketball. Then shrink it to the size of a pea. Now let it become whatever size it chooses to be. Usually it returns to the original size you visualized.

4. Begin to change the ball's color. Make it pink, then light green.

5. Now take the green ball and put it back where you originally saw it. At this point, notice whether or not your pain has been reduced.

6. As you open your eyes, you are now ready to resume your usual activities (p. 185).

Guided imagery can be used to promote recovery from other illnesses as well, including arthritis, hypertension, and ulcers. These authors describe imagery instructions given to patients with these types of illnesses as follows:

> As an example of how you can use mental imagery to deal with an illness other than cancer, if you have an ulcer, your mental picture of the ulcer might be a crater-type sore in the lining of the stomach or intestine, seeing it rough and raw. Picturing the treatment, visualize antacids coating the area, neutralizing the excess acid and having a soothing effect on the ulcer itself. Picture normal cells coming in and doubling, dividing, covering over the raw, ulcerated area. See your body's white blood cells picking up any debris and cleaning the area, making it a pink, healthy lining. The next step is to see yourself free from pain and healthy, able to deal with the stresses of life without producing ulcer symptoms.

If you have high blood pressure, you could use the imagery process to see the problem as little muscles in the walls of the blood vessels tightening down, so that it causes much higher pressure than necessary for the blood to be driven through. Now, see the medication relaxing those little muscles in the blood vessels, your heart pumping evenly, and with little resistance, and blood flowing smoothly through the vascular channels. See yourself as able to cope with the stresses of life without producing symptoms of tension.

If your illness is arthritis, first picture your joints very irritated and having little granules on the surfaces. Then see your white blood cells coming in, cleaning up the debris, picking up the little granules, and smoothing over the joint surfaces. Then see yourself active, doing what you like to do, free of joint pain (pp. 123–124).

Practice. The last step in guided imagery is to instruct patients to close their eyes and to practice visualizing the various images described above that are appropriate for their illness. Patients should practice guided imagery three to four times a day after completing relaxation exercises. It may be helpful for them to have the instructions tape-recorded. The recording will ensure that they do not omit any part of the process.

LEARNING ACTIVITIES

Emotive Imagery

This learning activity is designed to be completed with a partner who assumes the role of a patient while you assume the role of a health professional. The patient should identify a painful or uncomfortable situation to which he or she is exposed.

According to Chapter Objective 4, the health professional will be able to do the following:

1. Provide an explanation to the patient about the emotive imagery procedure and how it may be beneficial.

2. Determine the imagery potential of the patient by probing for details about the intensity of the patient's imagery.

3. Develop two imagery scenes that promote calmness and elicit a variety of pleasant sensations for the patient.

4. Instruct the patient to imagine these scenes as vividly and intensely as possible. Each scene should be imagined for about 30 seconds. During the use of imagery, the interviewer could simulate discomfort by describing a painful situation to the patient or by having the patient hold an ice cube for 30 seconds.

Guided Imagery

Following the instructions for guided imagery described below (from Simonton et al., 1980, p. 123), try to cope with an illness or pain you may have. Or use the guided imagery procedure with a real patient or a role-play patient.

Instructions for Guided Imagery for Pain or Illness

1. Create a mental picture of any ailment or pain that you may have, visualizing it in a form that makes sense to you.

2. Picture any treatment you are receiving and perceive it either to eliminate the source of the ailment or pain or strengthen your body's ability to heal itself.

3. Picture your body's natural defenses and natural processes eliminating the source of the ailment or pain.

4. Imagine yourself healthy and free of the ailment or pain.

5. Visualize yourself proceeding successfully toward meeting your goals in life.

6. Give yourself a mental pat on the back for participating in your recovery. See yourself doing this relaxation/mental imagery exercise three times a day, staying awake and alert as you do it.

7. Let the muscles in your eyes lighten up, become ready to open your eyes, and become aware of the room.

8. Now let your eyes open and you are ready to resume your usual activities.

Stress Inoculation Training

Stress inoculation training involves teaching patients both physical and cognitive coping skills. Meichenbaum and Turk (1976) describe stress inoculation as a type of psychological protection that is analogous to a medical inoculation providing protection from disease. According to these authors, stress inoculation gives the person "a prospective defense or set of skills to deal with future stressful situations. As in medical inoculations, a person's resistance is enhanced by exposure to a stimulus strong enough to arouse defenses without being so powerful that it overcomes them" (p. 3). Stress inoculation training involves three major components: (1) educating the patient about the nature of stressful reactions; (2) having the patient rehearse various physical and cognitive coping skills; and (3) helping the patient apply these skills during exposure to stressful or painful situations. Of these three components, the second, which provides coping-skills training, seems to be the most important (Horan, Hackett, Buchanan, Stone, & Demchik-Stone, 1977).

Stress inoculation training has been used to help patients cope with pain-related stress and to help patients tolerate physiological pain and tension headaches. It has also been used with cancer patients to help them overcome a fear of needles and the vomiting associated with chemotherapy. Other authors report the use of stress inoculation to help young children cope with unpleasant dental procedures (Siegel & Peterson, 1980) and with the discomfort and stress associated with tonsillectomies (Peterson & Shigetomi, 1981).

Guidelines for Using Stress Inoculation Training

Stress inoculation training is designed to help patients cope more effectively with recurrent distressing, painful events or situations. Table 13-5 lists five steps associated with stress inoculation.

Purpose and overview. The first step is to provide information about stress inoculation with a rationale and overview of the procedure. The health

Table 13-5
The Five Steps of Stress Inoculation Training

1. Information about procedure
   a. Rationale
   b. Overview
2. Education of patient
   a. Framework for patient's reaction
   b. Phases of stress reaction
   c. Coping strategies
3. Acquisition and practice of coping skills
   a. Collecting and giving information
   b. Physical relaxation
   c. Cognitive relaxation
   d. Four phases of cognitive coping
4. Instruction to apply all of the coping skills to distressing situation
5. Follow-up
   a. Assessment of how it is working
   b. Instruction to keep a record

care provider might explain the purpose of the procedure for a patient suffering from recurring pain as follows:

> You appear to be suffering greatly from recurrent pain and seem to be having difficulty in managing your feelings about it. The procedure known as stress inoculation may help you learn to cope with your pain and help you manage the intensity of your feelings or emotions about the pain each time the pain occurs. The procedure will help you feel more in control of your pain.

The health professional may then give the patient a brief overview of the procedure.

> First, we will try to help you understand the nature of your feelings and how the pain elicits certain thoughts and feelings. Next, you will learn some ways to manage the distress caused by your pain. After you learn these coping skills, we will practice using them each time the pain occurs.

Patient education. The second step is to educate patients about the framework of their reaction to the stressful or painful situation, the phases of stress reactions, and various coping strategies. Rybstein-Blinchik (1979) offers this explanation for the patient's reaction to pain:

> Research has shown that your experience of pain involves experiencing a state of heightened arousal that might include increased heart rate, sweaty palms, rapid breathing, or bodily tension. You have learned to call this state of arousal "pain." You have also learned to experience, at the time you feel this arousal, certain thoughts and images; and you are saying things to yourself at this time (p. 97).

The health professional could add to this explanation:

> The expectations, thoughts, and images that occur during pain influence your distressful reactions and emotions to each painful episode.

To help patients conceptualize their reactions, the health professional can explain that typical reactions to painful or stressful situations follow four specific stages: (1) preparing for the stressful situation or painful event (*before* the situation); (2) confronting and handling the event or pain (*during* the situation); (3) coping with critical moments or feelings (*during* the situation); and (4) rewarding or reinforcing behaviors after the stress or pain, in recognition of the use of appropriate coping skills during the first three phases (*after* the situation). The health professional might say:

> When you feel pain, you may assume that it will persist for a continuous period of time. However, your reaction is probably composed of several smaller reactions instead of just one single response. The first reaction begins when you feel the first sign of pain and then you probably anticipate what will happen. At this point, you can learn to prepare yourself for handling the pain more effectively. The next stage comes when you're in the middle of a painful episode and you feel the intensity

of the pain. You can learn how to confront the pain in a constructive way. At times, at critical moments, the pain may get particularly intense—and you may feel yourself losing control. At these times, you can learn how to cope with those intense feelings. Then, after the pain has gone, you can learn to congratulate yourself for trying to cope with the pain instead of allowing it to overwhelm you.

Patients should also be informed that they will learn a variety of ways to deal with the distressful situation or event. Such strategies include both physical and cognitive coping strategies.

Coping skills. Step three is to teach the patient actual coping skills and strategies and to provide the opportunity to practice them. First, collect information from the patient about the specific characteristics of the stressful or painful situation. For example, how often does the pain usually occur? How long does it last? Where is it most intense? What is the intensity of the pain? What does the patient do when the pain occurs? What does the patient think about while the pain is occurring? This type of information may be helpful in applying the coping strategies. Also, as we mentioned previously, providing information to the patient may help to prepare him or her to deal more effectively with the situation. For example, prepared childbirth teaches women and their labor coaches that the experienced pain is actually a uterine contraction. Participants are provided information about the timing and stages of labor and the intensity of contractions and are instructed to think about or picture the contraction as a wave. Such factual information dispels many myths and misconceptions surrounding the process.

After providing pertinent information about the nature of the stressful situation, the patient is ready to learn the coping strategies that can help manage the stress. In teaching physical and cognitive coping skills, the health professional should emphasize the important role of these skills in reducing stress and pain. For example, it can be reiterated that pain is created and exacerbated by muscular tension, accumulation of waste products (for example, lactic acid), and lack of "fuel" (glucose and oxygen) in the muscles. Physical coping strategies help to reduce pain by relieving muscle tension, reducing waste-product accumulation, and providing more oxygen to the working muscles. Physical coping strategies include muscle relaxation and meditation, which we described earlier. Any of these procedures, if used properly, can help patients relax more fully and decrease sensations of pain.

Patients also need to learn cognitive coping strategies to counteract feelings of helplessness that may exacerbate the pain. Emotive and guided imagery, which we described earlier, are examples of cognitive coping strategies. Attention-diversion is another cognitive coping strategy. In this case, the patient is instructed to concentrate on something other than pain, such as slow, deep breathing, counting ceiling tiles, or doing mental arithmetic (Meichenbaum, 1977).

Another cognitive coping strategy is to help the patient conceptualize the painful situation in several small phases: (1) preparing for the pain (before it occurs); (2) confronting and handling the pain; (3) coping with feelings at critical moments, such as during increase of pain's intensity; and (4) reinforcing or congratulating oneself for having coped with the situation/pain. In addition, the health professional helps the patient compile a list of "coping statements" to use during each of the preceding four phases. Coping statements are sentences or phrases that the patient can say either aloud or silently. They represent a positive way of talking oneself through a difficult situation. Coping statements seem to help patients manage pain by controlling negative thoughts and images, by acknowledging and relabeling discomfort, by "psyching" oneself up to confront the situation, by coping with intense pain, and by congratulating oneself for having coped successfully.

Table 13-6 presents some examples of coping statements that Meichenbaum and Turk (1976) have used with patients for each of the four phases mentioned. Remember that these are just exam-

ples; coping statements seem to work best when they are tailored to the individual patient.

After the coping statements have been compiled, patients practice saying them aloud. The patients must feel comfortable with the statements, or they may not use them. If, after continued practice, patients do not feel comfortable with the statements, new ones should be developed with the assistance of the health professional.

Application. The fourth step in stress inoculation is to have patients apply the procedures to the stressful or painful situation. The health professional should review with patients how the physical coping procedures and the cognitive coping strategies will be used in each of the four phases of the situation. For example, if patients have been given stress inoculation training to use before, during, and after receiving chemotherapy, it is imperative that they actually apply the techniques when the chemotherapy occurs.

Follow-up. The fifth and final step of the procedure involves follow-up—that is, an assessment of how well stress inoculation training has equipped patients to manage or cope with problem situations. Patients who are repeatedly exposed to uncomfortable situations or procedures such as allergy or insulin injections, extensive dental work, radiation, or chemotherapy may wish to keep records of the use of this procedure and ratings of its effectiveness.

There is an abbreviated version of stress inoculation that may be helpful for patients who do not have the time or inclination to go through all of the previously described steps. Patients can be provided with appropriate coping statements to use before, during, and after stressful or painful situations or events (this abridged procedure corresponds to items 3(d) and 4 on Table 13-5). For example, children have been taught coping statements such as "Everything is going to be all right" or "I will be all right in just a while" to repeat to themselves before and during uncomfortable dental procedures and tonsillectomies (Peterson & Shigetomi, 1981, p. 4; Siegel & Peterson, 1980, p. 786).

Table 13-6
Some Coping Statements Used in Stress Inoculation Training

Preparing for the painful stressor

What is it you have to do?
You can develop a plan to deal with it.
Just think about what you have to do.
Just think about what you can do about it.
Don't worry; worrying won't help anything.
You have lots of different strategies you can call on.

Confronting and handling the pain

You can meet the challenge.
One step at a time; you can handle the situation.
Just relax, breathe deeply, and use one of the strategies.
Don't think about the pain, just what you have to do.
This tenseness can be an ally, a cue to cope.
Relax. You're in control; take a slow deep breath. Ah! Good!
This anxiety is what they said you might feel. That's right; it's the reminder to use your coping skills.

Coping with feelings at critical moments

When pain comes, just pause; keep focusing on what you have to do.
What is it you have to do?
Don't try to eliminate the pain totally; just keep it manageable.
You were supposed to expect the pain to rise; just keep it under control.
Just remember, there are different strategies; they'll help you stay in control.
When the pain mounts, you can switch to a different strategy; you're in control.

Reinforcing self-statements

Good, you did it.
You handled it pretty well.
You knew you could do it!
Wait until you tell someone about which procedures worked best.

From "The Cognitive-Behavioral Management of Anxiety, Anger and Pain," by D. Meichenbaum and D. Turk. In P. O. Davidson (Ed.), *The behavioral management of anxiety, depression and pain.* Copyright © 1976 by Brunner/Mazel, Inc. Reprinted by permission.

In prepared childbirth, pregnant women learn to use coping statements such as "This is your baby" during the transition phase, "Think baby down and out" during the expulsion (pushing) phase, and "The baby is almost born now" when the contractions come very close together and are very powerful (Beals, 1980). In using this abbreviated stress inoculation procedure, patients must both rehearse and apply the coping statements during the uncomfortable or painful situation.

LEARNING ACTIVITIES

Stress Inoculation

Listed below are four situations involving uncomfortable or painful medical treatments. Select two of the four situations, and for each one identify in writing three possible coping statements a patient could use during each of the four phases: (1) preparing for the painful stressor (before situation); (2) confronting and handling the pain (during situation); (3) coping with pain at critical moments (during situation); and (4) reinforcing behaviors (after situation) (Chapter Objective 5).

Make the coping statements as specific as possible for each procedure. You may wish to contrast your examples with those given in Table 13-6 or share them with an instructor or colleague. The first one is completed as an example for you.

Situation A: A patient is about to have restoration of several teeth (for example, drilling).

1. Preparing for the stressor (before the dental appointment) coping statements:

    I'm going to control what I think about when I go for the appointment.

    I will stay calm in anticipating my appointment.

    It is never as bad as I imagine.

    It won't be bad—in fact, it is important for my dental health!

2. Confronting and handling the pain or discomfort (during the situation):

    I'm going to relax and tune out the noise.

    I can just relax when the chair is back like this. They will be finished in a while.

    I may perspire a little—just relax, everything is going to be fine.

3. Coping with pain at critical moments (during the situation):

    Just relax and take a deep breath.

    You are doing fine—pretty soon it will be over.

    Think about how important the work they are doing is for my mouth.

4. Reinforcing oneself (after the situation):

    I did pretty well after all.

    That wasn't as bad as I thought. Even the noise didn't bother me.

    Just think, it's over and my mouth is all fixed up. Wow!

Situations

B. A patient is scheduled to undergo a bone marrow aspiration.

C. A patient is due to have a baby in one month.

D. A patient must undergo a bladder catheterization.

E. A patient has to receive weekly chemotherapy injections.

Stimulus Control or Environmental Planning

Many human behaviors are habitual and are influenced by or patterned after events that precede those behaviors. Such events are called *antecedents*. Antecedents include situations, emotions, thoughts, images, behaviors, objects, or verbal instructions said aloud or to oneself. Stimulus control—also called environmental planning—involves reducing the number of antecedents associated with an undesirable behavior while simultaneously increasing the antecedents associated with desirable behavior (Mahoney & Thoresen, 1974; Thoresen & Mahoney, 1974).

Stimulus control or environmental planning is "rearranging or modifying environmental conditions that serve as cues or antecedents of a particular response" (Cormier & Cormier, 1979, p. 493). It has also been described as stimulus control in which patients are "taught to modify their physical or social environment...in order to change an undesirable behavior" (Melamed & Siegel, 1980, p. 52). Patients can learn to rearrange their environments so that undesirable health-related behaviors are decreased and desirable health-related behaviors are increased. For example, suppose a patient wanted to decrease his or her alcohol consumption. The patient could modify the environment by removing or locking up all alcoholic beverages in the home. Or he or she could modify the social environment by drinking only at social gatherings in the late afternoon or early evening.

To increase desirable behavior, Watson and Tharp (1981) recommend that patients "deliberately set up certain antecedents to stimulate a desired behavior" (p. 96). For example, consider patients who desire to increase their weekly exercise (for example, walking or jogging). They might decide to do the walking before breakfast, five days a week. By preparing exercise clothes and shoes at night before retiring, such patients could create or increase antecedents to support walking. Further, they could also ask their spouse to remind them of their commitment and to "applaud" their efforts. They could also encourage their spouse or a friend to join them as an exercise partner.

Decreasing Undesirable Behaviors

Table 13-7 enumerates the principles and cites examples of stimulus control techniques for decreasing undesirable health-related behaviors. The health professional helps patients reduce the number or frequency of cues or antecedents associated with undesirable behaviors. To decrease a behavior, the antecedent cues associated with it must be altered in terms of place and time of occurrence (Cormier & Cormier, 1979, p. 494). Carroll and Yates (1981) helped overweight patients to arrange cues in a way that made it difficult to execute the behavior (eating). For example, food in the refrigerator was to be placed in covered nontransparent bowls or in brown paper bags. The rationale for this stimulus control was that by reducing the environmental antecedent (the sight of food in the refrigerator), the food would be out of sight and thus would not induce eating between meals. Another example of rearranging or altering cues is to change the place where the behavior is to occur. Designating a particular place for drinking alcoholic beverages and limiting cigarette smoking to one place are other examples of arranging antecedents or cues to decrease undesirable health behaviors.

Table 13-7
Principles and Examples of Stimulus-Control Strategies

Principles of Change	Example
To decrease the frequency of a behavior:	
Reduce or narrow the antecedents associated with the behavior	
1. Prearrange or alter antecedents associated with the *place* of the behavior:	
a. Prearrange antecedents to make it cumbersome to execute the behavior.	Food in refrigerator kept in covered, nontransparent bowls, or in brown paper bags. Place food in high, hard-to-reach places.
b. Prearrange antecedents so that behavior is done only in a designated place and time.	Drink alcoholic beverages only at social events. Attend social events with spouse. Smoke only one cigarette at home, and only in one chair.
2. Alter the *time* or *sequence* (chain) between the antecedent cues and the resulting behavior:	
a. Break up or change the sequence.	Chew gum when urge to snack occurs. Substitute and engage in another activity when starting to go for a snack.
b. Build pauses into the sequence or chain.	Wait 10 minutes before getting snack. Purchase only foods that require preparation.
To increase the frequency of a behavior:	
1. Prearrange physical or environmental objects to act as antecedents or cues to increase the probability of performing the desired behavior.	Place back brace on bathroom sink to remind patient to wear it during the waking hours. Place medications on kitchen table to remind patient to take tablets with meals.
2. Self-instruction and imagining.	Patients imagine themselves doing exercises or instruct themselves on specific tasks or behaviors.
3. Place self-generated or written reminders in appropriate places.	Note on office desk to take medication. Alarm clock to remind child to empty bladder.
4. Build a chain or sequence as a clue or antecedent to the desired behavior.	Schedule low back exercises as part of morning exercise-shower-dress routine.
5. Acquire a social ally to encourage the desired behavior.	Get an exercise partner. Have a friend or relative cue patient to take medication.

Adapted from Cormier & Cormier, 1979, p. 495.

Stimulus control also helps reduce unhealthy behavior by "interrupting the learned pattern or sequence that begins with one or more antecedent cues and results in the undesired response" (Cormier & Cormier, 1979, p. 495). For example, a variety of behaviors make up the sequence of eating. When a person eats a snack between meals, there is a sequence or chain of behaviors that occurs. Before eating a snack, a person may be bored, think about food, get up and go toward the kitchen, look for a snack in the pantry, refrigerator, or kitchen cabinet, remove the snack container from where it is stored, and finally eat the snack.

A chain or sequence of behavior can be interrupted in one of two ways: either by breaking up the chain or building pauses into the chain (Watson & Tharp, 1981, pp. 113–118). Each of these techniques involves arranging or altering the time or sequence of the occurrence of the behaviors. Usually a chain of behaviors can be interrupted by the addition of another event or behavior to the sequence. For example, a patient who frequently snacks could interrupt the eating sequence by not going to look for a snack (early in the chain) and could substitute another behavior such as chewing gum or making a phone call when thinking about food or getting bored. Or, if a "snackaholic" typically eats at certain times, the usual order of events or behaviors leading up to the act of eating could be scheduled so that the snacker engages in another behavior at such times. Finally, the snacker could interrupt the chain by deliberately building pauses into the chain.

One way to handle habitual behavior is to pause before responding to an antecedent or a cue (Watson & Tharp, 1981, p. 114). For instance, whenever the snacker has an urge to get something to eat in response to a "want to eat" cue, a deliberate pause of 10 minutes could be interposed before actually going to search for food. This time interval could be gradually increased. With some behaviors, the pause may be strengthened by instructing the patient to take a few minutes and think about the benefits of not eating a snack. Another way to change habitual eating is to have no prepared foods available, thus forcing another pause (see Table 13-7 for other examples).

Increasing Health-Related Behaviors

There are several ways in which stimulus control can be used to increase health-related behavior. (Table 13-7 lists some principles and examples.) First, physical/environmental objects can be physically rearranged to act as antecedents to the desired behavior. For example, to increase wearing of a back brace, a patient could place the brace on the bathroom sink each night before retiring so that he or she would see it upon arising and be reminded to put it on. A patient wishing to meditate or do muscle relaxation exercises could arrange a special room or place for each session.

Leaving medicine in specific places around the house or workplace is an example of physically arranging antecedents for compliance in taking medication. (Of course, medication should never be left where children might find it.)

Another technique used to increase desirable behavior is to employ self-instruction or imagery as an antecedent or cue for the behavior. For example, patients might imagine themselves doing warm-up exercises such as leg stretches, sit-ups, toe-touching, push-ups, and running in place in preparation for a two-mile walking and jogging routine. Self-instruction may act as a cue for the desired behavior. Other patients may say to themselves "Don't buy junk foods; instead buy fresh or dried fruit," "Don't forget to schedule your exercises today," or "At four o'clock I need to practice my relaxation exercises and my imagery scenes."

A third technique is to have written reminders or messages in places where the patient will see them, such as the bathroom mirror, refrigerator door, dining room or kitchen table, or dashboard of the car. Patients starting a diet may carry a small pocket notebook listing things they are permitted to eat. A daily or weekly list can also be an effective reminder or cue. Alarm watches may be worn to remind patients to conform to medication schedules. Finally, combinations of any of the preceding techniques—for example, the use of self-instructional statements coupled with written reminders on daily calendars—may effectively stimulate desirable behaviors.

We mentioned previously that habitual behaviors are usually the end product of a chain or sequence of behaviors. Another technique that can increase desirable behavior is to build a chain that includes that behavior. One way to build such a chain is to schedule or plan the times at which the desired behavior is to occur. For example, if a patient is to take medication in the morning immediately after arising, he or she can be instructed to schedule the medicine taking at a particular time during the sequence of morning behaviors. For example, a patient may perform the following sequence of behaviors each morning: get out of bed, take off bed clothes, go to the toilet, shave, take a shower, get dressed, and proceed downstairs to eat breakfast. The patient can be instructed to take the medicine between dressing and eating breakfast. By scheduling it into this chain of routine behaviors, the patient increases the probability of taking the medication.

The last technique for increasing a behavior with stimulus control is to have a relative, spouse, or friend act as a "reminding" cue for engaging in the desired behavior. The social ally not only can act as an antecedent but also can provide positive reinforcement and encouragement for the patient's progress. The social ally can be anyone who has regular contact with the patient. His or her role is not to nag or punish the patient for lapses or errors but, rather, to provide subtle social cues and reinforcement. This technique can be combined with any or all of the procedures above. If a social ally is not available, any combination of the four other techniques may be a strong enough stimulus to increase the desirable behavior.

═══════════ LEARNING ACTIVITIES ═══════════

Stimulus Control

1. Choose a health-related behavior for yourself. Identify how you would use stimulus control techniques to increase and decrease antecedents related to this behavior.

2. Suppose an overweight patient needs to lose weight. According to Chapter Objective 6, you should be able to specify at least four stimulus control techniques you would recommend for decreasing each behavior specified below. Use Table 13-7 as a guide. Be very specific in your recommendations. An example of one behavior and recommendation are provided below. Feedback follows.

Behavior to Decrease: 1. Snacking between meals.
Recommendation: Buy only food that requires some time and effort to prepare.

Behavior to Decrease: 2. Eating high-calorie foods.
Recommendations:

Behavior to Decrease: 3. Multiple servings at meals.
Recommendations:

Feedback

Behaviors to decrease:
1. Snacking between meals.
Recommendations:

Buy only food that requires some time and effort to prepare.

Store food in inaccessible places and refrigerated food in opaque containers.

Limit eating to one room and one chair.

Do not participate in other activities while eating.

Eat at the same times every day.

Chew gum or substitute another activity when the urge to snack overpowers you.

Deliberately pause by delaying for ten minutes before reaching for snack food; gradually lengthen the pause.

2. Eating high-calorie foods

Do not shop when hungry.

Buy only foods on a prepared shopping list.

Eat larger portions of low-calorie foods (vegetables, fruits) to provide satiation.

3. Multiple servings at meal times

Use other people as reminders to help you avoid second helpings.

Prepare only single servings of food with no obvious leftovers.

Limit your servings to one helping of each food item.

Do not place serving dishes on the table.

Self-Monitoring

Self-monitoring is a process in which patients "observe and record specific things about themselves and their interactions with environmental situations" (Cormier & Cormier, 1979, p. 481). Self-monitoring by patients encourages them to assume a more active role in their own health care and also teaches them to make finer discriminations about their behavior (DiTomasso & Colameco, 1982). There are three ways self-monitoring can be used with patients.

First, the process can be used to gather information about problem health behavior. For example, if a patient suffers from pain, the patient can be instructed to record the intensity of the pain on a 10-point scale, the areas of the body in which the pain occurs, the time of day each pain episode occurs, the situation in which the pain occurs, and associated activities or thoughts that recur during each pain episode. This type of information can help the health professional make an accurate diagnosis and assessment of the problem and design effective treatment regimens.

When self-monitoring is used to gather information, it can be a reactive process. *Reactivity* refers to changes in behavior that occur as consequences of observing and recording. A second use of self-monitoring is as an intervention strategy. For example, patients with essential hypertension could be instructed to monitor their blood pressure daily, which may increase their compliance with the health care program. Although the reactivity to self-monitoring may create some confusion in information gathering, it can be an asset when the self-monitoring is used as an intervention strategy, in that it prompts change in the direction desired by the patient.

A third use of self-monitoring is for patients to record the times, frequencies, and reactions to other intervention strategies or treatment regimens. For example, patients could be instructed to keep a daily record of the number of times a muscle relaxation training audio-cassette tape was used, the time of day it was used, and their level of relaxation before and after exercises. Their use of self-monitoring should promote adherence to the required strategy or treatment.

Self-monitoring is the predominant intervention strategy in many weight-reduction programs. Overweight children and adults have used this strategy to self-monitor caloric intake, exercise, and weight change. Self-monitoring also has been used to decrease cigarette smoking. Hypertensive patients have self-monitored their blood pressure, and patients with insulin-dependent diabetes have monitored urine glucose. Self-monitoring also has been a valuable technique in promoting compliance with dental hygiene regimens.

Steps in Self-Monitoring

Thoresen and Mahoney (1974) have identified five steps in self-monitoring: (1) selection of a response (behavior to monitor); (2) recording of a response; (3) charting of a response; (4) display of charted data; and (5) an analysis of the data. Table 13-8 outlines these steps in more detail.

Selection of a response.   Selection of a response involves helping patients identify *what* to monitor. The target behavior to be monitored should be defined explicitly (DiTomasso & Colameco, 1982). It is also important for the health professional to help patients select appropriate types of behavior to monitor. For example, self-monitoring yielded greater weight loss for people who recorded their daily weight *and* daily caloric intake than for those who recorded only daily body weight (Romanczyk, 1974).

Generally, it is a good idea to have patients monitor the behaviors they most want to change. If patients successfully engage in self-monitoring one behavior, then more behaviors can be added.

Recording of the response.   After selecting and defining a behavior to monitor, patients and health professionals need to identify methods for recording the behavior. Systematic recording and instructions about the method of recording are important to the success of self-monitoring. Patients

Table 13-8
Steps of Self-Monitoring

1. Select and define target behavior.
   a. Write definition of behavior to change.
   b. Provide examples of behavior.
2. Record response or behavior.
   a. Specify the timing of self-monitoring.
      • Prebehavior monitoring to decrease undesired behavior.
      • Postbehavior monitoring to increase desired behavior.
      • Record immediately after behavior occurs.
      • Record when not distracted by the situation or by other competing responses.
   b. Select a method of recording (frequency, duration). Remember:
      • Frequency counts clearly separate occurrences of the behavior.
      • Duration measures responses that occur for a period of time.
   c. Select a device to assist in self-monitoring. Remember that the device should be:
      • Portable.
      • Accessible.
      • Economical.
      • Obtrusive enough to serve as a reminder to self-record.
   d. Engage in self-monitoring for at least two weeks. Then complete Steps 3, 4, and 5.
3. Chart behavior daily with a line graph.
4. Display data.
5. Analyze data. Compare data on the chart with stated desired behavior change.

Adapted from Cormier and Cormier, 1979.

need very specific instructions regarding both *when* and *how* to record behaviors. Listed below are four guidelines to help health professionals and patients to decide when to record.

1. If patients are using self-monitoring as a way to decrease an undesirable behavior, prebehavior monitoring may be more effective, since it seems to interrupt the response chain early in the process. For example, patients would record whenever they have the urge to eat a snack between meals but do not eat. Thus, the self-monitoring would consist of recording daily urges to snack between meals, but only when no snack was actually eaten.

2. If patients are using self-monitoring to increase desirable behavior, then post-behavior monitoring may be more successful. For example, patients may record each time they take anti-hypertensive medication during the week.

3. Record the instances of desirable behaviors immediately after they occur. Patients should record immediately after taking medication, after the urge to snack or smoke, or immediately after using imagery or relaxation to avoid pain.

4. Patients should be instructed and encouraged to self-monitor or self-record behaviors when not distracted by situations, by other people, or by competing responses (Cormier & Cormier, 1979, p. 485).

After patients have been instructed when to record the behaviors, the health professional needs to instruct them in *methods* for recording. McFall (1977) states that the method of recording can vary in a number of ways. He says:

> It can range from a very informal and unstructured operation, as when subjects are asked to make mental notes of any event that seems related to mood changes, to something fairly formal and structured, as when subjects are asked to fill out a mood-rating sheet according to a time-sampling schedule. It can be fairly simple, as when subjects are asked to keep track of how many cigarettes they smoke in a given time period; or it can be complex and time-consuming, as when they are asked

to record not only how many cigarettes they smoke, but also the time, place, circumstances, and affective responses associated with lighting each cigarette. It can be a relatively objective matter, as when counting the calories consumed each day; or it can be a very subjective matter, as when recording the number of instances each day when they successfully resist the temptation to eat sweets (p. 197).*

There are two methods patients may use to record or self-monitor:

1. Frequency count: Patients may record how many times a day they have used muscle relaxation or meditation or had an urge to snack. They may also record the number of coping statements or self-complimentary thoughts that have occurred.

2. Duration count: Patients may record how much time they spend eating each meal, performing exercises, meditating, or using the muscle relaxation techniques. It is also possible to combine the two methods. For example, the frequency of exercise and the duration of each exercise session could be recorded simultaneously.

After the method of self-monitoring has been determined, the health professional needs to help patients select a device for self-monitoring. A variety of devices can be used to help patients keep accurate records: wrist counter (golf counter), note cards, daily or weekly log sheets (graph paper), diaries, or a small audiocassette tape recorder. The device should be economical, portable, and accessible so that it is present whenever the behavior occurs (Watson & Tharp, 1981). Also, the device should be easy and convenient to use, unobtrusive if used in public but obtrusive enough to serve as a reminder for self-recording. Finally, the health professional should rehearse the recording procedures to ensure that patients will self-monitor

_____

*From "Parameters of self-monitoring," by R. M. McFall. In R. B. Stuart (Ed.), *Behavioral self-management: Strategies, techniques and outcomes.* Copyright © 1977 by Brunner/Mazel, Inc. Reprinted by permission.

accurately and should determine that patients are willing to engage in the process for at least two weeks.

Charting of the response. Cormier and Cormier (1979) suggest that the data recorded "with the aid of a recording device should be translated onto a more permanent storage record, as a chart or graph, that enables the patient to inspect the self-monitored device visually" (p. 487). The data can be charted on a line graph. For example, the frequency or duration of the self-monitored behavior is placed on a vertical axis and the horizontal axis represents the days. Figure 13-1 displays a self-monitoring chart kept by a patient to decrease snacking. Patients should receive instruction (verbal or written) on how to chart and graph the daily totals of the self-monitored behavior.

Display of the data. In addition to charting the self-monitored behavior, patients should be instructed to display the data in prominent places, such as the refrigerator or bathroom mirror. Charting and display of data are motivating tech-niques that may maintain continued adherence to use of this strategy.

Analysis of the data. Finally, patients should do an analysis of the self-monitored data and determine whether or not the data reveal that the behavior is within or outside the target limits. The health professional can help in data analysis. He or she should also periodically reinforce the patient for accurate and reliable self-recording, as this reinforcement can bolster the patient's motivation to self-monitor consistently and accurately (DiTomasso & Colameco, 1982). Remember, for a lengthy intervention, it is usually a good idea to have patients self-monitor problem health behaviors, application of the specific intervention strategy, or both. Self-monitoring can enhance patients' involvement in intervention and health care.

One problem with self-monitoring is that patients sometimes find it difficult to do on a regular basis. A health professional can increase the probability of patients' adherence to the procedure by keeping requirements for self-monitoring brief and simple.

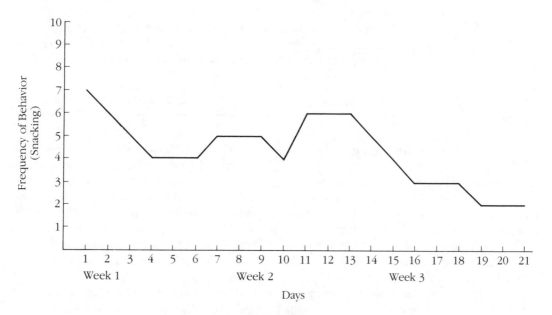

Figure 13-1
Self-Monitoring Chart

=== **LEARNING ACTIVITIES** ===

Self-Monitoring

This learning activity instructs you to use self-monitoring to increase or decrease a health-related behavior. According to Chapter Objective 7, you will be able to:

1. Select and define a target behavior.
   a. Specify one health-related behavior you would like to change (increase or decrease).
   b. Write a definition of this behavior.
   c. Provide some examples of this behavior. If this is difficult, make sure your definition reflects an observable outcome.
2. Record the behavior. Specify the timing of your self-recording. Remember, use prebehavior monitoring to decrease undesirable behavior and post-behavior monitoring to increase desirable behavior. Write down the timing method you will use.
3. Select a method of recording (frequency/duration). Remember, frequency counts for clearly separate occurrences of a behavior and duration counts for responses that occur for a period of time. Write down the method you will use.
4. Select a device to assist in self-monitoring that is portable, accessible, economical, and obtrusive enough to serve as a good reminder to self-record. List the device you'll use. (You may want to share your plan for Steps 1–4 with a colleague or an instructor before proceeding to Step 5.)
5. Engage in self-monitoring for at least two weeks. Then move to Step 6.
6. Chart your data by days on a simple line graph, and analyze any changes made over the weeks. Display the chart for appropriate encouragement from yourself or others.

Chapter Summary

This chapter has described a variety of intervention strategies useful for health maintenance or for patients with chronic or critical illnesses. These strategies have been used successfully with outpatients having chronic illnesses (COPE) as a part of their treatment regimen. Specifically, muscle relaxation, meditation, and self-monitoring have been used to reduce the severity of hypertension, tension headaches, insomnia, and other chronic conditions.

Other strategies described in this chapter have been used with patients suffering from acute but responsive illnesses that are easily diagnosed and treated (ACURE). For example, some of these patients have received preparatory information or have been taught physical and cognitive coping skills. These skills enable them to cope with diagnostic or surgical procedures or with other aspects of their illness.

Patients who have critical and recalcitrant illnesses (CARE), such as multiple sclerosis or cancer, have benefitted from the use of emotive and guided imagery strategies and from the stress reduction realized by regular practice of muscle relaxation or meditation.

This chapter also described how the various intervention strategies could be used not only as part of the treatment program for these types of patient but also by persons with no evident illness (PREP) as health-promoting or health-maintaining techniques. For example, the consistent use of muscle relaxation and meditation may bring about general stress reduction and promote calmness, and stimulus control and self-monitoring strategies may be useful for increasing or decreasing a variety of health-related behaviors, including exercise, good eating habits, smoking, and so on.

We also observed that these strategies are not useful for all patients. Patient adherence to the strategies is more likely if the strategy is presented as part of the overall treatment program rather than as something added as an "afterthought." Patients should receive a careful explanation about how and why a particular strategy will promote recovery and achieve health. Training in the use of the strategy and follow-up by the health professional are also essential for promoting patient adherence.

Suggested Readings _____

Benson, H. *The relaxation response.* New York: Avon, 1976. This book gives a good overview of the application and research associated with the relaxation response (respiratory meditation).

Carrington, P. *Learning to meditate: Clinically standardized meditation (CSM)—Course Workbook.* Kendall Park, N.J.: Pace Educational Systems, 1978. This is a very comprehensive self-instructional package for clinically standardized meditation (CSM). The instructor's kit includes three instructional tapes (audiocassettes) and three tapes on CSM applied to anxiety, stress-related illnesses, addictions, Type-A behavior, and exercise.

Carrington, P., Collings, G. H., Benson, H., Robinson, H., Wood, L. W., Lehrer, P. M., Woolfolk, R. L., & Cole, J. W. The use of meditation-relaxation techniques for the management of stress in a working population. *Journal of Occupational Medicine,* 1980, *22,* 221–231. This article provides a good illustration of the application of clinically standardized meditation as a prevention technique with telephone employees in New York.

Clark, C. C. *Enhancing wellness: A guide for self-care.* New York: Springer, 1981. The book is full of helpful assessment guides and practice exercises pertaining to wellness and health promotion. Suggestions for developing personal nutrition and physical fitness programs are included. Also discussed are topics about communication skills, stress reduction techniques, imagery, emotional health, and environmental sensitivity.

Cormier, W. H., & Cormier, L. S. *Interviewing strategies for helpers: A guide to assessment, treatment, and evaluation.* Monterey, Calif.: Brooks/Cole, 1979. The last half of this book provides step-by-step guidelines for applying muscle relaxation, stress inoculation, meditation, emotive imagery, self-monitoring, and stimulus control.

DiTomasso, R., & Colameco, S. Patient self-monitoring of behavior. *The Journal of Family Practice,* 1982, *15,* 79–83. This article describes various uses of self-monitoring by patients and offers ten practical suggestions for helping patients to implement a self-monitoring program.

Epstein, L. H., Beck, S., Figueroa, J., Farkas, G., Kazdin, A., Danemen, D., & Becker, D. The effects of targeting improvements in urine glucose on metabolic control in children with insulin-dependent diabetes. *Journal of Applied Behavior Analysis,* 1981, *14,* 365–375. This study examined the effects of preparatory information and self-monitoring on children with insulin-dependent diabetes.

Johnson, J. E., Rice, V. H., Fuller, S. S., & Endress, M. P. Sensory information, instruction in a coping strategy, and recovery from surgery. *Research in Nursing and Health,* 1978, *1,* 4–17. The article describes the effects of applying preparatory, procedural, and sensory information for surgical patients.

Meichenbaum, D., & Turk, D. The cognitive-behavioral management of anxiety, anger, and pain. In P. O. Davidson (Ed.), *The behavioral management of anxiety, depression and pain.* New York: Brunner/Mazel, 1976. This chapter describes the use of stress inoculation and provides an extensive list of coping statements that can be applied and used with managing pain.

Melamed, B. G., & Siegel, L. J. *Behavioral medicine: Practical applications in health care.* New York:

Springer, 1980. This book provides a description of the application of stimulus control, self-monitoring, and preparatory information to different patient concerns. It also describes factors that influence adherence.

Moore, K., & Altmaier, E. M. Stress inoculation training with cancer patients. *Cancer Nursing,* 1981, *5,* 389–393. These authors report the use of stress inoculation to help cancer patients cope with various medical treatments.

Nath, C., & Rinehart, J. Effects of individual and group relaxation therapy on blood pressure in essential hypertensives. *Research in Nursing and Health,* 1979, *2,* 119–126. The article describes the successful application of group and individual relaxation therapy in reducing blood pressure of hypertensive patients.

Sackett, D. L., Haynes, R. B., Gibson, E. S., Taylor, D. W., Roberts, R. S., & Johnson, A. L. Patient compliance with antihypertensive regimens. *Patient Counseling and Health Education,* 1978, *1,* 18–21. A classic study that investigates the use of self-monitoring as a way to improve compliance with an antihypertensive treatment regimen.

Shelton, J. R., & Rosen, G. M. Self-monitoring by patients. In G. M. Rosen, J. P. Geyman, & R. H. Layton (Eds.), *Behavioral science in family practice.* New York: Appleton-Century-Crofts, 1980. This chapter reviews self-monitoring methods and devices used in medical settings.

Simonton, O. C., Matthews-Simonton, S., & Creighton, J. *Getting well again.* New York: Bantam Books, 1980. This is a thorough presentation of relaxation, guided imagery, and other strategies used with cancer patients.

Turner, J. A., & Chapman, C. R. Psychological intervention for chronic pain: A critical review. I. Relaxation training and biofeedback. *Pain,* 1982, *12,* 1–21. This article is a recent review of the uses of muscle relaxation for pain control.

Wells, N. The effect of relaxation on postoperative muscle tension and pain. *Nursing Research,* 1982, *31,* 236–238. This study reported the effective use of muscle relaxation for cholecystectomy patients.

Ziesat, H. A. Behavior modification in the treatment of hypertension. *International Journal of Psychiatry in Medicine,* 1978, *8,* 257–265. The article describes use of self-monitoring, stimulus control, and direct social influence with essential hypertensive patients.

Ethical and Legal Issues in Health Care Interviewing

Objectives

After completing this chapter, you will be able to do the following:

1. Given a list of terms and their corresponding definitions, identify six legal terms pertinent to health professionals.

2. Given five case vignettes, identify the type of malpractice action most likely to ensue and provide an explanation for your choice.

3. Given a role-play consent interview, provide an oral explanation of a procedure or treatment to a patient that includes the six elements of informed consent.

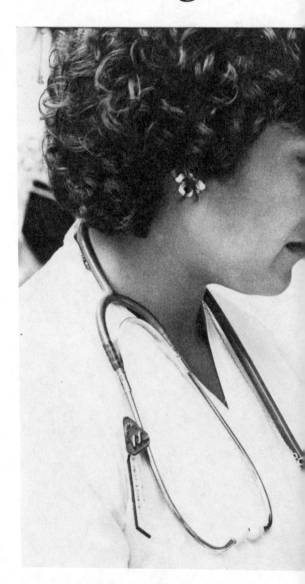

14

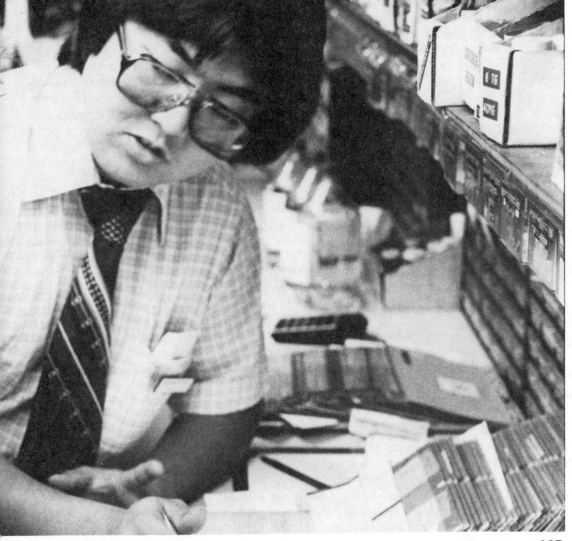

Out of the human rights movement of the past 20 years, there has emerged a model of *participatory health care*. As its name implies, this model of care recognizes not only the role of patients as consumers but also their right to be involved in making decisions that affect their health care. The participatory care model recognizes a desire and willingness on the part of patients to "get involved" and to assume some personal responsibility for their own good health. Further, this model allows an open discussion of strengths and weaknesses of various treatment approaches. The patient has some autonomy, and the professional is relieved of unilateral decision making and has the opportunity to "look beyond the narrow clinical evaluation of a patient's medical problem in an attempt to understand the problem in the context of the patient's life situation" (Shannon, 1981, p. 14).

In the participatory care model, professionals and patients are partners in the healing venture. As in other partnerships, the partners contribute their special talents to the resolution of problems but are considered as equals in all other matters. The *science* required to solve health problems falls within the health professional's domain. The *art* of applying that science to a specific problem is best comprehended by the patient. In short, the patient is the local expert or consultant regarding the personal aspects of the health problem. Whenever it is possible, the health professional incorporates the patient's suggestions and wishes into the treatment plan.

As this health care model has evolved, there has been a simultaneous evolution in the ethics of professional/patient interactions. Changes in ethics appear to follow a certain pattern. Over time an ethical problem becomes recognized and described by members of a profession because of the negative effects associated with it. Slowly but constantly pressure to ameliorate these negative effects increases. Eventually, concern becomes so great that a formal group of professionals and other concerned individuals, either appointed by law or self-appointed, investigates the matter and makes suggestions for change. These suggestions lead to tentative guidelines that are then tested for practicality.

Many such recommendations have arisen since the 1950s in the health care professions. Among them are the *International Code of Nursing Ethics,* adopted by the International Council of Nurses, July, 1953; *Statement on a Patient's Bill of Rights,* affirmed by the Board of Trustees of the American Hospital Association, November, 1972; and a Report of the Ad Hoc Committee of the Harvard Medical School to examine the definition of brain death, which was first published in the *Journal of the American Medical Association* in August, 1968.

Increasing ethical and legal pressures are now facing health professionals. Lawsuits to enforce or establish the concept of patient autonomy, to recognize the medical capabilities of certain lay persons, and to stimulate changes in the present health care system are more and more frequent and costly. Professionals have the option of resisting such change and risking the possibility of being forced out of the marketplace or accepting change and adapting their professional practices accordingly.

Most health professionals are beginning to "see the handwriting on the wall" and are making changes in their own practices. In the economy of supply and demand, they may attempt to please patients simply to recruit and retain more of them. As a result, there are fathers in labor rooms, birthing rooms, deliveries by midwives, increasing amounts of primary (ambulatory) care, patient educators, home dialysis units, consumer representatives on hospital boards and licensing boards, and so on. However, perhaps the single strongest impetus for change lies in the overt or covert threat of litigation. This threat is hardly a new development.

In 1374, the first civil malpractice action on record was brought before an English court. It alleged that the plaintiff's hand had been maimed due to inept treatment by a physician. The general proposition underlying this action and all malpractice claims is that the health care professional has a duty to act with reasonable care and skill in providing services to the public.

Malpractice has been defined specifically in many areas of legal case history. The criteria for its definition appear to change almost daily as new cases are decided. Classic definitions arose from caselaw early in this century. Creighton, in *Law Every Nurse Should Know,* cites "any professional misconduct, unreasonable lack of skill or fidelity in professional . . . duties, evil practice, or illegal or immoral conduct" (Creighton, 1981, p. 154) as constituting malpractice.

The basic allegation in most malpractice suits is negligence. Negligence is conduct "which falls below the standard established by law for the protection of others against unreasonably great risk of harm" (*Restatement of the Law, Second, Torts.* American Law Institute, 1967, sec. 282). In most situations in which negligence is invoked, there is no intent to cause harm. Rather, harm results from carelessness or lack of diligence by the practitioner. Increasingly, most experts in the malpractice field are quick to point out that negligence per se is not often the initial cause of the malpractice issue. Rather, the problem comes to light as a consequence of the poor end result or adverse outcome of a procedure or treatment regimen for which there was no guarantee of success and from which there should arise no liability. However, when patients face heavy financial obligations and a less-than-optimal solution to their health problem, they may attempt to recoup their financial and ego losses in the malpractice court.

The lack of a favorable or successful outcome has important implications for liability in malpractice suits. Whereas, in previous legal interpretation, compensation was not justified unless negligence or malpractice was proven, newer legal interpretations view compensation almost as a "right" for an unsuccessful outcome. Since no one party may be totally responsible, the compensation is usually paid by the professional perceived to be most able to pay. This "deepest pocket" logic applies particularly to physicians (James, 1980). However, in actual practice, any individual involved in the care of a patient with a less than optimal outcome may be at risk as a part of the "deepest pocket."

In general, the principles of law apply to all levels of health professionals. A dental assistant, an anesthetist, a nursing student, and so on would all be held responsible or liable in proportion to their level of education, training, and experience. In other words, any individual with some education, training, or experience in a particular area of expertise will be held more responsible and "a higher degree of care will be expected [from that person] . . . than from an ordinary person" (Creighton, 1981, p. 104).

According to Holder (1978):

Non-physician health professionals are held to the standard of skill, care, and knowledge possessed and used by the "reasonably prudent member" of their professional group as long as the activity undertaken is one commonly performed by members of the group. A nurse usually performing a function usually performed by other nurses, such as giving injections, is held to the standard of care of the "reasonably prudent nurse." On the other hand, if she undertakes to diagnose a condition and prescribe medication, she would be held to the standard of the reasonably prudent physician, since those activities are usually considered "practicing medicine," not "practicing nursing" (p. 47).

Therefore, the general principles of law discussed in this chapter apply to all health professionals, regardless of their areas of training, but vary in their applicability with the extent or degree of training and authority the health professional has.

We do not intend in this chapter to summarize the volumes of case studies that are reported elsewhere. Rather, we will elucidate the principles of law that have a bearing on malpractice, thus providing the reader with an awareness of this problem. If, then, "forewarned is forearmed," you will be better prepared to enter the health care arena with a full awareness of your responsibilities and potential liabilities.

This chapter describes various types of malpractice suits and offers specific recommendations for health professionals to use as guidelines in malpractice prevention and protection.

Types of Law Affecting Health Professionals

The body of law in the United States falls into two major categories. The first of these is *criminal law*. Crimes are actions committed against the state for which the state desires retribution. Criminal acts, therefore, violate written legal codes or statutes that are duly constructed by state legislative bodies. Proof of the commission of a crime, then, requires that an act be: (1) illegal (in defiance of written state law or code) and (2) performed with the intention of breaking the law (Creighton, 1981, p. 197).

An example is a nurse in an ICU who "cuts" morphine injections with sterile water and then appropriates the unused morphine to support her personal drug habit. Obviously, this practice violates written (state and federal) law and was done with deceptive intentions. Consequently, the act was a criminal act and would be dealt with as a crime. Although criminal offenses may certainly occur among health professionals, criminal law is outside the purview of this chapter and will not be discussed in further detail.

The other large body of common law in the United States is known as *civil law*. Civil law applies to the resolution of disputes between parties that are not specifically addressed in the written law devised by legislative actions. Civil law derives from statutes, constitutional and common law, or case law precedents. Civil law differs from criminal law in that it pertains to acts offensive to an individual and not to society in general. The vast majority of suits against health professionals are founded on civil law.

Two categories of civil law form the basis for most malpractice claims: (1) contract law and (2)

torts. *Contract law* involves the resolution of disputes over contracts, which are defined as legally binding agreements between parties to either perform or refrain from performing certain actions. Failure to comply with the terms of a contract is known as a breach of contract and may provide the basis for some civil suits involving health professionals.

Torts involve a "civil wrong, other than breach of contract, for which the court will provide a remedy in the form of an action for damages" (Black's Law Dictionary, 1979, p. 1335). If an individual feels that he or she has been wronged in some matter involving a personal interaction and feels entitled to compensation as a consequence of the predicament, he or she may bring an action of tort.

Torts may be either intentional or unintentional, and both types may form the basis for a malpractice suit brought against a health professional. *Intentional torts* include infliction of mental distress, fraudulent misrepresentation, invasion of privacy, and defamation of character. However, the most common *intentional* tort action brought against health professionals is assault and/ or battery—that is, the threat of or actual harmful or offensive touching or other contact of a person without his or her expressed consent. Of the *unintentional torts,* the most frequent type of action relevant to health professionals is negligence— that is, whether the practitioner acted with reasonable care or in a negligent fashion.

The remainder of this chapter will consider the types of malpractice cases that are commonly brought against health professionals as either contract breaches, assault and battery, or negligence. We will also discuss some specific recommendations for preventing and/or defending against these types of malpractice claims.

LEARNING ACTIVITIES

Definition of Legal Terms

In the preceding pages we have mentioned a number of important legal terms. Check your understanding of these terms by matching the legal terms listed in the left-hand column with their appropriate definition found in the right-hand column (Chapter Objective 1). The first one is completed as an example. Feedback follows the learning activity.

Legal Terms	*Definition of Terms*
1. Malpractice __f__	a. Applies to resolution of disputes between parties that are not specifically addressed by the written law devised by legislative actions.
2. Negligence _____	b. Legal action brought to provide compensation for an individual who feels she or he has been wronged by the actions of another person.
3. Criminal law _____	c. Harm or injury to patient resulting from carelessness or lack of diligence by a practitioner.
4. Civil law _____	d. Resolution of disputes over legally binding agreements between two or more persons.
5. Contract law _____	e. Acts committed against society or the state.
6. Torts _____	f. Professional misconduct; failure to act with care and skill in providing services to the public.

Feedback

2. Negligence: c (harm or injury to patient resulting from carelessness or lack of diligence by a practitioner).

3. Criminal law: e (acts committed against society or the state).

4. Civil law: a (applies to resolution of disputes between parties that are not specifically addressed by the written law devised by legislative actions).

5. Contract law: d (resolution of disputes over legally binding agreements between two or more persons).

6. Torts: b (legal action brought to provide compensation for an individual who feels she or he has been wronged by the actions of another person).

Breach of Contract

Contracts, as they apply to health professionals, can be established between any individuals who are competent and who are willing to provide consent. In addition, there must be some valid service, cause, motive, price, or influence considered of mutual value. For example, a healthy 23-year-old pregnant woman could contract with a nurse midwife to provide her prenatal and obstetrical care with the intention of having a home delivery. Assuming that both parties involved in this agreement are competent to make the decision to contract, then the valid consideration is the services of the midwife during the prenatal period and delivery of those services in exchange for a specified sum of money.

Contracts may be formal and explicit (wherein the provisions are spelled out in detail and in writing), or they may be implicit (wherein the considerations are implied by the nature of the contract and as a matter of common sense). In the example of the nurse midwife, the contract could be set down explicitly in writing and signed by both parties, or it could be established on a verbal and implicit basis. Most health care contracts are implied. They are similar to sales agreements in which it is implicit that a service will be provided in exchange for a given sum of money.

Implicit Contracts

Implicit contracts are established in a number of ways. Often health professionals fail to realize that they are establishing implicit contracts by their actions, if not by their words. Once treatment of any form begins, it is presumed that an implicit contract has been established (Holder, 1978, p. 3). Consider the following example, a situation not at all unfamiliar to medical interns and residents.

> A 78-year-old gentleman with long-standing heart disease is admitted to a coronary care unit with severe heart failure, following a myocardial infarction. The resident in the coronary care unit discusses his dismal prognosis at once with the man's spouse and realizes that she is extraordinarily anxious and distraught by the sudden turn of events. Twenty-four hours later, the patient suffers a second heart attack and dies. The spouse, in tears and on the verge of hysteria, requests the resident to provide her with a sedative so that she will be able to cope better with her grief, function more appropriately while making funeral arrangements, and so on. The resident complies with her request "out of the goodness of his heart" and provides her with a

prescription for a mild sedative without taking a history or performing an examination.

Although the resident had no intention of establishing a formal contract with the woman, she or he would undoubtedly be held responsible for the woman's care, at least so far as it related to the anxiety surrounding the death of her husband. The resident is considered responsible because she or he had commenced a treatment plan. The frightening fact is that medical professionals may give such prescriptions to patient's families out of compassion, without doing a proper evaluation. Consequently, there is much room for error in drug choice, untoward drug reactions, and so on, which may eventually lead to litigation.

Implicit contract making can also occur through telephone contact with a patient. The courts may interpret that an implied contract exists on the basis of a single telephone call (Holder, 1978, p. 3). The health professional may be requested to "call the pharmacy" (a common request of office receptionists) or "renew the prescription" or provide advice because the patient claims "it is impossible for me to come into the office right now." Many such calls are made for patient convenience or because the professional is "too busy" or too lazy to examine patient charts properly. Many minor tranquilizers are prescribed in this fashion for patients who are "doctor shopping" to avoid detection of a drug dependence. Such circumstances involve implied contracts and may lead to liability.

Reasonable Expectations

Health professionals may prevent suits based on breach of contract not only by being aware of how they implicitly establish contracts with patients but also by providing patients with as clear-cut and reasonable an oral contract as possible (or, better still, with a written contract), without providing false hopes, unreasonable expectations, and guaranteed outcomes. In a study of health care relationships, Green (1982) noted that there was:

> a common misunderstanding about the allocation of responsibility between doctor

and patient that was essential to making the relationship work. The tenor of expectations on the part of patients was that their health was now the responsibility of their doctor. There was no discussion of roles or complementary responsibilities that might have led to an appreciation of medical services as purely diagnosis and treatment of pathology; nor was there any understanding of the patient's responsibility for the dynamics of health that were within individual control, and not really amenable to medical control. Consequently, the working relationship broke down; the reason for seeking care remained unfulfilled or was negated by the complications and a lawsuit was the obvious expression of unfulfilled expectations (p. 6).

The establishment of clear-cut oral contracts can be facilitated by a frank discussion of patient and practitioner roles and expectations. As Chapter 3 emphasized, such a discussion should occur in the beginning phase of every health care interview. Initial interviews with patients are extremely important in this respect because they set the tone of the relationship and may create lasting first impressions.

In discussing expectations, health professionals should be certain to create *reasonable* expectations about what a given health care procedure or treatment can and cannot do for the patient. It is important to note the distinction, however, between providing the patient with the background for a positive "expectancy effect" and a "guarantee" of a favorable outcome. Notice the difference in the following examples of how a physician talks to a patient prior to coronary arteriography.

> Mr. Smith, if you will consent to this coronary arteriogram I will be able to find the cause of your chest pain. Then, I can operate on your heart, and after surgery your pain will be gone. I've done hundreds of these operations, just like yours, and all of my patients feel just like new after the operation. **Or** Mr. Smith, if you will consent to this coronary arteriogram, an X-ray of the blood vessels in your heart, I may be able to find a blockage in the blood

vessel of your heart that could cause your pain. Once I have a better idea of what the blood vessels are like, it may be possible to do surgery and relieve that pain, at least to some degree.

Notice that, although the physician in the second case left the patient with the understanding that there was a diagnostic and treatment regimen known for his particular problem (chest pain) and that frequently the treatment was beneficial, the physician did not provide a "money-back guarantee." The physician was being optimistic in helping the patient develop a positive expectancy effect but also was realistic and did not encourage unrealistic expectations.

The preceding paragraphs have concentrated on litigation against health professionals on the basis of unfulfilled contracts. Although a number of actions are based on such alleged breaches in contract, these actions constitute only a portion of the total number of malpractice actions that are filed. The remainder of these actions are filed not as breaches of contract but as violations of tort law and commonly consist of either assault and battery or negligence.

Intentional Torts: Assault and Battery

One of the fundamental guarantees of freedom in the United States is the freedom from threat of or actual personal contact from other individuals without consent. On occasion, actions for *assault* (threat of contact) and/or *battery* (actual contact) may occur in the health care setting. Even though a patient has consented to hospitalization and treatment in that hospital setting, he or she may object to or refuse to participate in any portion of such prescribed care. For example, a patient confined to a Stryker frame for immobilization following a back injury may refuse to agree to treatments by enema. Under such circumstances, if a member of the health care team should approach that individual with an enema bottle as if he or she were going to administer the enema, that team member could be potentially liable for an action of assault, as his or her actions constituted a threat to the largely immobilized patient. Further, if the enema was administered to the patient against his or her will, then battery has been committed, and once again the health professional may be liable.

In another example, if a physical therapist, acting on the orders of a physician, should insist upon range-of-motion exercises for a patient when the patient has specifically indicated that he or she does not desire such exercises, that patient may file an intentional tort action based on battery.

Implied or actual sexual contact with a patient or touching of certain parts of a patient's anatomy without consent also may provide grounds for a tort suit based upon assault and/or battery.

There are several recommendations the health professional can follow to reduce the likelihood of this type of suit. First, be aware of even typical procedures involving touch that may require patient consent. For example, a physical examination, X-ray, and drug injections are forms of touching or contact that require prior consent (Schwitzgebel & Schwitzgebel, 1980). Second, the critical factor in this type of suit is patient consent. Remember that the unconsented threat of or actual touching of a person may be grounds for this legal action, even though the contact is for the patient's welfare and is intended to benefit the patient. Patient consent must supercede even supervisor orders. Third, keep in mind that consent, once given, is never absolute or unlimited. In other words, touch or contact must not exceed that which was consented to by the patient (Schutz, 1982). Finally, avoid the use of threat or coercion as a means of persuading a patient to consent to a procedure or treatment.

Unintentional Torts: Negligence

Most malpractice actions are predicated on negligence. For example, an orderly could be sued for failing to deflate the balloon on a Foley catheter prior to the removal of the device. Under such circumstances, the court attempts to determine whether or not the defendant acted in a negligent fashion. In deciding the verdict, the jury uses the criterion of "doing what a reasonably prudent person would not do or failing to do what a reasonably prudent person would do under the same or similar circumstances" (Wade, 1980, p. 16).

Traditionally, four key elements have been necessary to prove a malpractice claim based on negligence:

1. That a patient/health professional relationship existed (substantiated by appointments, records, bills for services, and so on).

2. That the health professional did not render an acceptable standard of care to the patient (substantiated either by expert witnesses, by common sense, or by common knowledge under the legal doctrine *res ipsa loquitur* ("the act speaks for itself").

3. That this lack of care was the *proximate* or *sole* cause of injury to the patient without any independent, intervening causes (substantiated by proving that the patient did nothing to break the chain of causality between the professional's acts and the resulting injury—that is, a lack of contributory negligence).

4. That an actual injury was, in fact, sustained by the patient (substantiated by exacerbation of presenting symptoms, appearance of new symptoms, or other related damages).

Of these four elements, items 2 and 3 (standard of care and proximate cause) are the most critical in proving or defending against a malpractice claim based on negligence.

As we mentioned above, one of the key elements in a malpractice claim is proving that the health professional did not provide an acceptable standard of care to the patient. As applied to a member of an established profession, the standard of care can be divided into four aspects: diligence, competence, judgment, and superior abilities (Wade, 1980).

The first aspect of the standard of care involves diligence, attention, alertness, or caution (Wade, 1980). A member of the health professions who fails to apply such diligence, caution, and so on then acts in a careless or negligent fashion. Carelessness may extend to any failure to pay attention to detail, whether this encompasses a monitoring of body functions, a failure to maintain adequate records, or poor personal hygiene (for example, failure to scrub for surgery) if any of those failings should contribute to increased morbidity or mortality.

The second aspect of care has to do with the "exercise of special competence—possession of the skill, training, education, or experience" (Wade, 1980, p. 17) that the health professional would be expected to have. In other words, a dental assistant who fails to properly sterilize instruments, an X-ray technician who fails to adequately shield the gonads from radiation exposure, or a nurse or physician who gives blood to the wrong patient would all be construed by the law as not exercising the special competence expected of their profession by virtue of education, training, or experience.

The third aspect of care relates to the principle of "reaching a sound professional judgment" (Wade, 1980, p. 17). Whether or not the judgment is absolutely accurate is not usually the point of contention. The facts that are considered relate to the method by which data were obtained and used to arrive at the final professional judgment. The professional is not liable for a "mere error in judgment" (Wade, 1980, p. 17) if he or she has exercised due skill, care, diligence, and judgment in arriving at the mistaken conclusion.

A fourth aspect of care involves the requirement that an individual who possesses "superior abilities" must use them in application to the problem at hand. "If he has greater strength than the average person, keener eyesight, or greater dexterity, or more extensive knowledge or experience, it is not sufficient for him to meet the capabilities of the average person and a failure to use his superior qualities may amount to negligence" (Wade, 1980, p. 17).

In instances involving complex and specialized treatments and procedures, the standard of care may have to be established by the use of expert witnesses rather than laypersons. This restriction requires that a qualified expert in a particular field be the only individual who can present evidence suggesting negligence. Increasingly, such expert witnesses must be able to testify to accepted practice on a national level. The "locality rule" holding a health practitioner only to the standard of practice in his or her community has been replaced largely by a national standard of acceptable practice. In other cases, there is no need for expert medical testimony if the point of contention is easily judged by a layperson. Such cases are based on the legal doctrine of common knowledge, or *res ipsa loquitur,* which means "the thing speaks for itself." For example, a skin burn in the exact size, shape and location of a diathermy unit would easily "speak for itself" as to its cause and verify probable negligence (Wade, 1980, p. 19). A third way of determining the acceptable standard of care without expert medical testimony is based on the doctrine of informed consent, which includes that information required to appropriately establish the risks and benefits of a given procedure or treatment. Consent is discussed in detail later in this chapter.

A legal strategy available to health professionals as a defense against negligence is *idiosyncrasy.* An idiosyncratic effect is a totally unpredictable and unexpected effect from a drug or treatment modality that cannot be anticipated or predicted from usual and customary practice, tests, and so on. The peculiarity depends on some innate characteristic of the patient that is unknown, unpredictable, undescribable, and unexpected. As long as it can be shown that the therapy was administered in accordance with generally accepted and approved procedures and in a competent fashion, the possibility of idiosyncratic reaction may help a health professional establish that an acceptable standard of care was, in fact, provided despite the outcome (Creighton, 1981, p. 117).

Another key element used to prove malpractice by negligence is *proximate cause*—that is, the establishment of reasonable cause-and-effect relationship between the alleged negligent treatment and the untoward outcome. For example, if a young woman was involved in an automobile accident precipitated by a fainting spell occurring within an hour after an IUD insertion, it is quite likely that a jury would consider the IUD insertion a proximate cause of her fainting spell and thus of the collision. However, if such an accident occurred after she had had the IUD for six months, it is unlikely that proximate cause could be established (Creighton, 1981).

A legal defense strategy available to health professionals against proximate cause is *contributory negligence*. Contributory negligence describes irresponsible conduct on the part of the patient that may contribute to an injury. For example, in the incident described above, if there was corroborative evidence that the woman had specifically been instructed to bring another person with her for the express purpose of driving her home after the IUD insertion and she had failed to do so, the woman would probably be judged guilty of contributory negligence and the case against the health professional dismissed. Similarly, failure to follow a health professional's instructions concerning follow-up care or other restricted activities, which later contributed to an untoward outcome, should not result in liability to the health professional (Creighton, 1981, pp. 17–18).

================================ LEARNING ACTIVITIES ================================

Breach of Contract, Assault and Battery, and Negligence

In the following five vignettes, you are to read the case study, choose the appropriate term to describe the type of malpractice action most likely to ensue, and then explain why you chose that particular term (Chapter Objective 2). Feedback follows the exercise. The first one is completed as an example.

1. A 48-year-old female gives birth to a child with a chromosome abnormality that is relatively common in women of her age and that could have been detected before birth by using amniocentesis (taking a sample of the fluid from the uterus). She decides to sue her obstetrician. Her complaint will likely allege that her physician was guilty of:

_____ battery

_____ breach of contract

__√__ negligence

_____ assault

Why? He failed to recommend a prenatal test that could have detected the chromosomal abnormality of the fetus in utero.

2. A physical therapist attempts to carry out a physician's order to provide range-of-motion exercises for an elderly man who is recovering from surgery. He refuses to allow her to proceed. If she insists on performing the therapy, if sued, she may be found guilty of:

_____ assault

_____ battery

_____ negligence

_____ breach of contract

Why? _____

_____

3. A pregnant woman arranges for prenatal care to be followed by a home birth with a nurse midwife. The nurse midwife provides six months of prenatal care and then informs the patient she no longer can provide the remaining care or facilitate the home delivery. The patient would be most likely to sue on which of the following grounds?

_____ battery

_____ assault

_____ breach of contract

_____ negligence

Why? _____

_____

4. A pregnant woman in her second trimester is scheduled for a routine dental checkup and examination. After the dentist observes it is time for a set of routine dental X-rays, the patient refuses. The dentist replies that dental X-rays during the second trimester pose no risk to the mother or the fetus and attempts to perform the X-rays anyway. Even if the patient manages to dissuade the dentist at this point, if sued, the dentist may be found guilty of:

_____ breach of contract

_____ assault

_____ negligence

_____ battery

Why? _____

_____

5. A nurse administers the wrong I.V. to a patient recovering from a coronary by-pass operation. The patient goes into cardiac arrest within minutes after the improper I.V. was given. If sued, the patient or the patient's representative will probably allege that the nurse was guilty of:

_____ battery

_____ breach of contract

_____ negligence

_____ assault

Why? _____

_____

Feedback

Case 2: Battery (A patient retains certain rights to his or her body. If these are violated, as in this case by touching, an action for battery may be justified.)

Case 3: Breach of contract (The nurse midwife had an implicit contract with the patient and by providing partial treatment or care had initiated the terms of the contract. Because she failed to complete the actions understood in the contract, the midwife could be sued on the basis of breach of contract.)

Case 4: Assault (A patient must give consent for certain procedures, including X-rays, which involve contact or touch. If the patient refuses and the dentist threatens or attempts to administer the procedure anyway, the dentist would be committing an assault.)

Case 5: Negligence (A health professional has a duty to act carefully and skillfully in providing service to patients. By carelessly administering an improper I.V., the nurse is being negligent.)

Malpractice Prevention

The suggestions that follow are offered as "malpractice prophylaxis" for health professionals. If these suggestions are followed, they may help prevent the occurrence of a malpractice suit. General categories of malpractice prophylaxis to be discussed in this section are (1) effective communication and interpersonal skills, (2) accessibility, (3) fees, (4) ancillary staff, (5) due care, (6) informed consent, and (7) patient rights.

Communication and Interpersonal Skills

Virtually every authority on the subject agrees that the cause of the upsurge in malpractice litigation is due primarily to the deterioration of the health professional/patient relationship. When the distance between the health provider and the patient increases, whether through technical advances, geographic separation, or lack of interpersonal skills, malpractice action becomes more likely. The

history of common law supports the reluctance of people to sue those with whom they have strong favorable emotional ties (James, 1980, p. 219).

The development of such emotional ties, called *rapport* in the health professional/patient relationship, can be effected through the use of a number of well-developed and well-recognized techniques. These are discussed in some detail throughout this book; you probably recognize use of proper names, introductions, handshakes, small talk, and so on as devices that help initiate and cement a satisfactory patient/professional relationship. Politeness is another important factor in establishing rapport.

In no other portion of the practice of health care will the emphasis on communication skills be more relevant. Numerous studies have shown that principles of good communication can be taught and learned. This concept tends to contradict those who feel that communicators are born and not made. *Communication success* is the key to malpractice prevention. An analysis of a large series of malpractice actions stemming from emergency room interactions found that health professionals at highest risk are younger (relatively more impulsive, overconfident, and less mature, brash, without humility, and so on), have language problems (especially those not speaking the primary language of the patient), fail to provide adequate chart documentation (lazy, "keep it all in their heads," less conscientious with attention to detail), and have genuine communication problems. There are four factors that make a good health care provider: availability, affability, ability, and the willingness to communicate.

Of all the communication and interpersonal skills discussed in this book, the ability to listen carefully is probably the most important. Substandard care is often the product of misdiagnosis. In such cases, the health professional often fails to hear the patient's description of his or her symptoms, which may be the obvious clue to a correct diagnosis. Too often, there is the tendency on the part of the professionals to respond with the mentality of Procrastes—the legendary Greek who either added to or subtracted from the height of his victims so that they would fit his guest bed. Professionals must be able to listen to all of a patient's complaints and then establish relative priority of diagnoses, rather than listening to the first complaint, making a complete diagnosis, and then fitting the remainder of the complaints to the preconceived illness.

Accessibility

Health professional accessibility is another component of good service. Nothing is more frustrating than to wait for interminable hours for an appointment. During such waits, patients feel as if they exist for the convenience of the professional and as if they have no personal rights whatsoever. Consequently, the health professional should make every possible effort to stay "on schedule." If there are unavoidable delays, as there seem to be in virtually every practice, the patient should receive an apology and an explanation. Such an explanation might consist of "I am sorry to be so far behind with my appointments this morning. However, the patients who were here earlier took more time than I had anticipated. I hope that you will understand and also feel reassured that if you need more time than has been scheduled I will be happy to provide you with the same courtesy" (Umhau, 1982, p. 42).

Accessibility via the telephone is also important. On the one hand, telephone contacts can save time and are very convenient. On the other hand, there are many inherent traps in telephone use that must be constantly avoided (that is, telephone use involves implicit contract and leaves much room for misdiagnosis and improper treatment). Telephone calls should be returned at the earliest possible moment; failure to return calls or long delays suggest lack of interest and may lead to patient dissatisfaction.

All contacts with patients must convey concern and compassion. Enough time must be allowed and abrupt interactions avoided at all cost. If an emergency or some other pressing duty necessitates abrupt termination of an appointment, then the patient deserves an explanation and an opportunity to continue the appointment at the earliest possible time. Whether or not the professional is "swamped" with other patients, is in the midst of traumatic personal problems, or is just "having a bad day," patients must feel that during the interaction they are the single most important concern of the professional. Patients must be allowed time to express themselves, to receive satisfactory answers to their questions, to be allowed to enjoy their time with the health professional, and to achieve the ultimate satisfaction, relief, assurance, and compassion that can be administered.

Fees

Another major contributing factor to lawsuits is the bill that appears to be unjustifiably high. Particularly when treatments or procedures are unsuccessful, patients are disturbed to receive bills for services that did not bring about the end that they were expecting. Probably no bill is more distressing than the bill for services in an intensive care unit during a prolonged illness that ended in the patient's death. Other examples are the bills associated with extensive disfiguring surgery, palliative radiation therapy, prosthetic limb construction, private duty nursing care, and physical therapy services for the purpose of preventing limb contractures. Bills for what patients believe is an excessive number of laboratory studies, for multiple consultants, and for the numerous hidden charges associated with hospitalizations (such as added room charges for oxygen, bedside commodes, blood and I.V. administration, room humidifiers, egg-crate mattresses, and so on) are another area of contention (Ficarra, 1979, p. 307).

One solution to such problems is to discuss the charges personally with the patients. A recommended procedure is to post the usual fee schedule in an office so that the patient can do "comparison shopping." If patients raise questions about fees, these should be discussed openly and without hesitation (Umhau, 1982, p. 44). What to do about fees that patients believe are exorbitant is another problem. Some professionals suggest that since fees and the dunning letters associated with their collection are so often the cause of litigation, attempts to collect them are best forgotten (Ficarra, 1979, p. 309). Others have advocated asking the patients to "pay what you think my services have been worth," and still others may adjust fees according to family income, socioeconomic status, and so on. Still another alternative is to encourage the patient to pay something on the bill in the hope that it will eventually be paid off completely. Whatever the solution, certainly frank and open discussion of fees is as much a part of professional practice as any other subject and, if done properly, may serve as a major component of a risk management program.

Ancillary Staff

In addition to the attitudinal aspect of the health professional/patient relationship, there are several other factors that can reduce malpractice liability. There is no substitute for pleasant, affable, and accommodating ancillary personnel. From the secretary/receptionist who answers the phone, through the aide, assistant, technician, nurse associate, dentist, pharmacist, or physician, each individual potentially contributes to patient satisfaction or dissatisfaction. Ancillary personnel should be closely supervised by an appropriately designated staff supervisor. In addition, they should always define their roles and the part they will play in a given treatment regimen so that there is no confusion in the patient's mind.

Unless they are directly involved with a specific aspect of patient care, ancillary staff should refrain from voicing comments or opinions about patients' ailments (Regan, 1956, p. 493). The professional who does not see the total picture concerning a patient is unable to give good advice regarding a particular problem. Although many individuals may be involved with a patient's care, the "double messages" the patient receives as a result of asking the same question to many people may confuse him or her. They may also imply incompetence on the part of the professional, because there appears to be no consensus of opinion regarding treatment. Consequently, the wise professional refers specific questions to the responsible individual rather than attempting to provide all the answers.

All members of the health care team should work together and support one another. It is important to avoid discussing other health professionals with patients (Regan, 1956, p. 493). Very often, remarks made in passing about the work of other professionals may have a profound and detrimental effect. Liability may result from the suggestion that another health professional is providing inadequate care. Since it is difficult to establish rapport under the best of circumstances, certainly it is counterproductive to undermine rapport that has been established by another professional. If you are concerned that errors in judgment have been made, do not discuss this matter with a patient but, rather, refer it either directly to the individual concerned, to an appropriate professional society, to the hospital credentials board, and so on.

Due Care

There are several aspects to providing "due care" that help ensure that carelessness or oversights do not lead to negligence or unfavorable outcomes. First, the health provider should use practices that are recognized by at least a "respectable minority" in treating given illnesses. Unless he or she uses treatment modalities that are generally accepted, the professional may be conducting "experimental treatments." In general, when patients are injured under such circumstances, the professional is seen as negligent (Holder, 1978, p. 48).

Due care may also necessitate the use of consultants and ancillary personnel in various other aspects of treatment. When a given treatment modality fails to work or is not acceptable to the patient, it is the responsibility of the professional either to use additional methods of therapy or to refer the patient to others who may use alternate treatment methods or who may possess particular expertise (Holder, 1978, p. 49).

After having established a professional/patient relationship, the health professional must follow up on the progress of his or her patients and provide for the transfer of health care to other professionals as required (Holder, 1978, p. 54). Either the professional or the patient may terminate a contract at any time, provided that both parties are allowed sufficient time to make appropriate adjustments. Failure to provide the patient with an alternative source of treatment or a reasonable period of time in which to seek an alternative source of treatment may be considered abandonment. By the same token, if the professional office is moved or closed, patients must be notified that such a process is underway and that their records may be obtained and/or transferred to other sources of care (Jonsen, Siegler, & Winslade, 1982, p. 100).

Finally, all health professionals must be cautious in the suggestions or prescriptive statements they make to patients (Holder, 1978, p. 155). Paraprofessionals may make suggestions but should always be sure that their suggestions are supported by the professional in charge of the patient's care. Even a simple suggestion such as "Try two aspirin tablets," although very harmless on the surface, implies that the prescriber is knowledgeable and experienced in the management of the illness for which the aspirin was recommended.

Consequently, the person who makes such a statement would be held liable under the law for any side effects or drug interactions that occurred.

Informed Consent

The principle of informed consent is based on the legal doctrine *volenti non fit injuria,* which translates as "No wrong is done to one who is willing." In other words, it would be difficult for a person to file a complaint of battery as the basis for a malpractice action if he or she consented beforehand to a recommended procedure or treatment. Prior to the 1960s, the degree of disclosure of risks, complications, potential for success, and possible outcomes had to be verified in the courts by *expert witnesses,* professionals required to testify as to the possible shortcomings of their colleagues. It was difficult to obtain a decision in favor of the plaintiff (usually the patient) because such witnesses were frequently unwilling or unavailable. Further, because the tort battery implies an antisocial act, the courts were reluctant to press the accusation (Johnson, 1980, p. 284). Since the case of *Woods vs. Brumlop* in 1962, expert witnesses have no longer been needed to determine the adequacy of informed consent. This case established the so-called minority rule. According to the minority rule:

> The physician has the duty to make a full and frank disclosure to the patient of all pertinent facts relative to the illness, treatment, surgery, or therapy prescribed or recommended. Therefore, if the physician fails to so advise the patient, and afterwards the patient would have refused the treatment, surgery, or therapy performed, the physician has committed an act of malpractice and is liable for all harmful consequences which follow a proximate cause of the failure to disclose. Because of the relationship that exists between the physician and the patient, expert medical testimony is not necessary to show what a reasonable medical practitioner would have disclosed under the same or similar circumstances in a community (Johnson, 1980, pp. 285–286).

As we mentioned earlier, unsatisfactory or less-than-expected end results are often the cause of malpractice actions. The woman who has lost teeth in an automobile accident may be reasonably satisfied with a set of dentures if they are comfortable and good-looking and work satisfactorily. On the other hand, if the dentures are uncomfortable, unattractive, and not functional, she will be less than satisfied with the results. However, an unsatisfactory end result does not in itself create liability, as long as the patient has been advised beforehand of the risks and possible outcomes.

For informed consent to be effective as a legal protection to health professionals, it must meet two criteria: patient *competence* and *voluntariness*. Patients must be competent, or able to understand the information being given to them. If the patient is a minor (under 18) or has a diminished capacity to understand the information, consent must be obtained from the legal guardians or representatives. Consent also must be given by patients voluntarily and not under duress. If possible, the patient should have at least 48 hours following the consent interview to "think it over" (Schwitzgebel & Schwitzgebel, 1980).

To comply with the spirit of the doctrine of informed consent, health professionals must give information to patients that includes:

1. A fair explanation of the procedures to be followed, their purposes, and the identification of any procedures that are experimental.

2. A description of any attendant discomfort and risks reasonably to be expected.

3. A description of any benefits reasonably to be expected.

4. A disclosure of appropriate alternative procedures that might be advantageous for the patient.

5. An offer to answer any inquiries about the procedure.

6. An instruction that the person is free to withdraw consent and discontinue participation in the project or activity at any time without prejudice to the patient (Creighton, 1981, p. 202).

It is essential that this information be presented to patients in language that is nontechnical and comprehensible. As Schutz (1982) observes, "the duty to disclose is not satisfied merely by spewing out of facts, but must be a dialogue culminating in the patient's understanding" (p. 24).

Informed consent appears on the surface to be a very reasonable and attainable goal. However, a number of studies have shown that it is difficult to satisfy the patients' "need to know" and at the same time assure no legal loopholes. One study of the consent forms used by a number of hospitals revealed that the reading level required to understand the forms was equivalent to at least an advanced undergraduate, if not a graduate, education level (Grundner, 1980). Other studies have shown that more than half of patients do not understand or recall the content and implications of informed consent. " . . . Three factors were related to inadequate recall: education, medical status, and the care with which patients thought they had read their consent forms before signing" (Cassileth, Zupkis, Sutton-Smith, & March, 1980, p. 896).

Since the determination of adequate informed consent has been transferred from the province of the expert witness to that of the jury, and since patient recall of information appears to be so unreliable, each individual involved in patient care must be sure not only that the six categories of information comprising informed consent are discussed with the patient but also that there is good and thorough documentation of the patient's instruction. Then, if untoward results occur, the professional has performed her or his moral, legal, and ethical duty in properly informing the patient and has taken steps to diminish her or his own liability.

Documentation of informed consent can take a variety of forms, including the use of audiotapes of the consent interview and written consent forms. The written consent forms are signed by patients or guardians and should also be witnessed by an uninvolved or disinterested third party (Schutz, 1982). Even a few correctly answered multiple-choice questions following the consent interview can substantiate the patients' understanding (Schwitzgebel & Schwitzgebel, 1980). Providing and documenting informed consent may be enhanced by use of the Checklist for Obtaining Consent for Treatment (Schwitzgebel & Schwitzgebel, 1980) found in Table 14-1.

Table 14-1
Checklist for Obtaining Consent for Treatment

_____ Is the patient competent to consent?

_____ If the patient is not competent, is there a logical representative to grant consent?

_____ Is there any reason to suspect that the representative is not competent to consent?

_____ Should more than one representative give consent? For example, if both parents of a minor child are available, both signatures should be obtained.

_____ If the patient's representative(s) consent(s), does the patient offer any protest?

_____ Does the explanation of information needed to get consent from a surrogate, who is not the patient's parent, violate any rights of privacy of the patient?

_____ Is consent given voluntarily and free of any institutional coercion? Is any threat implied if the patient or his/her representative does not consent?

_____ Is there an explanation of the overall purpose of the activity and why she/he has been asked to participate?

_____ Is the procedure going to involve research or treatment or a combination of both?

_____ Is there an explanation of other appropriate alternative strategies for dealing with the problem and an offer to implement any one of them chosen by the patient?

_____ As much as possible, are the explanations of the innovative procedure, treatment, and alternatives offered in writing in nontechnical and objective language?

_____ Is the patient given the name of someone or some group who has (have) experienced the procedure and could freely discuss its benefits and disadvantages? (If not actual contact, is the client at least given an article to read that argues both sides of the proposed approach?)

_____ Are steps explained to guarantee there will be a system for early detection, minimization, and correction of harms? Is there an explanation of how the patient will be compensated, if at all, for any loss due to a harm suffered?

_____ Are procedures to preserve confidentiality explained, along with limitations (that is, types of data to be collected, length of retention, persons or agencies with access, publications)?

_____ Are any material inducements being offered to participate in the program?

_____ Is there a clear offer to answer any inquiries? (Sometimes the inquiries and their responses are written or a tape recorder is used.)

_____ Is there a clear instruction that the patient is free to withdraw his/her consent at any time without punishment? (There may be limitations if there is a physical or mental danger to the person; if so, state such conditions.)

_____ Is there a notation of the time the information was given and the consent given? (Allow at least 48 hours if possible to give the person time to "think it over.")

_____ How is the consent acknowledged? (At minimum, the person should sign underneath a statement reading "I have read and understand the above explanation." A few correctly answered multiple-choice questions would give even more manifest evidence of the person's understanding.)

_____ Is there a signature of an uninvolved third party who can serve as a witness to the consent process?

LEARNING ACTIVITIES

Informed Consent

According to Chapter Objective 3, you will be able to provide an oral explanation of a procedure or treatment to a role-play patient that includes the six elements of informed consent. We suggest you complete this activity in triads, with one person taking the role of a health professional, one person taking the patient's role, and one person being the observer. The health professional should conduct a 15-minute role-play consent interview with the patient and provide a description of a particular treatment or procedure that includes the six elements of informed consent. The patient can present one of the problem situations listed below. The observer should determine whether the professional included all of the six elements of informed consent as listed on p. 312. Here are the suggested patient situations:

1. You are a 45-year-old male patient who has just undergone a routine dental examination. The dentist has discovered an abscess above two of your upper left teeth and suggests a root canal. You have no idea what a root canal is.

2. You are a 24-year-old female with a darkly pigmented, flat, skin lesion on your left thigh. The physician's assistant has been requested to excise the lesion. The physician was concerned that the lesion could be an early skin cancer.

3. You are an 82-year-old black woman complaining that you have been vomiting up blood. A radiology technician is designated to perform an upper GI (gastrointestinal) series since the physician suspects the problem to be cancer of the stomach.

4. You are an 18-year-old high school student who was found to have a heart murmur during a routine physical examination for preseason football camp. The ECG (electrocardiographic) technician is requested to perform an electrocardiogram on you.

Participatory Care and Patient Rights

As we discussed at the beginning of this chapter, in recent years the traditional health professional/patient relationship has evolved from one of total authoritarianism through paternalism to a system of participatory health care. Such participatory care, in requiring patients to become educated about their health and illness, provides a degree of assurance for the professional that patient consent will indeed be "informed." If patients participate in making regular decisions about their care, it is unlikely that they will be faced with a major health care decision about which they have not already been educated or had considerable experience. Many lawsuits are filed because patients do not assume any responsibility for their own health care, and thus, patient participation is a major factor in malpractice prevention. A number of documents have substantiated the concept of patient rights. Probably the most well known of these is the Patient Bill of Rights adopted by the American Hospital Association.

If it is assumed that patients do have "rights," then they must be encouraged to take an active part in their own care. The VD National Hot Line, in an article titled "Patient Effectiveness" (1980) lists a number of ways in which patients can take part in their health care.

1. Make a problem list before going for an appointment.

2. Ask questions.

3. Get a second opinion before consenting to proposed surgical procedures.

4. Make your own decision, an informed one, regarding treatment plans or alternative medications.

5. Let the practitioner know how you felt about the interaction—good or bad.

6. Check out referral sources for up-to-date information.

7. Write down instructions or suggestions given to you (p. 4).

These behaviors not only contribute to informed consent but also reinforce patients' sense of responsibility for their health care. For example, Clark (1981) provides a list of questions to be used by patients if surgery is suggested:

_____ 1. What is the diagnosis, and how did you arrive at it?

_____ 2. In what percentage of cases does the surgery help?

_____ 3. In what percentage of cases does the surgery fail?

_____ 4. What is the worst that can happen if I do not have surgery?

_____ 5. What alternative treatments could be tried first?

_____ 6. What complications are expected as a result of the surgery?

_____ 7. What percentage of people get these complications?

_____ 8. What is the death rate associated with this operation?

_____ 9. What will be removed, repaired, or added to my body during surgery?

_____ 10. How long will it take to recuperate from the operation?

_____ 11. What anesthesia is planned?

_____ 12. Can local anesthesia, self-hypnosis, or acupuncture be used instead of general anesthesia?

_____ 13. Who will be administering the anesthesia, and are they qualified?

_____ 14. Where will the operation be done?

_____ 15. Could I have out-patient surgery rather than stay in a hospital?

_____ 16. Are you board-certified as a surgeon?

_____ 17. Are you a member of the American College of Surgeons?

_____ 18. How many times a week do you operate?*

Another way in which patients participate in their own health care is by having access to their medical records. Various military and federal agencies, as well as some health professionals, have long followed a policy of making patients responsible for the care, updating, and maintenance of their personal medical records (Schade, 1976, pp. 75–81). Over the years there has been a change in the way the courts have viewed the personal records of health professionals. In general, the position now held by most courts is that, although

---

*From Carolyn Clark, *Enhancing wellness*, p. 32. Copyright © 1981 by Springer Publishing Company, Inc., New York. Used by permission.

the health professional is the "owner" of the records, the patient should have free access to those records and their contents. Consequently, professionals should keep records that are easy to understand. Hirsh and Bromberg (1979) say that readily accessible patient records imply that the professional has "nothing to hide" and that access to such records reduces the patient's tendency to sue. They also suggest that records should be made readily available to patients without the necessity of a court subpoena and that the contents of records should be openly discussed with patients if questions arise. Time should be scheduled for this specific purpose as required.

Chapter Summary

This chapter has attempted to define the most common causes of malpractice actions brought against health professionals and to examine some of the ethical and legal issues presented by these suits. Specific types of suits we examined included breach of contract, assault and battery, and negligence. Since laws vary from state to state and jurisdiction to jurisdiction, it is impossible to provide specific legal information for any given area of the country. However, the basic principles that we have described are well established in the common law at the present time.

We also discussed how health professionals can prevent and protect themselves from malpractice litigation. Of these, due care, informed consent, and patient participation in health care are among the most critical.

Above all, we emphasized that most malpractice suits occur because of a deterioration in the health professional/patient relationship. Patients are more likely to sue professionals whom they do not like, do not trust, and cannot talk to easily and openly. Effective communication is the best way to reduce the likelihood of a malpractice suit. As we have emphasized throughout this book, effective communication is the cornerstone of patient interviewing and is the foundation on which superior health care rests.

Suggested Readings

Annas, G. J. *The rights of hospital patients.* New York: Avon, 1975. This useful handbook discusses the origin of the patient rights movement and other pertinent issues directly affecting both patients and health professionals, including confidentiality and privacy, consultation and referral, records, and informed consent.

Creighton, H. *Law every nurse should know.* Philadelphia: Saunders, 1981. This outstanding reference manual has multiple legal citations regarding malpractice law as it applies to the nursing profession.

Hirsch, C., Morris, R., & Moritz, A. *Handbook of legal medicine.* St. Louis: Mosby, 1979. A summary in handbook format of the major topics concerned with medicolegal problem areas. There are few specific case citations, but Chapter 32, "Medical Professional Liability," presents several very lucid but simple descriptions of major problem areas with the use of illustrations and a question/answer format.

Holder, A. *Medical malpractice law.* New York: Wiley, 1978. This book is well organized, with extensive legal citations. Especially useful are Chapter I, "Creation of the Physician-Patient Relationship" and Chapter II, "The Duty of Care."

James, A. *Legal medicine with special reference to diagnostic imaging.* Baltimore: Urban and Schwarzenberg, 1980. This book takes a scholarly and philosophical approach to medicolegal matters, showing the development of malpractice law and posing suggestions to resolve the present crisis. Particularly relevant are the chapters "The Relationship Between Law and Medicine," "A Survey of the Common Law Basis of Liability for Medical Practice," "Medical Malpractice Insurance: What Went Wrong?", and "An Overview of Informed Consent: Majority and Minority Rules."

Schuchman, H. Confidentiality: Practice issues in new legislation. *American Journal of Orthopsychiatry,* 1980, *50,* 641–648. This article offers guidelines to health care providers on preserving confidentiality of health care records, amidst differing policies of statutes, consumer groups, and health care ethical standards.

ROS Glossary

The following glossary defines in common terms all of the underlined terminology in A Review of Systems on page 174.

acholic Free from bile; a very light-colored stool frequently seen with gall bladder disease; "clay-colored" stool.

acne Pimples; comedones; an inflammation of the hair follicles in the skin.

albumin A simplest protein found in the human body; may be excreted in the urine in some renal diseases.

allergic rhinitis A seasonal allergic response of the lining of the nose characterized by a watery discharge, itching, and sneezing; "hay fever."

amnesia Forgetfulness; lack of memory.

anesthesia Loss of sensation to pain; numbness.

anorexia Loss of appetite.

anxiety An unexplainable feeling of fear or apprehension that may cause rapid heart rate, sweating, or palpitations.

aphasia Loss of the power of speech, writing, and understanding of written or spoken language; usually caused by injury or disease of certain areas of the brain.

arthritis Inflammation of the joints of the body.

asthma Disorder of the breathing apparatus characterized by recurrent attacks of spasm in the airways producing shortness of breath, difficulty in breathing, and wheezing.

ataxia Usually describes an inability to walk or run without stumbling; generally refers to any difficulty caused by improper muscle/movement coordination.

biopsy The removal of a portion of tissue from the body to allow microscopic examination for the purpose of establishing a definite diagnosis.

cataract Deterioration of the transparent lens of the eye so that the lens becomes opaque and vision is reduced.

chills Shivering of the body usually related to fever and associated with a sensation of being cold.

cholelithiasis Stones in the gall bladder.

claudication Pain or discomfort, usually in the lower extremities, provoked by exercise and due to a lack of sufficient oxygen in the muscles concerned as a consequence of reduced blood flow.

colic Acute, intermittent, frequently agonizing pain caused by spasms in the smooth muscle of internal organs and blood vessels (for example, renal colic or biliary colic).

constipation Difficulty or inability to have bowel movements.

cyanosis A bluish discoloration of the skin due to an inadequate amount of oxygen in the blood.

defecation The passage of stool from the rectum.

delusion A false idea or impression that will

Glossary definitions have been adapted from Dorland's *Illustrated Medical Dictionary,* 25th edition, W. B. Saunders, Philadelphia, 1974.

not be relinquished despite logical arguments (for example, "I am Napoleon Bonaparte.").

dentures False or artificial teeth used to replace missing natural teeth.

depression Depressed mood or marked loss of interest and pleasure in usual activities and pastimes often accompanied by low personal esteem, lack of motivation, inability to execute tasks and frequently accompanied by weight loss, lack of interest in sexuality, crying spells, and dejection.

dermatitis An inflammation of the skin; may be caused by allergy, infection, sun or chemical exposure, or reduced circulation.

diabetes A general term relating to disorders in which there is increased urine production; usually refers to diabetes mellitus, a disorder of carbohydrate metabolism due to lack of the hormone insulin.

diarrhea An increase in the frequency and water content of bowel movements.

dribbling Leaking of urine; frequently associated with coughing, sneezing, and prostate gland abnormalities.

dyspareunia Painful or difficult sexual intercourse.

dysphagia Difficulty in swallowing.

dyspnea Difficulty in breathing; shortness of breath.

dysuria Difficulty or pain with the passage of urine; burning sensation.

eczema A term used to designate an inflammation of the skin in which there is usually itching, redness, weeping, oozing, and crusting of tissue fluids; a type of dermatitis.

edema Swelling due to the accumulation of fluids in body tissues.

electrocardiogram (ECG) A graphic tracing depicting electrical activity of the heart.

enuresis Unconscious and involuntary loss of urine; bed-wetting.

epistaxis Nosebleeds.

exanthem A skin rash frequently associated with viral illnesses (for example, measles, roseola).

exophthalmos Abnormal protrusion of the eyeball; frequently associated with thyroid disease.

fever An increase in the body temperature above normal—that is, above 98.6° F.

frequency Term used to denote an increase in the number of occurrences of a particular function; frequently used to indicate an increased need to urinate at short intervals.

furuncle A common skin infection usually caused by staphylococci or streptococci and containing a "core"; boil.

galactorrhea Any milk-like secretion from the breast other than normal lactation; does not include pus or bloody secretions.

gingiva(e) The gum of the mouth; the mucous membrane that surrounds the base of the teeth.

glycosuria The presence of an abnormal amount of glucose in the urine; glucosuria; frequently observed with diabetes mellitus.

gout A type of arthritis characterized by the presence of uric acid crystals in the affected joint; frequently affects the great toes (podagra).

gustation The sense of taste.

hallucination The perception or imagination of a sight, sound, smell, taste, or touch of some object when the object is not physically present or apparent.

hematemesis Vomiting of blood.

impotence The inability, in the male, to achieve and maintain an erection.

insomnia The inability to go to sleep or to remain asleep for adequate periods of time.

insulin Hormone secreted by the pancreas that regulates carbohydrate metabolism; inadequate production is associated with diabetes mellitus.

jaundice Yellow discoloration of the skin due to the accumulation of bile pigments in the skin; usually associated with liver or gall bladder disease; also called icterus.

lacrimation The production and excretion of tears.

larynx The voice box; the upper part of the trachea; contains the vocal cords.

libido The sexual desire or drive.

melena   Dark, tarry-colored stools usually associated with the passage of blood through the digestive tract.

menarche   The onset of menstrual periods.

menopause   The cessation of menstrual periods.

murmur   A sound heard during auscultation over the heart and attributed to turbulence in the blood flow; usually a short, intermittent, swooshing sound.

nausea   An uncomfortable, unpleasant sensation with associated abdominal or epigastric discomfort that frequently precedes vomiting.

nephritis   An inflammation of the kidneys.

night sweats   Soaking sweats occurring during sleep; frequently associated with infection, especially tuberculosis.

olfaction   The sense of smell.

oliguria   A relative reduction in the amount of urine produced when compared to the fluid intake.

oral agents   Medication taken by mouth, but, especially those used in the treatment of diabetes mellitus in distinction to insulin, which must be injected.

orthopnea   Shortness of breath or labored breathing in the recumbent position; usually associated with heart or lung disorders.

otorrhea   Discharge from the ear.

palpitation   Rigorous, rapid heart action that is detected by patients; may consist of one or more regular or irregular beats.

paralysis   Loss or impairment of motor function caused by disorders of the muscles or nervous system.

paresthesia   An abnormal, usually disagreeable sensation (for example, burning, pins and needles).

paroxysmal nocturnal dyspnea   Shortness of breath or a smothering sensation occurring during recumbency and sleep; usually associated with cardiac or respiratory disease.

pharynx   The posterior portion of the mouth and throat.

phobia   An unexplainable, unrealistic fear of an object, person, or situation such as fear of riding in elevators.

pleurisy   An inflammation of the pleura, the membranes surrounding the lungs; characteristically produces pain and restriction of inspiration.

pneumonia   An inflammatory process involving the lungs.

polydipsia   Increased thirst culminating in an increased consumption of fluids; commonly seen with diabetes mellitus.

polyphagia   Increased appetite and craving for all types of foodstuff; commonly seen with diabetes mellitus.

polyuria   The production of large volumes of urine during a given time period; frequently associated with diabetes mellitus.

pruritis   Itching.

regurgitation   A reversal of the usual direction of flow (for example, the contents of the stomach during the process of vomiting or the flow of blood backward through an incompetent cardiac valve).

retention   The process of holding back against the usual pattern (for example, urinary retention due to prostatic enlargement).

scotoma   An area of reduced vision; a blind spot.

seizure   An episodic, transient disturbance of brain function resulting in loss of consciousness, loss of concentration, abnormal body movements, or incontinence; epilepsy.

sequela   Any residual impairment remaining after an illness or injury.

shingles   A viral infection usually localized to one or two dermatomal segments producing redness, itching, vesicle formation, and frequently residual intractable pain; Herpes zoster.

sputum   The mucous material "spat up" from the lungs, bronchi, and trachea; phlegm.

strabismus   An abnormal deviation of the eye from the normal visual axis; frequently associated with squinting; a "lazy eye."

stone   A hard mass or concretion developing in tissue or various body organs [for example, gall bladder stones, (frequently cholesterol), kidney stones (frequently calcium oxalate or phosphate)].

stricture A reduction in the diameter of a tubular organ resulting from injury or illness (for example, urethral stricture).

syncope A temporary loss of consciousness resulting from a reduction in blood availability to the brain; fainting.

tenesmus Straining, usually ineffectively, to accomplish a bowel movement.

tinnitus The presence of distracting sounds in the ears; ringing, buzzing, roaring, and so on.

tonsils A small mass of lymphoid tissue in the pharynx.

tumor Any new growth of tissue where the cell division is uncontrolled and progressive.

ulcer A local defect on the surface of an organ or tissue (for example, gastric ulcer, aphthous ulcer).

urgency The need to perform a bodily function with dispatch (for example, urgency to defecate).

urticaria A transient affliction of the skin frequently associated with allergic phenomena and consisting of a wheal and flare reaction and itching; hives.

varicosity A permanently distended structure (for example, varicose veins).

venereal disease A group of diseases spread through sexual intercourse or intimate interpersonal contact; more properly termed *sexually transmitted diseases* (for example, syphilis).

vertigo A sensation perceived that the individual is spinning in space or that the external world is spinning around the individual.

vision The sense of sight.

vomiting The forcible expulsion of the stomach contents through the mouth.

wheezing The high-pitched whistling sounds occurring during episodes of asthma or in chronic lung disease; generally caused by reduction in the caliber of the airways due to spasm in the smooth muscle of the airway walls.

References _____

Aguilera, D., & Messick, J. *Crisis intervention theory and methodology*. St. Louis: Mosby, 1974.

Andreasen, N., & Norris, A. Long-term adjustment and adaptation mechanisms in severely burned adults. *Journal of Nervous and Mental Disease*, 1972, *154*, 352–362.

Andreasen, N., Norris, A., & Hartford, C. Incidence of long-term psychiatric complications in severely burned adults. *Annals of Surgery*, 1971, *174*, 785–793.

Annas, G. J. *The rights of hospital patients*. New York: Avon, 1975.

Anstett, R., & Collins, M. The psychological significance of somatic complaints. *The Journal of Family Practice*, 1982, *14*, 253–259.

Bakal, D. A. *Psychology and medicine*. New York: Springer, 1979.

Beals, P. *Parents' guide to the childbearing year* (7th ed.). Minneapolis: The International Childbirth Education Association, 1980.

Belkin, G. S. *An introduction to counseling*. Dubuque, Iowa: William C. Brown, 1980.

Benson, H. Your innate asset for combating stress. *Harvard Business Review*, July–August, 1974, *52*, 49–60.

Benson, H. *The relaxation response*. New York: Avon, 1976.

Bernstein, D. A., & Borkovec, T. D. *Progressive relaxation training: A manual for the helping professions*. Champaign, Ill.: Research Press, 1973.

Bernstein, L. & Bernstein, R. S. *Interviewing: A guide for health professionals* (3rd ed.). New York: Appleton-Century-Crofts, 1980.

Blackham, G. J. *Counseling: Theory, process, and practice*. Belmont, Calif.: Wadsworth, 1977.

Black's law dictionary (5th ed.). St. Paul, Minn.: West, 1979.

Blocher, D. H. *Developmental counseling*. New York: Ronald Press, 1966.

Blum, R. H. *The management of the doctor-patient relationship*. New York: McGraw-Hill, 1960.

Brammer, L. M., & Shostrom, E. L. *Therapeutic psychology: Fundamentals of counseling and psychother-apy* (4th ed.). Englewood Cliffs, N.J.: Prentice-Hall, 1982.

Brockopp, G. W. Crisis intervention: Theory, process and practice. In D. Lester & G. W. Brockopp (Eds.), *Crisis intervention and counseling by telephone*. Springfield, Ill.: Charles C Thomas, 1973.

Buggs, D. C. *Your child's self esteem*. New York: Double-day, 1975.

Burton, G. *Interpersonal relations: A guide for nurses* (4th ed.). New York: Springer, 1977.

Caplan, R., Robinson, E., French, J., Caldwell, J., & Shinn, M. *Adhering to medical regimens*. Ann Arbor: Insti-tute for Social Research, University of Michigan, 1976.

Carkhuff, R. *Helping and human relations*. Vol. 1: *Selec-tion and training*. New York: Holt, Rinehart & Win-ston, 1969. (a)

Carkhuff, R. *Helping and human relations*. Vol. 2: *Prac-tice and research*. New York: Holt, Rinehart & Win-ston, 1969. (b)

Carkhuff, R., & Anthony, W. *The skills of helping: An introduction to counseling*. Amherst, Mass.: Human Resource Development Press, 1979.

Carkhuff, R., Pierce, R., & Cannon, J. *The art of helping III*. Amherst, Mass.: Human Resource Development Press, 1977.

Carrington, P. *Learning to meditate: Clinically stan-dardized meditation (CSM)—Course workbook*. Kendall Park, N.J.: Pace Educational Systems, 1978.

Carrington, P., Collings, G. H., Benson, H., Robinson, H., Wood, L. W., Lehrer, P. M., Woolfolk, R. L., & Cole, J. W. The use of meditation-relaxation techniques for the management of stress in a working population. *Journal of Occupational Medicine*, 1980, *22*, 221–231.

Carroll, L. J., & Yates, B. T. Further evidence for the role of stimulus control training in facilitating weight reduction after behavioral therapy. *Behavior Ther-apy*, 1981, *12*, 287–291.

Cartwright, A. *Human relations and hospital care*. Lon-don: Routledge and Kegan Paul, 1964.

Cassileth, B. R., Zupkis, R. V., Sutton-Smith, K., & March, V. Informed consent—Why are its goals imperfectly realized? *The New England Journal of Medicine,* 1980, *302,* 896–900.

Clark, C. *Enhancing wellness: A guide for self-care.* New York: Springer, 1981.

Clark, M. *Health in the Mexican American culture.* Berkeley and Los Angeles: University of California Press, 1970.

Corey, G., Corey, M., & Callanan, P. *Professional and ethical issues in counseling and psychotherapy.* Monterey, Calif.: Brooks/Cole, 1979.

Cormier, W. H., & Cormier, L. S. *Interviewing strategies for helpers: A guide to assessment, treatment, and evaluation.* Monterey, Calif.: Brooks/Cole, 1979.

Cousins, N. *Anatomy of an illness as perceived by the patient.* New York: Norton, 1979.

Creighton, H. *Law every nurse should know* (4th ed.). Philadelphia: Saunders, 1981.

DeGowin, E. L., & DeGowin, R. L. *Bedside diagnostic examination* (3rd ed.). New York: Macmillan, 1976.

Diagnostic and statistical manual of mental disorders (3rd ed.). Washington, D. C.: American Psychiatric Association, 1980.

DiTomasso, R., & Colameco, S. Patient self-monitoring of behavior. *The Journal of Family Practice,* 1982, *15,* 79–83.

Doster, J. A. Effects of instructions, modeling, and role rehearsal on interview verbal behavior. *Journal of Consulting and Clinical Psychology,* 1972, *39,* 202–209.

Duff, R. S., & Hollingshead, A. B. *Sickness and society.* New York: Harper & Row, 1968.

Egan, G. *The skilled helper: A model for systematic helping and interpersonal relating.* Monterey, Calif.: Brooks/Cole, 1975.

Egan, G. *The skilled helper: Model, skills, and methods for effective helping* (2nd ed.). Monterey, Calif.: Brooks/Cole, 1982.

Ekman, P., & Friesen, W. Head and body cues in the judgment of emotion: A reformulation. *Perceptual and Motor Skills,* 1967, *24,* 711–724.

Elder, J. *Transactional analysis in health care.* Menlo Park, Calif.: Addison-Wesley, 1978.

Enelow, A., & Adler, L. Basic interviewing. In A. Enelow & S. Swisher (Eds.), *Interviewing and patient care* (2nd ed.). New York/Oxford: Oxford University Press, 1979.

Enelow, A. J., & Swisher, S. N. *Interviewing and patient care* (2nd ed.). New York/Oxford: Oxford University Press, 1979.

Engel, G. L., & Morgan, W. L. *Interviewing the patient.* London: Saunders, 1973.

Epstein, L. H., Beck, S., Figueroa, J., Farkas, G., Kazdin, A., Danemen, D., & Becker, D. The effects of targeting improvements in urine glucose on metabolic control in children with insulin dependent diabetes. *Journal of Applied Behavior Analysis,* 1981, *14,* 365–375.

Epstein, L. H., & Masek, B. J. Behavioral control of medicine compliance. *Journal of Applied Behavior Analysis,* 1978, *11,* 1–10.

Ficarra, B. J. Prophylaxis against medical negligence. In C. H. Wecht (Ed.), *Legal medicine annual: 1978.* New York: Appleton-Century-Crofts, 1979.

Fisher, D. *I know you hurt, but there's nothing to bandage.* Beaverton, Oregon: Touchstone Press, 1978.

Foley, R., & Sharf, B. The five interviewing techniques most frequently overlooked by primary care physicians. *Behavioral Medicine,* February 1981, 26–31.

Follette, W., & Cummings, N. Psychiatric services and medical utilization in a prepaid health plan setting. *Medical Care,* 1967, *5,* 25–35.

Froelich, R. E. & Bishop, F. M. *Clinical interviewing skills* (2nd ed.). St. Louis: Mosby, 1972.

Froelich, R. E., & Bishop, F. M. *Clinical interviewing skills* (3rd ed.). St. Louis: Mosby, 1977.

Froelich, R. E., Bishop, F. M., & Dworkin, S. F. *Communication in the dental office.* St. Louis: Mosby, 1976.

Fuller, S. S., Endress, M. P., & Johnson, J. E. The effects of cognitive and behavioral control on coping with an aversive health examination. *Journal of Human Stress,* 1978, *4,* 18–25.

Gazda, G. M., Asbury, F. R., Balzer, F. J., Childers, W. C., & Walters, R. P. *Human relations development: A manual for educators* (2nd ed.). Boston: Allyn & Bacon, 1977.

George, R., & Cristiani, T. *Theory, methods, and processes of counseling and psychotherapy.* Englewood Cliffs, N.J.: Prentice-Hall, 1981.

Gerrard, B., Boniface, W., & Love, B. *Interpersonal skills for health professionals.* Reston, Va.: Reston, 1980.

Gilbert, T. F. *Human competence: Engineering worthy performance.* New York: McGraw-Hill, 1978.

Goldman, R. H., & Peters, J. M. The occupational and environmental health history. *Journal of the American Medical Association,* 1981, *246,* 2831–2836.

Goldstein, A. P. *Structured learning therapy.* New York: Academic Press, 1973.

Goldstein, A. P. Relationship-enhancement methods. In F. H. Kanfer & A. P. Goldstein (Eds.), *Helping people change* (2nd ed.). New York: Pergamon Press, 1980.

Gordon, R. L. *Interviewing: Strategy, techniques and tactics.* Homewood, Ill.: Dorsey, 1969.

Graham, S. Social factors in relation to chronic illness. In H. E. Freeman, S. Levine, & L. F. Reeder (Eds.), *Handbook of medical sociology.* Englewood Cliffs, N.J.: Prentice-Hall, 1963.

Green, J. A. The health care contract: Key to minimizing malpractice risks. *Professional Liability Newsletter,* March 1982, *4*(1), 1; 6–8.

Grundner, T. M. On the readability of surgical consent forms. *The New England Journal of Medicine,* 1980, *302,* 900–902.

Hackett, T., Cassem, N., & Wishnie, H. The coronary care unit: An appraisal of its psychological hazards. *New England Journal of Medicine*, 1968, *279*, 1365–1370.

Hackney, H., & Cormier, L. S. *Counseling strategies and objectives* (2nd ed.). Englewood Cliffs, N.J.: Prentice-Hall, 1979.

Hackney, H., Ivey, A., & Oetting, E. Attending, island and hiatus behavior: A process conception of counselor and client interaction. *Journal of Counseling Psychology*, 1970, *17*, 342–346.

Hackney, H., & Nye, L. S. *Counseling strategies and objectives*. Englewood Cliffs, N.J.: Prentice-Hall, 1973.

Hainer, B. L. Recognition and management of the overly affectionate patient. *The Journal of Family Practice*, 1982, *14*, 47–49.

Haynes, R. B., Sackett, D. L., Gibson, E. S., Taylor, D. W., Hackett, B. C., Roberts, R. S., & Johnson, A. L. Improvement of medication compliance in uncontrolled hypertension. *Lancet*, 1976, *1*, 1265–1268.

Hein, E. C. *Communication in nursing practice* (2nd ed.). Boston: Little, Brown, 1980.

Hillman, R., Goodell, B., Grundy, S., McArthur, J., & Moller, J. *Clinical skills: Interviewing, history taking, and physical diagnosis*. New York: McGraw-Hill, 1981.

Hirsch, C., Morris, R., & Moritz, A. *Handbook of legal medicine* (5th ed.). St. Louis: Mosby, 1979.

Hirsh, H. L., & Bromberg, J. Physician responsibilities in keeping medical records. *Malpractice Digest*, November–December 1979, 1–3. (Published by St. Paul Fire and Marine Insurance Co., St. Paul, Minn.)

Holder, A. R. *Medical malpractice law* (2nd ed.). New York: Wiley, 1978.

Horan, J. J. Coping with inescapable discomfort through in vivo emotive imagery. In J. D. Krumboltz & C. E. Thoresen (Eds.), *Counseling methods*. New York: Holt, Rinehart & Winston, 1976.

Horan, J. J., Hackett, G., Buchanan, J. D., Stone, C. I., & Demchik-Stone, D. Coping with pain: A component analysis of stress inoculation. *Cognitive Therapy and Research*, 1977, *1*, 211–221.

International code of nursing ethics. In T. M. Beauchamp & L. Waters (Eds.), *Contemporary issues in bioethics*. Belmont, Calif.: Wadsworth, 1978.

Ivey, A. E. *Microcounseling: Innovations in interview training*. Springfield, Ill.: Charles C Thomas, 1971.

Ivey, A. E., & Authier, J. *Microcounseling: Innovations in interviewing, counseling, psychotherapy, and psychoeducation* (2nd ed.). Springfield, Ill.: Charles C Thomas, 1978.

Ivey, A. E., & Gluckstern, N. *Basic influencing skills, Participant manual*. North Amherst, Mass.: Microtraining Associates, 1976.

Ivey, A. E., & Simek-Downing, L. *Counseling and psychotherapy: Skills, theories, and practice*. Englewood Cliffs, N.J.: Prentice-Hall, 1980.

Jacobson, E. *Progressive relaxation*. Chicago: University of Chicago Press, 1929.

James, A. E., Jr. Medical malpractice insurance. In A. E. James, Jr. (Ed.), *Legal medicine with special reference to diagnostic imaging*. Baltimore, Md.: Urban and Schwarzenberg, 1980.

Jessop, A. L. *Nurse-patient communication: A skills approach*. North Amherst, Mass.: Microtraining Associates, 1979.

Johnson, B. A. An overview of informed consent. In A. E. James, Jr. (Ed.), *Legal medicine with special reference to diagnostic imaging*. Baltimore, Md.: Urban and Schwarzenberg, 1980.

Johnson, D. W. *Reaching out: Interpersonal effectiveness and self-actualization* (2nd ed.). Englewood Cliffs, N.J.: Prentice-Hall, 1981.

Johnson, J. E., Kirchhoff, K. T., & Endress, M. P. Altering children's distress behavior during orthopedic cast removal. *Nursing Research*, 1975, *75*, 404–410.

Johnson, J. E., & Leventhal, H. Effects of accurate expectations and behavioral instructions on reactions during a noxious medical examination. *Journal of Personality and Social Psychology*, 1974, *29*, 710–718.

Johnson, J. E., Morrissey, J. F., & Leventhal, H. Psychological preparation for an endoscopic examination. *Gastrointestinal Endoscopy*, 1973, *19*, 180–182.

Johnson, J. E., Rice, V. H., Fuller, S. S., & Endress, M. D. Sensory information, instruction in a coping strategy, and recovery from surgery. *Research in Nursing and Health*, 1978, *1*, 4–17.

Jonsen, A. R., Siegler, M., & Winslade, W. J. *Clinical ethics: A practical approach to ethical decisions in clinical medicine*. New York: Macmillan, 1982.

Kagan, N. Counseling psychology, interpersonal skills, and health care. In G. C. Stone, F. Cohen, & N. E. Adler (Eds.), *Health psychology: A handbook*. San Francisco: Jossey-Bass, 1979.

Kahn, R. L., & Cannell, C. F. *The dynamics of interviewing*. New York: Wiley, 1957.

Kasl, S. V. Issues in patient adherence to health care regimens. *Journal of Human Stress*, 1975, *1*, 5–17.

Kirscht, J., & Rosenstock, I. Patients' problems in following recommendations of health experts. In G. C. Stone, F. Cohen, & N. E. Adler (Eds.), *Health psychology: A handbook*. San Francisco: Jossey-Bass, 1979.

Knight, P. H., & Bair, C. K. Degree of client comfort as a function of dyadic interaction distance. *Journal of Counseling Psychology*, 1976, *23*, 13–16.

Koos, E. L. *The health of regionville*. New York: Hafner, 1967.

Kozier, B., & Erb, G. *Fundamentals of nursing*. Menlo Park, Calif.: Addison-Wesley, 1979.

Lahiff, J. M. Interviewing for results. In R. C. Huseman, C. M. Logue, & D. L. Freshley (Eds.), *Readings in interpersonal and organizational communication* (2nd ed.). Boston: Holbrook Press, 1973.

Leigh, H., & Reiser, M. F. *The patient: Biological, psychological, and social dimensions of medical practice.* New York: Plenum, 1980.

Leventhal, H., & Johnson, J. E. Laboratory and field experimentation: Development of a theory of self-regulation. In P. Wooldridge, R. Leonard, J. Skipper, & M. Schmitt (Eds.), *Behavioral science and nursing theory.* St. Louis: Mosby, 1981.

Lewis, G. K. *Nurse-patient communication* (3rd ed.). Dubuque, Iowa: William C. Brown, 1978.

Ley, P. Toward better doctor-patient communications. In A. E. Bennett (Ed.), *Communication between doctors and patients.* London: Oxford University Press, 1976.

Lipkin, M. *The care of patients: Concepts and tactics.* New York: Oxford University Press, 1974.

Long, L., & Prophit, P. *Understanding/responding: A communication manual for nurses.* Monterey, Calif.: Wadsworth, 1981.

Mahoney, M. J., & Thoresen, C. E. (Eds.). *Self-control: Power to the person.* Monterey, Calif.: Brooks/Cole, 1974.

Major, R. H., & Delp, M. H. *Physical diagnosis* (6th ed.). Philadelphia: Saunders, 1963.

Matthews, D., & Hingson, R. Improving patient compliance. *Medical Clinics of North America,* 1977, *61,* 879–889.

McFall, R. M. Parameters of self-monitoring. In R. B. Stuart (Ed.), *Behavioral self-management: Strategies, techniques and outcomes.* New York: Brunner/Mazel, 1977.

McGuire, D., Thelen, M., & Amolsch, T. Interview self-disclosure as a function of length of modeling and descriptive instructions. *Journal of Consulting and Clinical Psychology,* 1975, *43,* 356–362.

McGuire, P. Teaching essential interviewing skills to medical students. In D. J. Oborne, M. M. Gruneberg, & J. R. Eiser (Eds.), *Research in psychology and medicine* (Vol. 2). London: Academic Press, 1979.

Medio, F. *Teaching interpersonal communication skills to medical students: A comparison of four methods.* Unpublished doctoral dissertation, West Virginia University, 1980.

Mehrabian, A. Communication without words. *Psychology Today,* September 1968, 53–55.

Meichenbaum, D. *Cognitive behavior modification.* New York: Plenum, 1977.

Meichenbaum, D., & Turk, D. The cognitive-behavioral management of anxiety, anger, and pain. In P. O. Davidson (Ed.), *The behavioral management of anxiety, depression and pain.* New York: Brunner/Mazel, 1976.

Melamed, B. G., & Siegel, L. J. *Behavioral medicine: Practical applications in health care.* New York: Springer, 1980.

Minuchin, S. *Families and family therapy.* Cambridge, Mass.: Harvard University Press, 1974.

Minuchin, S., Rosman, B., & Baker, L. *Psychosomatic families: Anorexia nervosa in context.* Cambridge, Mass.: Harvard University Press, 1978.

Moore, K., & Altmaier, E. M. Stress inoculation training with cancer patients. *Cancer Nursing,* 1981, *5,* 389–393.

Nath, C., & Rinehart, J. Effects of individual and group relaxation therapy on blood pressure in essential hypertensives. *Research in Nursing and Health,* 1979, *2,* 119–126.

Okun, B. F. *Effective helping: Interviewing and counseling techniques.* North Scituate, Mass.: Duxbury, 1976.

Okun, B. F. *Effective helping: Interviewing and counseling techniques* (2nd ed.). Monterey, Calif.: Brooks/Cole, 1982.

Padilla, G. V., Grant, M. M., Rains, B. L., Hansen, B. C., Bergstrom, N., Wong, H. L., Hanson, R., & Kubo, W. Distress reduction and the effects of preparatory teaching films and patient control. *Research in Nursing and Health,* 1981, *4,* 375–387.

Parsons, T. *The social system.* New York: The Free Press, 1951.

Passons, W. R. *Gestalt approaches in counseling.* New York: Holt, Rinehart & Winston, 1975.

Patient effectiveness. *VD National Hotline,* Spring 1980, p. 4 (newsletter published by the American Social Health Association, Palo Alto, Calif.).

Patterson, C. H. *Theories of counseling and psychotherapy* (3rd ed.). New York: Harper & Row, 1980.

Pepinsky, H., & Pepinsky, P. *Counseling: Theory and practice.* New York: Ronald Press, 1954.

Peterson, L., & Shigetomi, C. The use of coping techniques to minimize anxiety in hospitalized children. *Behavior Therapy,* 1981, *12,* 1–14.

Potter, S. Language and society. In P. Hazard & M. Hazard (Eds.), *Language and literacy today.* Chicago: Science Research Associates, 1965.

Pratt, L., Seligmann, A., & Reader, G. Physicians' views on the level of medical information among patients. *American Journal of Public Health,* 1957, *47,* 1277–1283.

Puryear, D. A. *Helping people in crisis.* San Francisco: Jossey-Bass, 1979.

Raths, L., & Simon, S. *Values and teaching.* Columbus, Ohio: Merrill, 1966.

Raush, H., & Bordin, E. Warmth in personality development and in psychotherapy. *Psychiatry,* 1957, *20,* 351–363.

Regan, L. J. *Doctor and patient and the law* (3rd ed.). St. Louis: Mosby, 1956.

Reiser, D. E., & Schroder, A. K. *Patient interviewing.* Baltimore, Md.: Williams & Wilkins, 1980.

Restatement of the law, Second, Torts. Philadelphia: American Law Institute, 1967, sec. 282.

Rogers, C. *Client-centered therapy.* Boston: Houghton-Mifflin, 1951.

Rogers, C. The necessary and sufficient conditions of therapeutic personality change. *Journal of Consulting Psychology,* 1957, *21,* 95–103.

Romanczyk, R. G. Self-monitoring in the treatment of obesity: Parameters of reactivity. *Behavior Therapy,* 1974, *5,* 531–540.

Rosen, J. & Wiens, A. Changes in medical problems and use of medical services following psychological intervention. *American Psychologist,* 1979, *34,* 420–431.

Rosenthal, R. S. Malpractice: Cause and its prevention. *Laryngoscope,* 1978, *88,* 1–11.

Rotter, J. B. Generalized expectancies for interpersonal trust. *American Psychologist,* 1971, *26,* 443–452.

Russell, R. K., & Sipich, J. F. Treatment of test anxiety by cue-controlled relaxation. *Behavior Therapy,* 1974, *5,* 673–676.

Rybstein-Blinchik, E. Effects of different cognitive strategies on chronic pain experience. *Journal of Behavioral Medicine,* 1979, *2,* 93–101.

Sackett, D. L., Haynes, R. B., Gibson, E. S., Taylor, D. W., Roberts, R. S., & Johnson, A. L. Patient compliance with antihypertensive regimens. *Patient Counseling and Health Education,* 1978, *1,* 18–21.

Satir, V. *Peoplemaking.* Palo Alto, Calif.: Science and Behavior Books, 1972.

Schade, H. I. My patients take their medical records with them. *Medical Economics,* March 8, 1976, *53*(5), 75–81.

Schmidt, L. D., & Strong, S. R. Expert and inexpert counselors. *Journal of Counseling Psychology,* 1970, *17,* 115–118.

Schuchman, H. Confidentiality: Practice issues in new legislation. *American Journal of Orthopsychiatry,* 1980, *50,* 641–648.

Schutz, B. *Legal liability in psychotherapy.* San Francisco: Jossey-Bass, 1982.

Schwitzgebel, R. L., & Schwitzgebel, R. K. *Law and psychological practice.* New York: Wiley, 1980.

Seay, T., & Altkreuse, M. Verbal and nonverbal behavior in judgments of facilitative conditions. *Journal of Counseling Psychology,* 1979, *26,* 108–119.

Seer, P., & Raeburn, J. M. Meditation training and essential hypertension: A methodological study. *Journal of Behavioral Medicine,* 1980, *3,* 59–71.

Shannon, T. A. The physician-patient relationship: Where to now? *Colloquy: The Journal of Physician-Patient Communications,* February 1981, 1–2; 14.

Shapiro, D. H. Instructions for a training package combining formal and informal Zen meditation with behavioral self-control strategies. *Psychologia,* 1978, *31,* 70–76.

Shelton, J. R., & Rosen, G. M. Self-monitoring by patients. In G. M. Rosen, J. P. Geyman, & R. H. Layton (Eds.),

Behavioral science in family practice. New York: Appleton-Century-Crofts, 1980.

Sheppe, W., Jr. & Stevenson, I. Techniques of interviewing. In H. I. Lief, F. V. Lief, & N. R. Lief (Eds.), *The psychological basis of medical practice.* New York: Hoeber, 1963.

Shertzer, B., & Stone, S. *Fundamentals of counseling* (2nd ed.). Boston: Houghton-Mifflin, 1974.

Shulman, J. Current concepts of patient motivation toward long term oral hygiene: A literature review. *Journal of American Society of Preventive Dentistry,* 1974, *4,* 7–15.

Siegel, L. J., & Peterson, L. Stress reduction in young dental patients through coping skills and sensory information. *Journal of Consulting and Clinical Psychology,* 1980, *48,* 785–787.

Sierra-Franco, M. *Therapeutic communication in nursing.* New York: McGraw-Hill, 1978.

Simmons, O. Implications of social class for public health. In E. G. Jaco (Ed.), *Patients, physicians and illness.* Glencoe, Ill.: The Free Press, 1958.

Simonton, O. C., Matthews-Simonton, S., & Creighton, J. *Getting well again.* New York: Bantam Books, 1980.

Sleeth, C. K. *The clinical study of a patient: A problem-oriented approach.* Unpublished case study, Department of Family Practice, West Virginia University Medical Center, 1975.

Smith, C. K., & Leversee, J. H. Basic interviewing skills. In G. M. Rosen, J. P. Geyman, & R. H. Layton (Eds.), *Behavioral science in family practice.* New York: Appleton-Century-Crofts, 1980.

Smith, J. C. Meditation as psychotherapy: A review of the literature. *Psychological Bulletin,* 1975, *82,* 558–564.

Smith, V., & Bass, T. *Communication for health professionals.* Philadelphia: J. B. Lippincott, 1979.

Stekel, S., & Swain, M. The use of written contracts to increase adherence. *Hospitals,* 1977, *51,* 81–84.

Stillman, P., Sabers, D., & Redfield, D. The use of paraprofessionals to teach interviewing skills. *Pediatrics,* 1976, *57,* 769–774.

Stone, G., & Gotlib, I. Effect of instructions and modeling on self-disclosure. *Journal of Counseling Psychology,* 1975, *22,* 288–293.

Stone, G., & Morden, C. J. Effect of distance on verbal productivity. *Journal of Counseling Psychology,* 1976, *23,* 486–488.

Strong, S. Counseling: An interpersonal influence process. *Journal of Counseling Psychology,* 1968, *15,* 215–224.

Strong, S., & Schmidt, L. Expertness and influence in counseling. *Journal of Counseling Psychology,* 1970, *17,* 81–87.

Stuart, R. B., & Davis, B. *Slim chance in a fat world.* Champaign, Ill.: Research Press, 1972.

Susser, M., & Watson, W. *Sociology in medicine.* London: Oxford University Press, 1971.

Svarstad, B. Physician-patient communication and patient conformity with medical advice. In D. Mechanic (Ed.), *The growth of bureaucratic medicine*. New York: Wiley, 1976.

Thoresen, C. E., & Mahoney, M. J. *Behavioral self-control*. New York: Holt, Rinehart & Winston, 1974.

Thoresen, C., Telch, M., & Eagleston, J. Approaches to altering the Type A behavior pattern. *Psychosomatics*, 1981, *22*, 472–482.

Truax, C., & Carkhuff, R. *Toward effective counseling and psychotherapy*. Chicago: Aldine, 1967.

Turner, J. A., & Chapman, C. R. Psychological intervention for chronic pain: A critical review. I. Relaxation training and biofeedback. *Pain*, 1982, *12*, 1–21.

Tyson, G. A., & Kramer, D. The primacy-recency effect in counselor response. *Journal of Clinical Psychology*, 1981, *37*, 88–90.

Umhau, J. F. Handling patients' complaints with finesse. *Physician's Management*, 1982, *22*(6), 43–49.

Vaughn, M., & Marks, J. Teaching interviewing skills to medical students: A comparison of two methods. *Medical Education*, 1976, *10*, 170–175.

Verwoerdt, A. Psychopathological responses to the stress of physical illness. In Z. J. Lipowski (Ed.), *Advances in psychosomatic medicine*. Vol. 8: *Psychosocial aspects of physical illness*. Basel, Switzerland: S. Karger, 1972.

Volicer, B. J., Isenberg, M. A., & Burns, M. W. Medical-surgical differences in hospital stress factors. *Journal of Human Stress*, 1977, *3*, 3–13.

Wade, J. W. A survey for the common law basis of liability for medical malpractice. In A. E. James, Jr. (Ed.), *Legal medicine with special reference to diagnostic imaging*. Baltimore: Urban and Schwarzenberg, 1980.

Waitzkin, H., & Stoeckle, J. The communication of information about illness. In Z. J. Lipowski (Ed.), *Advances in psychosomatic medicine*. Vol. 8: *Psychosocial aspects of physical illness*. Basel, Switzerland: S. Karger, 1972.

Walker, H. K., Hall, W. D., & Hurst, J. W. *Clinical methods*. Boston: Butterworth, 1976.

Watson, D., & Tharp, R. G. *Self-directed behavior: Self-modification for personal adjustment* (3rd ed.). Monterey, Calif.: Brooks/Cole, 1981.

Wells, N. The effects of relaxation on postoperative muscle tension and pain. *Nursing Research*, 1982, *31*, 236–238.

Whitlock, G. *Understanding and coping with real life crises*. Monterey, Calif.: Brooks/Cole, 1978.

Williams, R., Haney, T., Lee, K., Hong Kong, Y., Blumenthal, J., & Whalen, R. Type A behavior, hostility, and coronary atherosclerosis. *Psychosomatic Medicine*, 1980, *42*, 539–549.

Wishnie, H., Hackett, T., & Cassem, N. Psychological hazards of convalescence following myocardial infarction. *Journal of the American Medical Association*, 1971, *215*, 1292–1296.

Wittgenstein, L. *The philosophical investigations*. New York: Macmillan, 1958.

Zborowski, M. *People in pain*. San Francisco: Jossey-Bass, 1969.

Ziesat, H. A. Behavior modification in the treatment of hypertension. *International Journal of Psychiatry in Medicine*, 1978, *8*, 257–265.

Zifferblatt, S. M. Increasing patient compliance through the applied analysis of behavior. *Preventative Medicine*, 1975, *4*, 173–182.

Subject Index

Name Index